SECOND EDITION

Living a Healthy Life with Chronic Pain

Sandra LeFort, MN, PhD • **Kate Lorig**, DrPH
David Sobel, MD, MPH • **Diana Laurent**, MPH
Virginia González, MPH • **Marian Minor**, RPT, PhD
Maureen Gecht-Silver, OTD, MPH • **Francis Keefe**, PhD

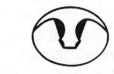

Bull Publishing Company
Boulder, Colorado

Published by Bull Publishing Company
P.O. Box 1377
Boulder, CO, USA 80306
www.bullpub.com

Library of Congress Cataloging-in-Publication Data

Names: LeFort, Sandra M., author.
Title: Living a healthy life with chronic pain / Sandra LeFort, MN, PhD, Kate Lorig, DrPH, David Sobel, MD, MPH, Diana Laurent, MPH, Virginia González, MPH, Marian Minor, RPT, PhD, Maureen Gecht-Silver, OTD, MPH, Francis Keefe, PhD.
Description: Second edition. | Boulder, CO : Bull Publishing Company, [2021] | Includes index. | Summary: "This book is designed to help readers manage their pain so that they can get on with living a satisfying, fulfilling life. Chronic pain includes many types of conditions from a variety of causes. Despite these differences, all readers of this book have one very important thing in common - they are living with pain every day. Acknowledging that overcoming chronic pain is a daily challenge, this book provides readers with proven self-management tools to help them meet that challenge"-- Provided by publisher.
Identifiers: LCCN 2021018146 (print) | LCCN 2021018147 (ebook) | ISBN 9781945188497 (paperback) | ISBN 9781945188503 (ebook)
Subjects: LCSH: Chronic pain--Popular works. | Chronic diseases--Popular works. | Self-care, Health.
Classification: LCC RB127 .L384 2021 (print) | LCC RB127 (ebook) | DDC 616/.0472--dc23
LC record available at https://lccn.loc.gov/2021018146
LC ebook record available at https://lccn.loc.gov/2021018147

Second Edition

27 26 25 24 23 22 21   10 9 8 7 6 5 4 3 2 1

Interior design and project management: Dovetail Publishing Services
Cover design and production: Shannon Bodie, Bookwise Design

This book is dedicated to the memory of Howard Montrose Genge for his courage in the face of pain; Mary Ellen Jeans, PhD, for believing in education for people in pain; Halsted Holman MD, who started us on this journey 40 years ago and has been a mentor every step of the way; and people of all ages and their families who struggle with pain in their lives.

Acknowledgments

MANY PEOPLE HELPED US write this book. Among the most important are the thousands of participants in the Chronic Pain Self-Management Program. The original study for this program was funded by the National Health Research and Development Program of Health Canada. Today we have participants around the world.

Many professionals also assisted us, including Lynn Beatie, PT, MPT, MHA, , Norman Buckley, MD, FRCPC, Beth Darnall, PhD, Sean Mackey MD, Emily Clairmont, MS, RD, CD, John W. Doyle, BA, Robin Edelman MS, RDN, CDE, Steven Feinberg, MD, Chaplain Bruce Feldman, MD, Shelley Gershman, RN, Peg Harrison, MSW, Noorin Jamal, RN, MN-NP, , Michael McGillion, PhD, RN, Patrick McGowan, PhD, Sean Mackey MD, PhD, Ronald Melzack, PhD, Yvonne Mullin, MSc, RD, , Catherine Regan, PhD, Ned Pratt, BFA, Richard Seidel, PhD, and Judith Watt-Watson, PhD, RN., Heather Zuercher, MPH. A special thanks to Nicolaj Holm Faber, Chief Consultant, Danish Committee on Health Education, whose support has been invaluable. To all of you, your help has been gratefully received.

A special thanks to Jon Peck, James Bull, and Erin Mulligan, who helped us every step of the way. Editors are unsung heroes of good books. We wish to acknowledge their fine contributions to making this a more readable, understandable book. We would also like to thank our T-Trainers, Master Trainers, and Leaders. There are now hundreds of you, and you all have made important suggestions that helped us craft this book.

We would like to thank DRx, publisher of The Healthy Mind, Healthy Body Handbook (also published as Mind & Body Health Handbook) by David Sobel, MD, and Robert Ornstein, PhD, for permission to adapt sections of their book.

Finally, many thanks to Jim Bull, Claire Cameron, and the team at Bull Publishing. Bull Publishing has been a strong supporter of health-related books for more than 40 years. Jim's support and encouragement have been essential to the development of this book. We couldn't have done it without you!

If you would like to learn more about our continuing research, online programs, trainings, and materials, please visit our website:

https://www.selfmanagementresource.com/

We are continually revising and improving this book. If you have any suggestions or comments, please send them to

SMRC@selfmanagementresource.com

Contents

17 Planning for the Future: Fears and Reality   357

A Note About Canadian Content

Throughout the book you will see material that is shaded. This material is of special interest to our readers in Canada. We would like to extend a special thanks to the Canadian health care community and the following individuals: Patrick McGowan, PhD; Yvonne Mullan, MSc, RD, CDE; Shayan Shakeraneh, MPH; and Sherry Lynch, BA, BSW, MSW.

Disclaimer

This book is not intended to replace common sense, professional medical or psychological advice. You should seek and get appropriate professional evaluation and treatment for problems—especially unusual, unexplained, severe, or persistent symptoms. Many symptoms and diseases require and benefit from specific medical or psychological evaluation and treatment. Don't deny yourself proper professional care.

- If your symptoms or problems persist beyond a reasonable period despite using self-care recommendations, you should consult a health professional. What is a reasonable period will vary; if you're not sure and you're feeling anxious, consult a health care professional.

- If you receive professional advice in conflict with this book, you should rely upon the guidance provided by your health care professional. He or she is likely to be able to take your specific situation, history and needs into consideration.

- If you are having thoughts of harming yourself in any way, please seek professional care immediately.

This book is as accurate as its publisher and authors can make it, but we cannot guarantee that it will work for you in every case. The authors and publisher disclaim any and all liability for any claims or injuries that you may believe arose from following the recommendations set forth in this book. This book is only a guide; your common sense, good judgment, and partnership with health professionals are also needed.

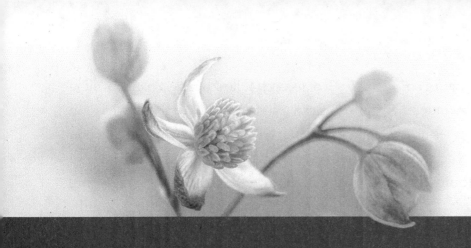

CHAPTER 1

Chronic Pain Self-Management: What It Is and How to Do It

CHRONIC PAIN IS PAIN THAT LASTS beyond three months. This is the time it takes most injuries to heal. Nobody wants to live with chronic pain. Unfortunately, roughly 25 percent of people worldwide live with chronic pain. Most pain is a result of an injury or illness. But some chronic pain has no known cause. What is known is that people with chronic pain often want to get their life back. In this book, we provide tools for you to explore and use to manage and lessen your pain so you can do the things you want and need to do.

Self-management may seem like a strange concept. All self-management really means is having the skills and confidence to get your life back and live with pain. And pain may not be the only problem. Arthritis, back pain, headache, fibromyalgia, and other chronic pain problems often cause fatigue. They can also result in a loss of physical strength and endurance. In addition, chronic pain can cause emotional distress, including frustration, anxiety, anger, and a sense of helplessness or even hopelessness. So how can you be healthy, and get your life back, when these things are happening to you?

Each of us must follow our own path but all of our paths can lead to healthier and full lives. You follow your best path by learning how to function at your best even when life presents challenges.

We can help you do this by suggesting many tools and tricks for living a more fulfilling, active, and enjoyable life. That is what this book is all about.

How to Use This Book

Before we go any further, let's talk about how to use this book. At the end of this chapter, on page 17, you will find a self-test. After you read this chapter, take the test and score it, and then read the suggestions about the parts of this book that can be most helpful to you. You do not need to read every word in every chapter. Instead, read the first two chapters (Chapter 1, *Chronic Pain Self-Management: What It Is and How to Do It*, and Chapter 2, *Becoming an Active Self-Manager*) and then use your self-test results (page 21), the table of contents, and the index to find the information you need from the other chapters. In every chapter and every section of this book, there are information and tools to help you learn and practice self-management skills. This is not a textbook. It is more like a workbook. Feel free to skip around and take notes right in the book. This will help you find and learn the skills you need to follow your own path.

In this book, you will not find any miracles or cures. Instead, you will find hundreds of tips and ideas to make your life easier. The advice comes from pain experts, including physicians, psychologists, physical therapists, occupational therapists, nurses, and people like you who are living with and actively managing their pain.

Please note that we talk about "actively managing." We use the word *managing* on purpose. Management is the key to the tools in this book. There is no way to avoid managing a chronic condition. If you choose to do nothing, that is one way of managing. If you only take medication and ignore other kinds of self-care, that is another management approach. There are many ways to manage your health. But research shows that people who choose to be active self-managers—those who follow the best treatments that health care professionals have to offer and are actively involved in daily monitoring and management—live healthier lives.

In this chapter, we discuss what pain is and how acute pain and chronic pain differ. We also discuss self-management. We introduce the most common problems people with chronic pain face, and we share the self-management skills to address those problems. It does not matter what specific conditions you have. These skills are useful not just for chronic pain, but for the management of any chronic condition and for living a healthier life. This is good news because people with chronic pain often have other health problems. And learning these common life-management skills allows you to successfully manage your life, not just a single condition. The rest of the chapters in the book give you the tools needed to become an active manager of both your chronic pain and the other parts of your life.

What Is Pain?

Pain is a part of being alive. It protects us from danger. You move away from a fire and stay away from stinging bees because of pain. Pain is universal. It is an experience almost humans share. At the same time, pain is a very personal experience. My pain is not the same as yours. Your pain is not the same as another person's. Throughout human history, humans have tried to understand pain. Because you can't see another person's pain, it seems invisible. But when you feel it yourself, pain is all too real. In this part of the chapter, we are going to discuss how research and information about pain has changed over the years. If this is not of interest to you, please feel free to skip to page 7.

The Gate Control Theory of Pain

For most of human history, people believed that the mind and body were separate and that pain was totally physical. By the late 1800s, scientists started to study pain. The idea that pain is purely physical just didn't fit the facts. But progress was slow. In 1959, two scientists—Dr. Ronald Melzack from McGill University and Dr. Patrick Wall from Oxford University—developed new ideas about pain called the gate control theory. Their ideas revolutionized pain research.

Nerve endings all over your body are sensitive to types of stimuli (prompts). Stimuli can be pleasurable, such as a warm shower or massage, or they can cause harm and signal danger, such as a hot stove. Stimuli and prompts, such as heat, cold, pressure, or chemicals, can trigger nerve impulses. If the stimuli are strong enough, the nerve impulses the stimuli trigger travel along the nerves to the spinal cord and up to the brain.

Imagine you just stubbed your toe. Within nanoseconds, the nerve endings in your toe respond and send nerve impulses along the nerves in your body from your toe, foot, leg, buttock, and up to the spinal cord in your back. The spinal cord is the part of the many-branched nerve highway that connects to your brain. There are several pathways for nerve impulses to travel to the brain. Your brain receives the impulses and asks, *"How dangerous is this?"* If your brain thinks the pattern of nerve impulses are dangerous, you feel pain. In other words, pain is not in your toe (although it sure feels like it is). *Pain is produced by your brain to tell you and your body to take action.* Because this is so fundamental, it bears repeating: *although the pain stimuli can come from any part of the body, all pain is processed in the brain.* This does not mean pain is not real. In fact, pain usually results from a very real prompt (like a stubbed toe). It just means that no matter where your pain comes from, you do not feel pain until the nerve impulses reach the brain.

Melzack and Wall said that there is a transmission station or "gate" in the spinal cord that affects the flow of nerve impulses to the brain. Think of it just like a gate you open or close to get to your apartment courtyard or your backyard. Two things can happen when nerve impulses (from somewhere like your toe) reach the gate:

- If the gate is open, the impulses pass through and continue up the spinal cord to the brain. If the brain senses danger, you experience pain.

- If the gate is closed or partially closed, then only some or none of the nerve impulses travel to the brain. If the brain interprets the signals as a little danger—not enough to worry about—or no danger, you experience little or no pain.

How and why does the gate open or close? The brain can send electrical messages down nerve pathways to close the gate and shut out or reduce the flow of nerve impulses to the brain. Other times, these electrical messages might open the gate. Many factors can open or close the gate.

Some of these factors come from your mind. They include your past experience, what you learned about pain from your culture and social environment, your fears, your beliefs about pain, the attention you direct toward the pain, and your emotions. A positive mood, distraction, or deep relaxed breathing can close or partially close the gate. Strong emotions, such as fear, anxiety, or expecting the worst, can open the gate.

Have you ever had pain that never seemed to go away? Imagine that this pain became even worse and you worried it might be serious,

maybe a sign of cancer, so you went to see a health care provider. You found out the pain is caused by a strained muscle. Even on the way home, you probably felt less pain. This is an example of how experience and fear can affect pain. When you thought you had cancer, the pain was unstoppable; once you found out you had a minor strain, the pain faded.

Research on the gate control theory indicates that pain results from many interactions at different levels of our nervous system—in billions of nerve cells, the spinal cord, and the brain. People's physical bodies, feelings and emotions, thoughts and beliefs, and other factors are all involved in the experience of pain. Our brains produce our pain and can help relieve pain. The mind and body are completely connected. They influence each other all the time.

The Neuromatrix Theory of Pain

But the story does not stop here. The gate control theory mostly explained what is happening when nerve impulses travel to the spinal cord. But what is going on within the brain itself? Several sources are helping health care researchers to answer that question. These sources include advanced brain imaging like MRIs, studies of the link between pain and genetics, research into the immune system and the body's response to stress, and Dr. Melzack's latest neuromatrix theory of pain.

Scientists know that at least seven (and probably more) areas of the brain are active when people feel pain. Some of these brain regions control emotions, others control thinking (cognitive function), and still others control the processing of body sensations. These areas of the brain are connected to each other through a large, complex network of nerve cells and neurochemicals (chemicals produced in the nervous system and the brain). Dr. Melzack calls this network of nerve cells and neurochemicals a neuromatrix network. This network organizes the huge amount of information coming into the brain. Genetics determine the makeup of each person's neuromatrix network just as genetics determines our hair color. But just as you can change your hair color, you can help your own network to better manage your pain.

Figure 1.1 shows there are at least three different sources of information that travel to the neuromatrix network in the brain. These sources are:

■ Thoughts, both positive and negative (memories of past experience, beliefs about pain, etc.)

■ Body sensations from all over the body—your skin, muscles, tissues, eyes, ears, etc. (heat, pressure, touch, etc.)

■ Emotions (fear, anxiety, etc.)

The neuromatrix network processes information to produce a pattern of nerve impulses. If your brain interprets this pattern to mean that your body is in danger, a number of things happen, including the following:

■ You feel pain.

■ You take actions to protect your body. In the case of a stubbed toe, for example, you might start hopping around, raising your foot, and rubbing your toe. You might sit down and decide not to walk on your foot until the pain is better. Often, actions are unconscious, including tensing your muscles or holding your breath. Movements that are reactions to pain can even occur while you are sleeping.

■ Your body releases many neurochemicals that help regulate pain and stress. These neurochemicals include adrenaline (which helps prepare the body for action), other immune system chemicals (which fight inflammation), endorphins (which decrease pain), and hormones such as progesterone and testosterone.

One of the most difficult things to understand is that pain is not disease or injury. Pain is the response to the brain's assessment of danger. That's why there is no exact relationship

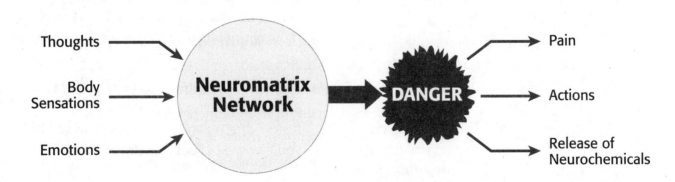

Figure 1.1 **Pain and the Brain**

between how strong a stimulus is, the amount of injury it causes, and the amount of pain a person feels. Two people can be in the same pain-producing situation but have very different experiences. One person may be in excruciating pain while the other feels little pain or discomfort. Or a person may feel extreme pain in one situation but not in another even when the amount of body tissue damage is exactly the same. That's because the central nervous system and brain interpret information and decide what it means at any given time. The brain decides if there is danger or no danger.

Pain is complex. That makes sense because the human brain is so complex. Scientists and health care professionals have to learn a lot more before we have all the answers about pain. But thankfully you don't have to wait for researchers to discover all the answers to start managing your pain. The information scientists already know about pain supports all the tools in this book. Research has shown that the tools you will learn about in this book help close the gate and influence the brain's response to stimuli.

Things to Know about Pain

- Pain is 100 percent in the brain. Your brain senses danger and wants you to do something about it.

- There is no single "pain center" in the brain. Billions of nerve cells in the spinal cord and in many areas of the brain are involved in processing pain.

- There is no single pathway for nerve impulses to travel to the brain to be interpreted as pain. There are several pathways. Some go up to the brain from the spinal cord and others travel down from the brain to the spinal cord.

- The central nervous system and the brain are "plastic." (This is termed *neuroplasticity*.) This means that the central nervous system and brain are changing and adapting to new information all the time. This, in turn, means that people *can influence their nervous systems and their brains*.

- At least 350 genes and probably more are thought to be involved in the regulation of pain.

- The immune system, and neurochemicals, play a big role in pain regulation.

- When the brain senses "danger," the body wants to protect you. This process works well with acute pain because you stop, rest, and let healing begin. With chronic pain, protective actions such as limiting movement and tensing muscles work against you. Healing has already happened as much as it is going to, and not moving is going to harm rather than help you.

- If you are interested in exploring concepts about pain beyond this brief introduction, review the multiple resources provided for you at www.bullpub.com/resources.

How Does Acute Pain Differ from Chronic Pain?

A common misconception is that chronic pain is the same as acute pain, except that chronic pain lasts longer. But there are many differences between acute and chronic pain. You can read more about these differences in Table 1.1. Understanding the differences between acute and chronic pain is a powerful step toward successful pain management for you and your family.

Table 1.1 **Acute and Chronic Pain: The Differences**

	Acute Pain	**Chronic Pain**
Duration	Short or time-limited	Long term; usually lasts more than three months (which is the typical time for healing)
Intensity	Often intense, depending on the cause	Varies in intensity, from mild to very severe
Location	Most often in one body area	Felt in one or many body areas
Purpose	Has survival value; warns of danger and harm and causes us to take action	Has little survival value; no longer warns of immediate danger or harm
Cause	Often due to tissue damage caused by injury or broken bones; biological mechanisms of acute pain such as inflammation are well understood	Biological mechanisms of chronic pain are complex compared with acute pain; the brain misinterprets nerve impulses as "danger" even after body tissues have healed or healed as much as they are going to
Emotional response	Associated with anxiety and worry, but these feelings go away	Often associated with ongoing irritability, fatigue, isolation, fear, helplessness, etc.; chronic pain is like a form of chronic stress
Diagnosis	Commonly accurate	Often difficult
Treatment	Treatments usually effective, and cure is common	Many treatments used with less consistent success; the goal of treatment is to calm the nervous system and retrain the brain
Role of activity and exercise in treatment	Rest is often best. Rest allows healing to begin	Activity and exercise, balanced with rest, are essential
Role of professionals	Diagnose and treat	Teach and partner
Role of person with pain	Follow treatment advice	Partner with health professionals; be responsible for daily management

Acute Pain

Everyone has experienced acute pain. Whether it is a stubbed toe, a sore throat, a toothache, or the aftereffects of surgery, acute pain usually has a known cause and normally goes away once healing has taken place. Acute pain is part of the body's defense against danger and harm. When acute pain strikes, you pay attention, take action, and do what you can to stop or lessen the pain.

The biological mechanisms of acute pain have been studied a lot and are well understood. Inflammation is the first response of the immune system and other body systems to an injury. White blood cells and other substances rush to the area, causing redness, heat, and swelling. Inflammation also reopens the gate in the spinal cord (see page 4) to allow nerve signals to go to the brain. Then we feel pain. At the same time, the brain and spinal cord release substances that start the healing process, reduce inflammation, and help us cope with the pain (see Figure 1.1 and page 5).

Because acute pain helps us survive, people manage it very differently from than chronic pain. In the early stages, acute pain can cause anxiety and worry. You may wonder: "What is the cause of the pain? How bad will the pain get? Will the pain go away?" The brain instructs the body to protect the injured area. Muscles can go into spasm. You may unconsciously hold muscles in tension. If it hurts enough, you stop, rest, and conserve energy. If, for example, you have had surgery or are feeling the aches and pains of flu, being too active can slow healing. You need to rest.

Once you understand the cause of the pain, seek treatment, and start to feel better, your anxiety usually lessens. As the pain and anxiety decreases and the healing happens, your body's protective mechanisms lessen. You gradually increase your activity, and your life gets back to normal.

When you have acute pain, your role and the role of your health care providers are clear. You go to your health care provider for a diagnosis and to get advice on how to treat your condition. For the most part, you follow that advice. You don't usually argue about whether you need a cast for a broken leg or whether you should take antibiotics for a severe chest infection. As a result, healing occurs, and the acute pain usually goes away.

But what if the pain does not go away? What if the brain network continues to interpret nerve impulses as "dangerous," even when there is no immediate danger? Then you may experience chronic pain.

Chronic Pain

Chronic pain is defined as pain lasting longer than three months. This is longer than the usual time it takes for the body to heal and recover from sickness or injury. There are different ways to classify chronic pain. In this book, we talk about two main kinds of chronic pain. One is pain associated with the symptoms of a chronic disease such as arthritis. The other kind of chronic pain is idiopathic chronic pain. You have probably heard a lot about disease-related pain, but you may not know what idiopathic pain is or you may not have even heard of it. So let's take some time now to understand this term.

Idiopathic means that we do not understand what causes the pain. Examples of idiopathic pain can include musculoskeletal pain (such as chronic neck, shoulder, and lower back pain), pain resulting from whiplash injuries, fibromyalgia, chronic regional pain syndromes, repetitive strain injury pain, postsurgical pain, phantom limb pain, chronic pelvic pain, and pain following a stroke. Persistent headache pain as well as pain from poorly understood chronic conditions such as irritable bowel syndrome, Crohn's disease, and interstitial cystitis are other examples. Initially, these pains may be triggered by an event such as a workplace injury, a minor fall, a surgical procedure, or a virus. Sometimes the pain may stem from nothing in particular or nothing specific. Often, idiopathic pain starts as acute pain that should have gone away but did not. Why? While there are no easy answers to this question, new research suggests that chronic inflammation along with many other factors play a role in many chronic pain conditions.

Chronic Pain Symptoms

When people experience acute pain, a full recovery is usually expected. Chronic pain, in contrast, usually leads to more symptoms. Many people assume that their symptoms are due only to one cause: their pain. But it is often more complex than that. Chronic pain can cause other symptoms, and each of these symptoms can make your other symptoms worse. For example, chronic pain can cause you to unconsciously hold tension in parts of your body, restricting movement of your muscles and joints. This can lead to fatigue. You may also take shallower breaths so that your body does not receive the oxygen it needs to function well. Pain-related stress and anxiety can also cause muscle tension, fatigue, and more pain. In addition, stress and anxiety can cause poor sleep and difficult emotions. Difficult emotions can leave you feeling frustrated, unhappy, and depressed. While pain can cause fatigue and poor sleep, so can depression. All these symptoms feed on each other. The interactions of symptoms make chronic pain complex to manage. It produces a vicious cycle that only gets worse unless you find a way to break the symptom cycle (see Figure 1.2 on page 10).

When the body is bombarded with chronic pain symptoms and intense signals that your brain interprets as pain, your nervous system eventually loses its ability to respond effectively. As a result, in people with chronic pain, areas of the spinal cord and brain change over time. The changes cause some people to become more sensitive to weaker signals. For example, these people may develop sensitivity to even mild touch that would typically not cause pain. Or pain that was once located in only one body part may seem to move to other areas, causing widespread pain. Also, the intensity or strength of the pain may begin to change from one day to the next. Just as soon as you have gotten used to one intensity or type or place for pain, the level or location or type changes.

People with chronic pain may have an increase in some neurochemicals and a decrease

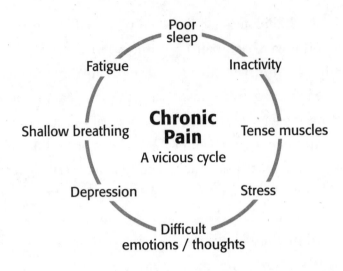

Figure 1.2 **The Vicious Cycle: Chronic Pain Symptoms**

in others (see page 5). For example, your body may release excess cortisol (a neurochemical released during stress). This release of cortisol can destroy tissues and cause more pain. Or your body may produce fewer endorphins (so-called feel-good neurochemicals), less serotonin (a neurochemical that plays a role in sleep and mood), and other neurochemicals that help regulate the body's response to pain, such as inflammation. It's as though your body can't keep up with the demand for helpful neurochemicals and instead makes too much of the harmful ones.

The emotional response to chronic pain is different from the response to acute pain. In a very real sense, chronic pain is a form of chronic stress. Chronic pain is associated with ongoing tension, fear, anxiety, fatigue, and difficult emotions such as frustration and anger. This can lead to feelings of helplessness, hopelessness, and depression.

When you feel this way, nagging questions arise: *Why me? Why is the pain not going away?*

What do I really have? How can I explain this to other people when I can't understand it myself? What does the future hold? All these questions and concerns are very real. But the big secret of dealing with chronic pain is that the answers to these questions don't really matter or help. The way to deal with chronic pain is not to look for causes but to move toward management. You may never know what causes your pain. Instead of obsessing about what causes your pain, be kind to yourself, learn and practice self-management, and resolve to get the most out of life.

The good news is that there are things you can do that may increase the levels of helpful neurochemicals, including exercise, relaxation and meditation, positive thinking, and even laughing. Throughout this book we examine ways to break the chronic pain symptom cycle by using self-management tools and skills and resolving physical and emotional helplessness. Exercise, for example, plays a key role in chronic pain management. Because exercise helps your body produce helpful neurochemicals, it is important to be active when you have chronic pain. This is another way chromic pain, which benefits from exercise, is unlike acute pain, which initially requires rest. In addition to generating helpful neurochemicals, exercise can help your brain reinterpret body movements as safe and not dangerous.

Understanding and Managing Your Chronic Pain

Throughout this book you will find tools to help you "close the gate," retrain the brain, and support the regulation of helpful neurochemicals. To get started with managing your pain and retraining your brain, you need to carefully observe how chronic pain and its treatment affect your physical and mental health. Chronic pain is different for every person. With experience, you can become an expert at knowing the effects of your condition and its treatment. You are the only person who lives with your chronic pain every minute of every day. Watching how it affects your life and making accurate reports to your health care providers are key parts of being a good self-manager.

Once you begin to observe your symptoms, you can start managing both symptoms and pain. The self-test and self-scoring at the end of this chapter on pages 17 and 21 are useful tools. They can help you learn more about your own pain, like how severe it is and how often it flares and what happens to your body and emotions when it flares. It is also useful to pay attention to what makes your pain better or worse. You will find some advice on how to keep a pain diary or pain activity sheet on pages 56 and 57.

When you develop a painful condition, you become more aware of your body. Minor symptoms that you ignored may now cause concerns.

For example, you may wonder if the pain in your leg is a sign that you should stop exercising. Is your pain spreading to other parts of your body, and if it is, what does that mean? Does the pain in your back mean there is something really serious going on with your spine? There are no simple, reassuring answers. There are also no fail-safe ways to sort out serious signals from minor symptoms that you can safely ignore. But we offer some guidelines in this book to help lessen the risk of missing more serious symptoms.

What Is Self-Management?

Self-management is the use of skills (tools) to manage the work of living with your chronic pain while continuing your daily activities. At the same time, you must deal with emotions brought about by your condition. Both at home and in the business world, managers are in charge. Managers don't do everything themselves; they work with others, including consultants, to get the job done. What makes them managers is that they are responsible for making decisions and making sure that their decisions are carried out.

As the manager of your chronic pain, your job is much the same. You gather information and hire a consultant or team of consultants (your doctor and other health professionals). Once your team members have given you their best advice, it is up to you to follow through. All chronic conditions need day-to-day management.

Managing chronic pain, like managing a family or a business, is a complex undertaking. Most chronic conditions take an up-and-down path. They do not follow a steady path, and they are not the same every day or every week. Chronic pain is like that too. There are many twists and turns, and you will need to make midcourse corrections to manage chronic pain. By learning self-management skills, you can ease the problems of living with your condition. The key to success in any undertaking is (1) defining the problem, (2) deciding what you want to do, (3) deciding how you are going to do it, and (4) learning a set of skills and practicing them until you master them. Success in chronic pain self-management is the same.

What Are Self-Management Skills?

This book is about self-management skills. You do not have to learn and use all these skills. You can just learn and practice the ones that are most useful for you. Also, you do not have to learn all these skills at once. Slow and steady wins the race. Some of the major skills include:

- problem solving and action planning to make positive changes in your life

- decision making about your health and wellness, such as when to seek medical help and what treatments to try

- maintaining a healthy lifestyle with regular exercise, healthy eating, good sleep habits, and stress management

- finding and using community and other resources

- observing, understanding, and managing your condition and your symptoms

- working effectively with your health care team

- using medications and assistive devices safely and effectively

- learning and practicing cognitive (thinking) and behavioral pain-management techniques such as challenging worst-case thinking, practicing relaxation, and pacing activities

- talking about your illness with family and friends

- adapting social activities

- managing your work life

Using Self-Management Skills and Tools

In this book, we describe many skills and tools to help relieve the problems caused by chronic pain. We do not expect you to use all of them. Pick and choose. Experiment. Set your own goals. What you do may not be as important as the sense of confidence and control that comes from successfully doing something you want to do. We have learned that knowing the skills is not enough. You need a way to use these skills in your daily life. Whenever you try a new skill, the first attempts may be clumsy, slow, and show few results. It is easier to return to old ways than to continue trying to master new, and sometimes difficult, tasks. The best way to master new skills is to go slow, practice, and evaluate the results.

What you do about something is largely determined by how you think about it. For example, if you think that having chronic pain is like falling into a deep pit, you may have a hard time motivating yourself to crawl out, or you may even think the task is impossible. The thoughts you have can greatly determine what happens to you and how you handle your health problems.

Good self-managers are people who have learned three types of skills to negotiate this path:

■ **Skills to deal with chronic pain.** Chronic pain, like any health condition, requires that you do new things to address your condition. These may include practicing relaxation techniques regularly, developing a fitness program, and monitoring your pain levels so you know when to take rest breaks. You may have more frequent visits with your health care providers. You may need to take medications or treatments on a daily basis. All of these are examples of the work you must do to manage your chronic pain condition and your health. This book discusses helpful pain-management skills in Chapter 4, *Understanding and Managing Common Symptoms and Problems*, Chapter 5, *Using Your Mind to Manage Pain and Other Symptoms*, Chapter 7, *Exercising and Physical Activity for Every Body*, Chapter 8, *Exercising to Feel Better*, Chapter 9, *Healthy Eating and Pain Self-Management*, Chapter 10 *Healthy Weight and Pain Self-Management*, Chapter 14, *Managing Your Treatment Decisions and Medications*, Chapter 15, *Understanding Medications and Other Treatments for Chronic Pain*, and Chapter 16, *Managing Specific Chronic Pain Conditions: Arthritis, Neck and Back Pain, Fibromyalgia,* *Headache, Pelvic Pain, and Neuropathic Pain Syndromes.*

■ **Skills to continue your normal life.** Chronic pain does not mean that life stops. Life goes on. There are still chores to do, jobs to perform, and relationships to continue. You may need to learn new skills or adapt the way you do things in order to keep doing the things you need and want to do. This book discusses helpful life-management skills in Chapter 2, *Becoming an Active Self-Manager*, Chapter 3, *Finding Resources*, Chapter 6, *Organizing and Pacing Your Life for Pain Self-Management and Safety*, Chapter 12, *Managing Pain during Employment and Unemployment*, and Chapter 17, *Planning for the Future: Fears and Reality.*

■ **Skills to deal with emotions.** When you are diagnosed with a chronic pain condition, your future changes. Your plans change and your emotions change. Many of your new emotions may be negative. They may include anger ("Why me? It's not fair"), fear ("I am afraid to move my body in case I hurt myself"), depression ("I can't do anything anymore, so what's the use?"), frustration ("No matter what I do, it doesn't make any difference. I can't do what I want to do"), isolation ("No one understands. No one wants to be around someone who is in pain all the time"), or thinking the worst ("I have cancer; they just haven't found it yet"). Negotiating the path of chronic pain means learning skills to work with negative emotions. This book discusses helpful emotional-management skills in Chapter 5, *Using Your Mind to Manage Pain and Other*

Symptoms, Chapter 11, *Communicating with Family, Friends, and Health Care Providers*, Chapter 12, *Managing Pain during Employment and Unemployment*, and Chapter 13, *Enjoying Sex and Intimacy*.

Same Condition, Different Responses

Self-management can make a real difference in how you live your life with chronic pain. Let's consider some examples. Brent suffers from chronic lower back pain. He is in pain most of the time and has difficulty sleeping. He took early retirement because of his pain and now, at age 55, he spends his days sitting at home watching TV or lying down resting. He avoids most physical activity because of his pain, weakness, and fatigue. Brent doesn't pay much attention to his diet. He has become very irritable. It even seems too much trouble when the grandchildren he adores come to visit. Most people, including his family, no longer enjoy Brent's company.

Josefa, age 66, also suffers from chronic lower back pain. Every day she manages to walk several blocks to the local library or the park. When the pain is severe, Josefa practices relaxation techniques and tries to distract herself. If the pain is still bad, she takes medication that her doctor has prescribed. She has learned to plan her activities around her condition so she can still do things she enjoys, like meeting her friends for coffee and visiting her grandchildren. Josefa even manages to take care of the grandkids sometimes when her daughter has to run errands. Her husband is amazed at how much zest she has for life.

Brent and Josefa both live with the same condition and similar physical problems. Yet their abilities to function and enjoy life are very different. Why? In part, the difference lies in their respective attitudes toward their chronic pain. Brent has allowed his quality of life and physical abilities to decline. Josefa has learned to take an active role in managing her pain. Even though she has limitations, *she* controls her life instead of letting the pain take control.

Why is it that two people with similar chronic pain conditions live their lives so differently? One may be able to minimize the effect of symptoms, while the other is always thinking about the worst and is extremely disabled. One may focus on healthy living, while the other is completely focused on the pain. We have all noticed that some people with severe physical problems get on well, while others with lesser problems seem to give up on life. The difference often lies in their management style. One of the keys that affects the impact of any disease is how engaged the person is in self-management.

Attitude alone cannot cure chronic pain. But a positive attitude and certain self-management skills can make it much easier to live a healthy life with a chronic pain condition. Research shows that pain, discomfort, and disability can be modified by beliefs, thoughts, mood, and the attention paid to symptoms. For example, with arthritis of the knee, a better predictor of how disabled, limited, and uncomfortable the person will be is his or her degree of depression rather than the evidence of physical damage to the knee visible on X-rays.

Research has also found excessive negative thinking and focusing attention on pain to be a strong contributor to increased levels of pain and disability in people with neck, shoulder, and back pain and different types of nerve pain. What goes on in a person's mind is at least as important as what is going on in the person's body. As one self-manager from our program says, "It is not mind over matter. It is that mind matters!"

Chronic pain can cause a change in lifestyle. Some people may decide to slow down at work and focus on their home life. They may decide to spend more time deepening relationships with family and friends, or they may pick up an old hobby they used to enjoy. For example, Melanie has had fibromyalgia for three years. She loves music and learned to play the guitar when she was younger, but she hadn't played for years because she was too busy. After her diagnosis, she started playing again and discovered a whole new network of friends where she lives as well as online. She feels her life is richer because of music and her new friends. So, although chronic pain is a difficult condition and may close some doors, you can, like Melanie, choose to open new ones.

David developed chronic hip and leg pain after a car accident 15 years ago. After four surgeries, he still has chronic pain. A few years back, he became involved in a support group as a way to handle his stress. Now he is the director of a local chronic pain association. He feels that before the accident he would never have thought he had the skills to be a leader. Chronic pain, he says, taught him to be persistent and work toward a goal. For him, "knowing that I'm involved and helping others" is the key.

Working with Health Care Providers to Manage Your Pain

This book focuses on self-management, but self-management does not mean managing your chronic pain condition alone. Get help or advice when you are concerned or uncertain. If a symptom is severe, lasts a long time, or begins after you start a new medication or treatment, check it out with your health care provider. Collaboration and partnership are the cornerstones of effective care (see Chapter 11, *Communicating with Family, Friends, and Health Care Providers*). Health care professionals are experts in health conditions, and they can be your most valuable consultants. But you are the expert about your own life and how pain affects your daily life. Because you are responsible for managing your condition day-to-day, the advice and lifestyle changes proposed by health professionals must be based on your needs.

Throughout this book, we give some specific examples of what actions to take if you have certain symptoms. Deciding when to take action when you experience symptoms is where your partnership with your health care providers becomes critical. Good treatment depends on good communication with health care providers. Let's look at an example: Suzanne, Jose, and Maya all have arthritis that affects their back, hands, and knees. They have been prescribed medicine for their condition, but so far their pain is no better.

■ Suzanne tells her doctor that she sometimes forgets to take her medicine and is not getting much exercise. She is overweight. Her doctor talks with her, and together they work out a plan to help her remember her medications, start an exercise program, and cut down on the amount of food she eats.

■ Jose reports in his wellness checkup that he takes his medications, is exercising, and is eating well. But he also mentions that sometimes the medication upsets his stomach. The doctor decides to change his medication because what he is currently on is not reducing Jose's pain and has unpleasant side effects.

■ Maya does not want to take her prescribed medication. She is doing everything she can to manage her pain: being physically active, using distraction and relaxation, and eating well. Still she finds that on some days she just stays in bed all day because the pain is too bad. The doctor talks to her about using her medication regularly so that she won't have so many bad days. In the end, she decides to try taking the medication daily for a month and then reporting back to the doctor about how things are going.

The management of arthritis varies for each of these people. Their treatment plans are different and depend on what each person is doing and what each one tells their health care team members. Effective pain management involves an observant person talking openly with health care providers.

Other Things to Know about Chronic Pain

■ You are not to blame. You are not responsible for causing your chronic pain or failing to cure it. Chronic pain conditions are caused by a combination of genetic, biological, environmental, and psychological factors. There are many things you can do that will help you manage your chronic pain condition. Remember, although you are not responsible for causing the pain, you are responsible for acting to manage it.

■ Don't do it alone. Isolation is often a side effect of chronic pain. As supportive as friends and family members may be, they often cannot understand what you feel as you struggle to make it through each day. However, there are others who know firsthand what it is like to live with a chronic pain condition. Remember at the beginning of the chapter, we noted that up to one in four people live with chronic pain. Connecting with other people with similar pain problems can reduce your sense of isolation and help you understand what to expect. Someone who has a chronic pain condition like yours can offer practical tips on how to manage symptoms and feelings on a day-to-day basis. Other benefits of reaching out to others include having the experience of helping them manage *their* illness. This can help you appreciate your strengths and inspire you to take a more active role in managing your own condition. Support can also come from learning how someone else lives with chronic pain—you may find real stories from real people anywhere: a book, website, blog, an Instagram account, or a Facebook group. Or it can come from talking with others on the telephone or in support groups, either online or in person.

■ You are more than your pain. Too often pain becomes the center of someone's life. But you are more than your pain—you are a person. And life is more than trips to the clinic and managing symptoms. It is vital to do the things you enjoy. Find ways to enjoy nature by growing a plant or watching a sunset, or indulge in the pleasure of a long, intimate chat or a tasty meal. Celebrate companionship with family or friends. Finding ways to introduce moments of pleasure is vital to chronic pain self-management. Focus on your abilities and strengths rather than disabilities and problems. Helping others is one way to increase your own sense of what you can do instead of focusing on what you can't. Celebrate small improvements. If chronic pain teaches anything, it is to live each moment more fully. Within the true limits of whatever pain condition you have, there are ways to enhance your function, sense of control, and enjoyment of life.

■ Illness can be an opportunity. As strange as it may sound, chronic pain can enrich lives. It can make you reevaluate what you care about, shift priorities, and move in exciting new directions that you may never have considered before.

Your Chronic Pain Self-Management Self-Test

The following self-test is a useful tool that can help you learn more about your own pain, like how severe it is and how it affects your body and emotions when it strikes. To take charge of your pain self-management, you need to know and understand your pain.

Chronic Pain Self-Management Self-Test

To help you with your pain self-management, please take this self-test. When you are finished, you can score yourself and, based on your score, find more information.

Fatigue (Tiredness)

Circle the *number* that describes your **fatigue** in the **past two weeks.**

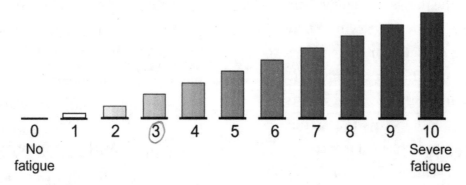

Scoring: Put your Fatigue Score here.   **My Fatigue Score** _____

Sleep

Circle the *number* that describes your **sleep** in the **past two weeks.**

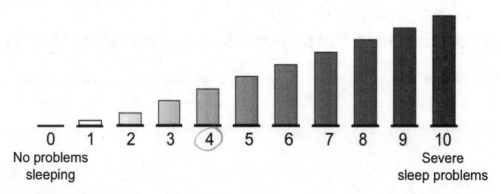

Scoring: Put your Sleep Score here.   **My Sleep Score** _____

Pain Intensity

Circle the *number* that best describes the intensity (strength) of your pain in the **past two weeks** from 0 (no pain) to 10 (severe pain).

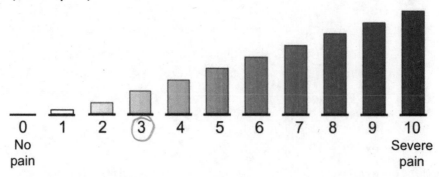

Scoring: Put your Pain Score here.   **My Pain Score** _____

Activity Interference

Circle the *number* describes how much pain has gotten in the way of your doing the things you need and want to do from 0 (not at all) to 10 (very much) in the **past two weeks.**

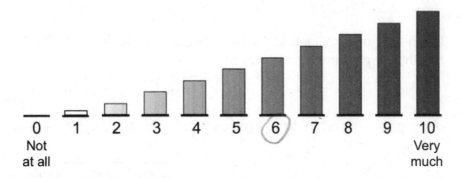

| 0 | 1 | 2 | 3 | 4 | 5 | 6 | 7 | 8 | 9 | 10 |

Not at all   Very much

Scoring: Put your Interference Score here.   **My Interference Score** _____

Health Worries

On scale of 0 to 4, how much time during the **past two weeks** (please *circle* one *number* for each question):

	None of the time	A little of the time	Some of the time	A good bit of the time	All of the time
1. Were you discouraged by your pain or health problems?	0	1	②	3	4
2. Were you fearful about your future health?	0	1	2	③	4
3. Was your health a worry in your life?	0	1	2	③	4
4. Were you frustrated by your pain or health problems?	0	1	2	③	4

Scoring: Add the four circled numbers to get your Worries Score.   **My Worries Score** __11__

Physical Activities

We would like to know more about your endurance exercise (cardiovascular or aerobic exercise). Endurance exercises include walking, running, dancing, swimming, rowing, bicycling, Nordic (cross-country) skiing, etc. Stretching is not considered endurance exercise.

Please fill in each space with 0 or the number of **total minutes of endurance exercise** you did each day last week. Be sure to total your daily minutes. The minutes can be spread out throughout the day.

Monday ____ Tuesday ____ Wednesday ____ Thursday ____ Friday ____ Saturday ____ Sunday ____

Scoring:

How many days did you exercise 10 minutes or less? _____

How many days did you exercise more than 10 minutes but less than 30 minutes? _____

How many days did you exercise 30 minutes or more? _____

Height and Weight

Your height: _5'_

Your weight: _133_

Are you overweight?

Yes   No   (If you are not sure, look at the Body Mass Index table on pages 234–235 to find the healthy weight for your height.)

Managing Pain

When you are feeling pain, how often do you (please *circle* one *number* for each question):

	Never	Almost never	Some-times	Fairly often	Very often	Always
1. Try to feel distant from the pain and pretend that it is not part of your body?	0	1	2	3	4	5
2. Think of it not as pain but as some other sensation, like a warm, numb feeling?	0	1	2	3	4	5
3. Play mental games or sing songs to keep your mind off the pain?	0	1	2	3	4	5
4. Challenge the way you think about the pain?	0	1	2	3	4	5
5. Practice visualization or guided imagery, such as picturing yourself somewhere else?	0	1	2	3	4	5

Scoring: Add the five circled numbers to get your Management Score. **My Management Score** _____

Medications

Are you now taking opioids for your pain?   Yes   No

Opioids include the following:

- hydrocodone (Vicodin®)
- oxycodone (OxyContin®, Percocet®)
- oxymorphone (Opana®)
- morphine (Kadian®, Avinza®)
- codeine
- fentanyl

Do you have any opioid medication in your home?   Yes   No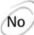

Chronic Pain Self-Management
Self-Test—What It Means

What Do Your Answers Mean?
For each category, refer to your scores from the self-test.

Fatigue (Tiredness)

If your score is:

0–4 Fatigue is probably <u>not your main concern</u>. Though you may want to work on fatigue management, you may want to start by addressing another issue that is more of a problem for you. The good news is that almost all the tools in this book, when used regularly, can help you fight fatigue.

5–7 Fatigue is probably an important concern for you. Your fatigue may be related to your pain. The good news is that by working at it day by day, you can do a lot to reduce your fatigue. Start by reading pages 67–68 and Chapter 4, *Understanding and Managing Common Symptoms and Problems.*

8–10 Fatigue is probably a major problem for you. You should let your health care providers know about your fatigue level. Pain and some medications can cause fatigue or make it worse. You might need to change your medications. Are you taking your medications as prescribed? If not, taking your medications correctly might help. The good news is that by working on it daily, you can do a lot to reduce your fatigue. Start by reading pages 67–68 and Chapter 4, *Understanding and Managing Common Symptoms and Problems.*

Sleep

If your score is:

0–4 Sleep is probably not your main concern. Though you may want to work on sleep management, you may want to start by addressing another issue that is more of a problem for you. The good news is that almost all the tools in this book when used regularly can help you get better sleep.

5–7 Sleep is probably an important concern for you. Pain and sleep problems are often related. They each make the other one worse. The good news is that by working at it day by day, you can do a lot to get better sleep. Start by reading pages 69–74 in Chapter 4, *Understanding and Managing Common Symptoms and Problems.*

8–10 Sleep is probably a major problem for you. You should let your health care providers know about your sleep problems. Pain and some medications can cause problems sleeping. You might need to change your medications. Are you taking your medications as prescribed? If not, taking your medications correctly might help. The good news is that by working on it daily and practicing good sleep self-management, you can get better sleep. Start by reading pages 69–74 in Chapter 4, *Understanding and Managing Common Symptoms and Problems.*

Pain

There are many ways to think about pain. Let's consider two of these. Sometimes people have a low pain level, but it interferes a lot with what they want to do.

First, what is your day-in and day-out level of pain? (Pain Intensity section on your self-test.) Second, how much does pain interfere with the things you want and need to do? (Activity Interference section on your self-test.)

If your total score for both Pain Intensity and Activity Interference is between 0 and 4:
Pain is not a major problem for you. This probably means that you are managing pain and your health well. However, there are always new things to learn.

If your total score for both Pain Intensity and Activity Interference is 5 or above:
Pain is an important concern for you. Pain is often related to fatigue, poor sleep, depression, and stress. Each one makes the others worse (see page 59). The good news is that by working at it day by day, you can do a lot to reduce your pain and how your pain interferes with what you want and need to do. You can start by learning a little more about pain in this chapter, and looking at your other scores to work on the pain-related areas where you score high.

If your score for Pain Intensity is between 0 and 4 and for Activity Interference is 5 or above:
Your score means that your day-to-day pain is not too intense, but pain interferes greatly in the things you want and need to do. Ask yourself why and how your pain interferes. Is it because you tire easily or overdo it sometimes?

If so, read about pacing yourself in Chapter 6, *Organizing and Pacing Your Life for Pain Self-Management and Safety*. Is your pain caused by sore muscles or joints? If so, start with the Moving Easy Program and exercises in Chapter 8, *Exercising to Feel Better*. These are very gentle and are designed to help get you moving without making pain worse. Are you afraid of falling? Then the balance exercises in Chapter 8 are a good place to start (see pages 166–169). If you are overweight, that may be a major cause of your pain. You can read about getting to and maintaining an appropriate weight in Chapter 10, *Healthy Weight and Pain Self-Management*.

Health Worries

If your score is:

0–4 You are probably dealing with very few or no difficult emotions. The good news is that no matter where you start in this book, your worries will probably become even fewer.

5–8 You are dealing with some difficult emotions. This is not unusual. Chronic pain can result in chronic stress and worry. You might want to start by reading about difficult emotions in Chapter 5, *Using Your Mind to Manage Pain and Other Symptoms*. No matter which chapter you decide to start with, the good news is that almost all the self-management activities in this book help you better handle your worries.

9–16 You are dealing with a lot of worries and difficult emotions about your pain and health conditions. These are probably serious enough for you to talk with your doctor, psychologist, or social worker. Seeking help is part of being a good self-manager. You do not need to feel so down. Get some help. You can start learning more by reading pages 97–112 in Chapter 5, *Using Your Mind to Manage Pain and Other Symptoms*. The good news is that there are many things that can help: self-management, talk therapy, and/or medications. Read Chapter 11, *Communicating with Family, Friends, and Health Care Providers* to prepare for your discussion with your health care professional.

Physical Activities

Physical activity and exercise are important for everyone but especially for people who experience pain. Often some of the pain is due to weak muscles and joints. Gentle exercise can help strengthen muscles and reduce pain.

If you exercised less than 10 minutes four or more days last week, you are not doing much exercise right now. The recommendation is that everyone exercise 30 or more minutes four to five days a week. There is no time like the present to start!

- Practice the Moving Easy Program (introduced on page 173) on your CD or MP3 player at least every other day. You will find pictures of all the exercises in Chapter 8, *Exercising to Feel Better*.

- As the Moving Easy Program becomes easier, add 5 to 15 minutes of walking four days a week. Read more about endurance exercise in Chapter 7, *Exercising and Physical Activity for Every Body*.

- If you are only able to do the Moving Easy Program, that is OK! Keeping your body moving will help you.

If you exercised more than 10 minutes but less than 30 minutes four or more days last week, you are already taking part in an exercise program. Congratulations! The recommendation is that everyone exercise 30 or more minutes four to five days a week. Consider building on your current exercise program. For the best results:

- Read Chapter 7, *Exercising and Physical Activity for Every Body*, and Chapter 8, *Exercising to Feel Better*.

- Do the Moving Easy Program (introduced on page 173) a few times. Pay attention to how the movements make you feel. You may find places in your body that need a little work on flexibility or strength.

- Do moderate endurance exercise on most days of the week (four or five days), working toward a total of 30 minutes for each exercise day.

- The 30 minutes does not have to be done all at once. For example, your goal can be to work up to 10 minutes at a time three times per day, most days ot the week.

- Also do flexibility and/or strengthening exercises most days of the week.

- Flexibility exercises before and after endurance exercise help prevent sore muscles and injury.

- Strengthening exercises help make your muscles stronger and more efficient.

- Do strengthening exercises no more often than every other day, two to three days per week.

If you exercised 20 minutes but less than 30 minutes four or more days last week, good work!

You are almost at the recommended amount. The recommendation is that everyone exercise 30 or more minutes four to five days a week. Just add a little more to what you are doing now, and you will be there. Remember that you do not have to do all your exercise at once. You can break it down into several sessions a day.

■ Consider doing the Moving Easy Program (introduced on page 173). Although this may seem easy, you may find a few spots that need some extra work.

■ You can also read Chapter 7, *Exercising and Physical Activity for Every Body,* and Chapter 8, *Exercising to Feel Better.*

If you exercised 30 minutes or more four or more days last week, *wow!* It looks like you are already doing a lot of endurance exercise! Congratulations on keeping your body moving!

■ It is important to spread out your endurance exercise to more days of the week. Doing about 30 to 60 minutes of endurance exercise most days of the week is the goal.

■ Remember, flexibility or strengthening exercises are also an important part of a complete fitness program. If you are not doing much of these, add some flexibility exercises before and after endurance exercise. Doing so helps prevent sore muscles and injury. You can start with the Moving Easy Program in Chapter 8, and read Chapter 7, *Exercising and Physical Activity for Every Body,* and Chapter 8, *Exercising to Feel Better.*

Weight

People often do not think about how excess weight can cause pain. However, being overweight makes your muscles, joints, and bones work much harder. Think about lifting three different bags, one with three apples (weighing one pound), one with nine apples (weighing three pounds), one with 18 apples (weighing six pounds), and finally one with 30 apples (weighing ten pounds). Each bag is probably a bit more difficult to lift than the previous one. You might also feel more and more pain in your back, arms, shoulders, hips, knees, or feet. When you put the heavier bags down, the pain goes away.

If you are overweight, losing weight can help decrease pain. Use your height and weight to find your body mass index (BMI) on pages 234–235 in Chapter 10, *Healthy Weight and Pain Self-Management.* Body mass index is one of the best indications of whether someone is underweight, healthy weight, or overweight. The information on page 232 can help you better understand BMI.

If your BMI is below 18.5, you are underweight. You will find information to help you gain weight on pages 243–244 in Chapter 10, *Healthy Weight and Pain Self-Management.*

If your BMI is between 18.5 and below 25, you are at a healthy weight. Good for you. You might want to review Chapter 9, *Healthy Eating and Pain Self-Management,* and Chapter 10, *Healthy Weight and Pain Self-Management.* Even if you are at a normal weight, you might not be getting all the benefits you could from healthy eating.

If your BMI is 25 or above, you are overweight. Excess weight may be adding to your pain. The good news is that losing just 5 to 10 percent of your weight can make a big difference. (This is 10 to 20 pounds for someone who weighs 200 pounds.) Any weight loss is helpful. You will find out more about how to lose weight and keep it off in Chapter 10, *Healthy Weight and Pain Self-Management*. Chapter 9, *Healthy Eating and Pain Self-Management*, will help you make good decisions about healthy eating.

Managing Pain

When you have pain, your thoughts matter. Did you know that we do not feel pain until our nerves send a signal to our brains? The same part of our brain that tells us we have pain also tells us when we are angry or depressed. It is not surprising that by using the mind, we can often lessen our pain.

If your score is:

21–30 You are using your mind to manage your pain a lot. Good for you! You might find some more helpful hints in Chapter 5, *Using Your Mind to Manage Pain and Other Symptoms*. If your response to number 5 on your self-test for managing pain is below 4, be sure to read the content about Challenging Negative Self-Talk and Worst-Case Thinking (page 102) and listen to the relaxation CD or MP3. There you can find four different relaxation exercises from which to choose. (If you did not purchase a relaxation CD or MP3 with your book, you can order one from www.bullpub.com or use a relaxation recording or app of your choice.)

11–20 You are probably not using your mind as much as you could to help with your pain. It may be that you are only doing one or two things, or that the things you are doing are not working for you as well as they might. You might find some helpful ideas in Chapter 5, *Using Your Mind to Manage Pain and Other Symptoms*. If your response to number 5 on your self-test for managing pain is below 4, be sure to read the content about Challenging Negative Self-Talk and Worst-Case Thinking (page 102) and listen to the relaxation CD or MP3. There you can find four different relaxation exercises from which to choose. (If you did not purchase a relaxation CD or MP3 with your book, you can order one from www.bullpub.com or use a relaxation recording or app of your choice.)

0–10 You are not using one of your most valuable pain-management tools, or it may be that you are only using one or two techniques. We suggest that you read Chapter 5, *Using Your Mind to Manage Pain and Other Symptoms*, and choose one or two things to try. Remember, relief comes slowly, so give each tool a two-week trial before you decide it is not for you. If your response to number 5 on your self-test for managing pain is below 4, be sure to read the content about Challenging Negative Self-Talk and Worst-Case Thinking (page 102) and listen to the relaxation CD or MP3. There you can find four different relaxation exercises from which to choose. (If you did not purchase a relaxation CD or MP3 with your book, you can order one from www.bullpub.com or use a relaxation recording or app of your choice.)

Medications

Opioids are often very helpful for short-term pain such as that experienced immediately after surgery. But did you know that long-term use of opioids can cause more pain?

If you are currently taking opioids for pain or considering using opioids, read pages 329–333 in Chapter 15, *Understanding Medications and Other Treatments for Chronic Pain*. Reducing or stopping opioids is not something you should try on your own. You need a knowledgeable health professional to help you taper your use of these medications. Tapering usually takes many months and does not cause withdrawal symptoms or increased pain.

If you currently have any opioid medication at home, you are not alone. One study found that more than half of the people in the United States have opioids they are no longer using. These are usually sitting on a shelf or in a drawer waiting to be found by visitors, household help, children, or grandchildren. A major source of misused opioids is from homes. If you have opioids at home, please dispose of them safely (not down the toilet). Ask your pharmacist how to best dispose of them. You may be able to turn them in to your local police station or pharmacy. Or look for locked drug disposal boxes in your community.

■   ■   ■

We suggest you take this test and then start our self-management journey. Comeback and retake the test every two to three months to see your progress.

For a complete list of suggested further readings, useful websites, and other helpful resources, please see www.bullpub.com/resources.

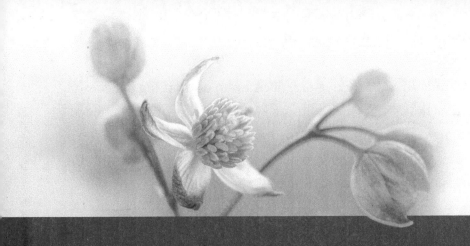

CHAPTER 2

Becoming an Active Self-Manager

Y OU ARE ALREADY A SELF-MANAGER. It is impossible to have a chronic pain condition without becoming a self-manager. How you live each day and the decisions you make affect you, your symptoms, and your quality of health and life. For example, some people with chronic pain conditions manage by withdrawing from life. They may stop doing their favorite activities, stay in bed, and socialize less. The pain becomes the center of their existence. Other people with the same condition and symptoms somehow manage to get on with life. They may have to change some of the things they do or the way they do them. We think of the self-manager who talks about the 90 percent of the things he can do rather than the 10 percent he cannot. Life can continue to be full and active, although people with chronic pain may need to make some changes in how they do things.

The difference between these two kinds of people is not the pain condition but rather how the people with chronic pain decide to manage their pain. Please note the word *decide*. Self-management is always a decision: a decision to be active or a decision to do nothing, a decision to seek help or a decision to suffer in silence. Since you are already a self-manager, you need to decide which kind of self-manager you want to be.

Self-Management Tasks and Your Self-Management Plan

The information and skills in this book are the tools you need to become an active self- manager. Being an active self-manager means you are ready and willing to:

- **Take care of your chronic pain and other health conditions.** When you are taking care of your health, you are following a treatment plan. You are taking the right kind of medicine and embracing healthy behaviors, such as exercising, changing worst-case thinking, and healthy eating. You are keeping informed about your health status, asking questions, and sharing information with health care providers, family, and friends. You actively take part in planning your treatment program by monitoring and reporting on your condition as well as sharing your preferences and goals with all members of your health care team.

- **Carry out your normal activities.** Your "normal activities" are the activities of life that are meaningful to you. They may include work, hobbies, socializing, volunteering, and being with family. Sometimes you may need to adjust the way you do these activities, but if you are an active self-manager, you continue to do most or all of them. As a self-manager, you are also willing to add new healthful activities into your daily life, such as exercising, eating more healthy foods, and taking time to calm your mind. You are also willing to eliminate unhealthy activities such as smoking.

- **Manage your emotions.** Chronic pain can cause emotional changes. You may experience anxiety, anger, uncertainty about the future, sadness due to changed expectations and unmet goals, and even depression. Chronic pain and the related emotions can also affect relationships with family and friends. These feelings are difficult, but they are also a part of the natural "ups and downs" in life. Self-managers know this and are committed to learning how to deal with their emotions.

You are the manager of your life, and like the manager of an organization or a household, you need information, a variety of helpful tools or skills, and an overall plan. This book gives you

Self-Management Tasks

- Take care of your chronic pain and other health conditions.
- Carry out your normal activities.
- Manage your emotions.

Self-Management Plan

1. Decide what you want to accomplish (your goal).
2. Look for various ways to accomplish your goal. This may include problem solving, decision making, and action planning as well as using one or more of the tools in this book.
3. Draft a short-term action plan or agreement with yourself. Make a schedule of where to start and what steps to take and when to take them.
4. Carry out the first part of your plan.
5. Check the results weekly.
6. Make changes as needed.
7. Reward yourself for each small success.

these things. A self-management plan features the steps you can find in the box above.

Although many self-management tools are discussed throughout this book, in this chapter we start by presenting the three most important tools: problem solving, decision making, and taking action. These are the tools that help you to decide which of the other tools work best for you as well as when and how to use the tools successfully.

Problem Solving: Finding Ways to Do Things

Awareness of problems sometimes start with a general feeling of uneasiness. Let's say you are unhappy but not sure why. Upon closer examination, you find that your pain limits your contact with some relatives who live far away. With the problem identified, you decide to take a trip to visit these relatives. You know what you want to accomplish, but now you need to make a list of ways to solve the problem.

In the past you always drove to see these relatives, but now making the trip in one day of driving is too painful and tiring, so you consider other options. You consider leaving at noon instead of early in the morning and making the trip in two days instead of one. You consider asking a friend to come along to share the driving. There is also a train that stops within 20 miles of your destination. Or you could travel by air. You decide to take the train.

The trip still seems overwhelming because there is so much to do to prepare. You decide to write down all your ideas for steps to take to make the trip a reality. These include choosing a good time to go, buying your ticket, figuring out how to handle luggage, finding a ride to and from the station, deciding if you can make it up and down the stairs to get on the train, and determining if you can walk on a moving train to get food or go to the bathroom.

You come up with a few problem-solving ideas to get started. First, you decide that you will call and find out just how much the railroad can help. You also decide to start taking a short walk each day, including walking up and down a few steps so that you will be steadier on your feet. The next day, you call the railroad and start your walking program.

A week later you check the results of your actions. Looking back at all the steps to be accomplished, you see that a single call answered many questions. The railroad office told you that they help people who have mobility problems and they have ways of dealing with many concerns. However, you are still worried about walking. Even though you are walking daily and doing better, you are still unsteady. You make a change in your plan by consulting a physical therapist, who suggests using a cane or walking stick. Although you don't like using it, you realize that a cane will give you the extra security you need on a moving train.

You have just engaged in problem solving to achieve your goal of taking a trip. Let's review the specific steps in problem solving.

1. **Identify the problem.** This is the first and most important step in problem solving. It is also usually the most difficult step. It can be hard to figure out exactly which problem you need to solve. But it just may take a little more thinking. You may know, for example, that stairs are a problem, but with a little more effort, you can determine that the real problem is your fear of falling.

2. **List ideas to solve the problem.** You may be able to come up with a good list yourself. You may also want to call on friends, family, members of your health care team, or community resources. These are your

consultants. One note about using consultants: These folks cannot help you if you do not describe the problem well. For example, there is a big difference between saying that you can't walk because your knee hurts because of arthritis and saying that you can't walk because your feet hurt because you cannot find walking shoes that fit properly.

3. **Pick an idea to try.** As you try something new, remember that new activities are usually difficult. Be sure to give your potential solution a fair chance before deciding it won't work.

4. **Check the results.** After you've given your idea a fair trial, figure out how you are doing with your problem. If all goes well, your problem may even be solved.

5. **Pick another idea if the first didn't work.** Make changes as needed. If you still have the problem, pick another idea from your list and try again.

6. **Use other resources.** Ask your consultants for more ideas if you still do not have a good solution.

7. Finally, if you have gone through all the steps until all ideas have been exhausted and the problem is still unsolved, you may have to accept that your problem may not be solvable right now. This is sometimes hard to do. If a problem can't be solved right now, that doesn't mean that you can't solve it later. That also doesn't mean that other problems you have cannot be solved now. Even if your path is blocked, there are probably alternative paths. Don't give up. As the British say, "Keep calm and carry on."

Problem-Solving Steps

1. Identify the problem.
2. List ideas to solve the problem.
3. Pick one idea to try.
4. Check the results.
5. Pick another idea if the first didn't work.
6. Use other resources.
7. Accept that the problem may not be solvable now.

Decision Making: Weighing the Pros and Cons

Making decisions is another important tool in our self-management toolbox. Some of the steps in decision making are like the problem-solving steps we just discussed. These steps can help you solve problems and make decisions.

1. **Identify the options.** For example, you may have to make a decision about getting help in the house or continuing to do all the work yourself. Sometimes the options are to change a behavior or to not change at all.

2. **Identify what you want.** You may want to continue your life as normally as possible, to have more time with your family, or not have to shovel the walkways, cut the grass, or clean the house. What is most important to you? Your values are the things you think are valuable and meaningful in your life. (We discuss more about values in Chapter 5, *Using Your Mind to Manage Pain and Other Symptoms.*) Sometimes identifying your deepest values (such as spending time with family) helps set priorities and increases your motivation to change.

3. **Write down pros and cons for each option.** List as many positives and negatives as you can for each option. Don't forget the emotional and social effects.

4. **Rate each pro and con** on a 5-point scale, with 1 indicating "not important" and 5 indicating "extremely important."

5. **Add up the ratings** and compare the pros and the cons for each option. If the pro column has the higher total for an option, it is a good option. If the con column has the higher total for an option, it is not as good of an option. If the totals are close or you are still not sure, go to the next step.

6. **Apply the "gut test."** For example, if you are trying to make a decision about work, ask yourself, does going back to work part-time feel right to you? If it feels right, you have probably reached a decision. If it doesn't, the way you feel should probably win out over the math from steps 4 and 5. When your feelings don't agree with the scores, it helps you understand that the reasons for your decision are emotional. You also may decide that you are not ready to decide yet. You may need to explore your feelings more, gather more information, or

perhaps discuss it with someone else such as your health care team, family, or friends.

Decision-Making Example

Should I get help in the house?

Pro	Rating	Con	Rating
I'll have more time	4	It's expensive	3
I'll be less tired	4	It's hard to find good help	1
I'll have a clean house	3	They won't do things my way	2
		I don't want a stranger in the house	1
Total	11		7

Add the points for the pro column and then add the points for the con column. Your decision in this option would be to get help because the pro score (11) is significantly higher than the con score (7). If this option feels right in your gut, you have the answer.

Here is an example of how to apply the decision-making process yourself:

Now it's your turn! Try making a decision using the following chart. It's OK to write in your book.

The key to successful problem solving and decision making is to take action. We talk about this next.

Decision to be made

Pro	Rating	Con	Rating
Total			

Decision-Making Steps

1. Identify the options.
2. Identify what you want.
3. Write down the pros and cons for each option.

4. Rate each pro and con.
5. Add up the ratings.
6. Apply the "gut test."

Taking Action: Making Things Happen

So far in this chapter we have introduced the steps to both problem solving and decision making. But knowing what you want to do and need to do is not always enough. You now have to take action. We suggest that you start by doing one thing at a time.

Sometimes we reject options without knowing much about them. In the earlier example, our traveler was unable to make a long driving trip but wrote a list of alternative travel arrangements and then chose the train.

Setting Your Goals

Before you can take action, you must decide what you want to do first. Be realistic and specific when setting your goal. Think about what you would really like to do. One self-manager wanted to join her family for a holiday meal in her daughter's home that had 20 steps leading up to it. Another wanted to overcome fatigue and attend evening social events. Still another wanted to continue to ride his motorcycle even though he could no longer lift his 1,000-pound (450 kg) bike.

Living with Uncertainty

Living with uncertainty can be hard. However, it is something that most of us simply have to do sometimes. Uncertainty is one of the causes of emotional ups and downs. Chronic pain takes away some of your sense of security and control. It can be frightening. You are following your life path, and suddenly you are forced to detour to a different, unwanted path. And even as you work with health professionals and start new treatments, this uncertainty continues. Of course, everyone has an uncertain future, but most people do not think about this. When you have pain, however, this becomes a big part of your life. You are uncertain about your future health and perhaps about your ability to continue to do the things you want, need, and like to do. Many people find it very challenging to make decisions while accepting uncertainty. The tools in this chapter can help you make decisions even in the face of uncertainty.

One of the problems with goals is that they often seem like dreams. They are so far off, big, or difficult that it is easy to be overwhelmed and not even try to accomplish them. We discuss this problem next. For now, take a few minutes and write your goals below (add more lines if you need to).

Goals

_____

_____

_____

_____

Put a star (✩) next to the goal you would like to work on first.

Don't reject a goal until you have thought about possible alternatives to achieve it.

Exploring Your Options

There are many ways to reach any specific goal. For example, our self-manager who wanted to climb 20 steps could start off with a slow walking program and climb just a few steps each day, or she could ask to have the family gathering at a different place. The man who wanted to manage his fatigue so he could attend social events could plan rest periods during the day, go on shorter outings, ask a friend to go along to help with driving, or talk to his health care team about other ways to manage fatigue. Our motorcycle rider could buy a lighter motorcycle, ride in a fellow biker's sidecar, put "training wheels" on his bike, or buy a three-wheeled motorcycle.

As you can see, there are many options for reaching most goals. List all the options you can think of and then choose one or two to try out.

Throughout the book you will see lines of text that are shaded. This material is of special interest to our readers in Canada.

Sometimes it is hard to think of all the options yourself. If you are having problems listing options, it is time to use a consultant, just as you do in problem solving. Share your goal with family, friends, or health professionals. Don't ask someone else to decide what you should do. Rather, ask for suggestions. It is always good to add to your list of options by getting fresh ideas from someone or somewhere new. Call organizations such as the American Chronic Pain Association, the Chronic Pain Association of Canada, or the organization specific to your condition such as the Arthritis Foundation in the United States or the Arthritis Society in Canada. Local community or senior centers may also have good information. Search trusted sites on the internet.

A note of caution: people may never seriously consider many options because they assume they don't exist or are unworkable. Never make this assumption until you have thoroughly investigated an option. One woman we know had lived in the same town all her life and felt that she knew all about the community resources. When she was having problems with her health insurance, a friend from another city suggested contacting an insurance counselor. The woman dismissed this suggestion because she was certain that this service did not exist in her town. It was only when, months later, the friend came to visit and called the Area Agency on Aging (which exists in most counties in the United States) that the woman learned that there were three insurance counseling services nearby. (In Canada, similar services are provided by Programs and Services for Seniors.) Our motorcycle rider thought that training wheels on a Harley was a crazy idea but investigated the idea when a worker at a bike shop suggested it. He added 15 years to his riding life using training wheels. In short, never assume anything. Assumptions are the enemies of good problem solving and decision making.

Write the list of options for how you might reach your main goal here. Put a star (☆) next to the two or three options you want to research further and pursue.

Options: Possible Ways to Reach Your Goal

_____

_____

_____

_____

_____

Making Short-Term Plans: Action Planning

Once a decision has been made and your goal has been set, you have a pretty good idea of where you are going. However, your goal may still seem overwhelming. How will I ever move, how will I ever be able to paint again, how will I ever be able to _____ (you fill in the blank)? The secret to succeeding is *not* trying to do everything at once. Instead, first look at one thing you can realistically expect to accomplish within *the next week*.

This approach to moving toward your goal is *action planning*. An action plan is short-term and doable, and it sets you on the road toward achieving your goal. Your action plan should be about something you *want* to do or accomplish. It should help you solve a problem or reach a goal. It is a tool to help you do what *you* wish. Do not make action plans to please your friends, family, or health care provider.

Action plans are probably your most helpful self-management tool. Most of us are able to do things that will make us healthier, but we fail to do them. For example, most people with chronic pain can walk—some just across the room, others for half a block. Most can even walk several blocks, and some can walk a mile (one and a half kilometers) or farther. However, few people have a regular walking exercise program.

An action plan can help you do the things you know you *should* do. But to create a successful action plan, it is better to start with what you *want* to do. It can be *anything*! Let's go through the steps for making a realistic action plan.

Creating Your Realistic Action Plan

First, decide what you will do this week. For a person who wants to be a better step climber, this might be climbing three steps on four consecutive days. A person who wants to continue riding a motorcycle might spend half an hour on two days researching lighter motorcycles and motorcycle training wheels.

Make very sure that your plans are "action-specific." Don't decide "to lose weight" (which is not an action but the result of an action). Instead, decide to "drink tea instead of soda" (which is an action).

Next, make a specific plan. Deciding what you want to do will get you nowhere without a plan to do it. The plan should answer the following questions:

- Exactly *what* are you going to do? Are you going to walk? How will you eat less? Which relaxation technique will you practice when you are tense?

- *How much* will you do? Answer this question with details about time, distance, portions, or repetitions. Will you walk one block each day, walk without sitting down for 15 minutes three times this week, eat half portions at lunch, or do relaxation exercises for 15 minutes four days this week?

- *When* will you do this? Again, be specific: before lunch, in the shower, as soon as you come home from work. Connecting a new activity with an old habit is a good way to make sure it gets done. Consider what comes right before your action plan that could prompt the new behavior. For example, brushing your teeth can remind you to take your medication. Or decide you will do a 15-minute relaxation exercise in the evening right after washing the dinner dishes. Another trick is to incorporate your new activity right before an old favorite activity. You may decide to walk around the block before reading the paper or watching your favorite TV show.

- *How often* will you do it? This is a bit tricky. You might want to do a new healthy activity every day, but that is not always possible. It is usually best to decide to do an activity three or four times a week to give yourself "wiggle room" in case something comes up. If you do it more often, that's even better. However, if you are like most people, you will feel less pressure if you complete your activity three or four times a week and still feel successful. (Note that taking medications is an exception. This must be done exactly as directed by your health care team members.)

Take the following steps when creating your action plan:

1. First, *start where you are*. In other words, start small or start slowly. If you can walk for only one minute, start your walking program by walking one minute every hour or two, not by trying to walk an entire block. If you have never done any exercise, start with just a few minutes of warm-up. A total of 5 or 10 minutes is enough. If you want to lose weight, set a goal based on your existing eating behaviors, such as eating half portions at lunch and snacks. For example, "losing a pound (about half a kilogram) this week" is not an action plan because it does not involve a specific action. "Not eating after dinner four evenings this week," by contrast, is a fine action plan.

2. Second, *schedule some time off*. All people have days when they don't feel like doing

anything. That is a good reason for saying that you will do something three times a week instead of every day.

3. Third, once you've made your action plan, *ask yourself* the following question: "On a scale of 0 to 10, with 0 being not at all sure and 10 being absolutely sure, how sure am I that I can complete this entire plan?" If your answer is 7 or above, your action plan is probably reasonable. If your answer is below 7, you should revisit your action plan. Ask yourself why you are unsure. What problems do you expect to encounter? Then see if you can change your plan to make yourself more confident of success.

4. Once you have made a plan you are happy with, put your plan in writing and post it where you will see it every day. Thinking through a weekly action plan is one thing. Writing it down makes it more likely you will take action. Keep track of how you are doing and the problems you encounter. (There is a blank action-planning form at the end of this chapter. Make photocopies so you can use them weekly.)

Carrying Out Your Action Plan

If your weekly action plan is well written and realistically achievable, you should be able to complete it without too much trouble. The following are a few extra steps you can take to make completing your plan easier:

■ Tell people about your plan and ask family or friends to check in with you on how you are doing. Having to report your progress is good motivation.

A Successful Action Plan

A good action plan:

■ is something *you* want to do

■ is achievable (something you can expect to be able to accomplish in a week)

■ is action-specific

■ answers the questions *What? How much? When?* and *How often?*

■ is something you are sure that you will complete entirely with a confidence level of 7 or higher (on a scale from 0 = not at all sure to 10 = absolutely sure)

■ Keep track of your daily activities while carrying out your plan. Many successful self-managers make lists of what they want to accomplish.

■ Check things off as you complete them. This will tell you how realistic your planning was and will be useful in making future plans.

■ Make daily notes, even of the things you don't understand at the time. Later these notes may be helpful in problem solving.

At the end of each week, check to see if you completed your action plan and if you are any nearer to accomplishing your goal. Are you able to walk farther? Have you lost weight? Are you less anxious? Monitoring your progress is important. You may not see progress day by day, but you should see little positive changes each week. If you are having problems, this is the time to use the problem-solving steps (page 31).

For example, our stair-climbing friend didn't climb any stairs for the first few weeks of her

Success Improves Health

The benefits of lifestyle change go beyond the rewards of adopting healthier habits. Yes, you feel better when you exercise, eat well, keep regular sleeping hours, stop smoking, and take time to relax. But there's also evidence that the feelings of self-confidence and control over your life that come from making any successful change also improve your health as well.

As people age or develop a chronic pain condition, physical abilities and self-image may decline. For many people, it is discouraging to find that you can't do what you used to do or want to do. By changing and improving one area of your life, whether it is boosting your physical fitness or learning a new skill, you regain a sense of optimism and energy. By focusing on what you can do rather than what you can't do, you're more likely to lead a more positive and happier life.

plan. Each day something stopped her from taking action: no time, fatigue, cold weather, and similar things. When she looked back at her notes, she realized she was coming up with lots of reasons not to climb. She began to realize that the real problem was her fear of falling with no one around to help her. She decided to use a cane while climbing stairs and to do it when a friend or neighbor was around. This midcourse correction got her on track and helped her complete her action plan.

Making Midcourse Corrections (Back to Problem Solving)

When you are trying to overcome obstacles, your first action plan may not always be a workable one. If your planned action doesn't work, don't give up—try something else. Modify your short-term plans so that your steps are easier, give yourself more time to accomplish difficult tasks, choose different steps to get you to your goal, or check with your consultants for advice and assistance. If you are not sure how to go about this, go back and read pages 29–33.

One last note to consider: Not all goals are achievable. Having a chronic pain condition may mean having to give up some plans. If this is true for you, don't dwell too much on what you can't do. Rather, start working on another goal that you can and would like to accomplish.

Rewarding Yourself

The best part of becoming a good self-manager is the reward that comes from accomplishing your goals and living a fuller and more comfortable life. However, you don't have to wait until your action plan is complete and your goal is reached. Reward yourself frequently for your short-term successes. For example, decide that you won't read the paper or visit your favorite social media site until after you exercise. Thus, reading the paper or scrolling through new posts becomes your reward. One self-manager buys only one or two pieces of fruit at a time and walks the half mile (0.8 kilometer) to the supermarket every day or two to get more fruit. Another self-manager, who stopped smoking, used the money he would have spent

How People Change

Thousands of studies have been done to learn how people change—or why they don't change. Here's what researchers have learned:

- **Most people change by themselves, when they are ready.** Yes, physicians, counselors, spouses, and self-help groups coax, persuade, nag, and otherwise try to assist people to change their lifestyle and habits. But most people change when they are ready, and without much help from others.

- **Change is not an all-or-nothing process.** Change happens in stages. Most of us think of change as occurring one step at a time. Each step is an improvement over the one before it. Although a few people do make changes this way, it is rare. For example, more than 95 percent of people who successfully quit smoking do so only after a series of setbacks and relapses. In most cases, the path to change resembles a spiral more than a straight line. People often return to previous stages before moving forward ("two steps forward, one step back"). Relapses are not failures but setbacks, which are a normal part of change. Dealing with relapse helps people learn how to maintain change; it provides feedback about what doesn't work.

- **Making changes often depends on doing the right things at the right time.** People who are given strategies to change that do not match their readiness to change are less successful at changing than people who receive no assistance at all. For example, making an elaborate written plan of action when you really haven't decided you want to change is a prescription for failure. You're likely to get bored, discouraged, or frustrated before you even start.

- **Confidence in your ability to change is the key ingredient for success.** Your belief in your own ability to succeed is important. It predicts whether you will attempt change in the first place, whether you will persist if you relapse, and whether you will ultimately be successful in making the desired change.

on cigarettes to have his house professionally cleaned. There was even money left over to go to a baseball game with a friend. Rewards don't have to be fancy, expensive, or high in calories. There are many healthy pleasures that can add enjoyment to your life.

The Self-Management Toolbox

You can accomplish a lot with problem solving, decision making, and action planning. Now that you understand the meaning of self-management, the tasks involved with it, and these three key self-management tools, you are ready to learn about the other tools that will make you a successful self-manager. Most self-management tools work for all types of chronic pain conditions. The self-management tools discussed in this book include strategies for incorporating the following healthy, helpful practices into your life: exercise; balancing activity and rest; good nutrition; weight management; organization strategies; medication management; communication strategies; sex and intimacy; workplace strategies; strategies for finding resources; and planning for the future.

As you learn more about the tools in this book, keep these basic truths in mind:

- **Symptoms have many causes.** Because symptoms have many causes, there are many ways to manage most symptoms. When you understand the nature and causes of your symptoms, you are better able to manage them.

- **Not all management techniques work for everyone.** It is up to you to find out what works best for you. Be flexible. Experiment.

Try different techniques and check the results to determine which management tool is most helpful for which symptoms and under what circumstances.

- **Learning new skills and gaining control of the situation take time.** Give yourself several weeks to practice before you decide if a new tool is working for you.

- **Don't give up too easily.** New skills, including exercise and using your mind to manage health conditions, require both practice and time. It may be awhile before you notice the benefits. Even if you feel you are not accomplishing anything, don't give up. Be patient and keep on trying.

- **These techniques should not have negative effects.** If you become frightened, angry, or depressed when using one of these tools, do not continue to use it. Try another tool instead.

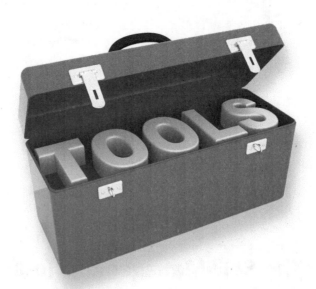

**For a complete list of suggested further readings,
useful websites, and other helpful resources, please see
www.bullpub.com/resources.**

Your Action Plan

When you write your action plan, be sure it includes the following:

1. What you are going to do (a specific action)
2. How much you are going to do (time, distance, portions, repetitions, etc.)
3. When you are going to do it (time of the day, day of the week)
4. How often or how many days a week you are going to do it

Example: This week, I will walk (what) around the block (how much) before lunch (when) three times (how many).

This week I will _____ (what)

_____ (how much)

_____ (when)

_____ (how often)

How sure am I that I can complete this plan

0	1	2	3	4	5	6	7	8	9	10

Not at   Absolutely
all sure   sure

Comments

Monday _____

Tuesday _____

Wednesday _____

Thursday _____

Friday _____

Saturday _____

Sunday _____

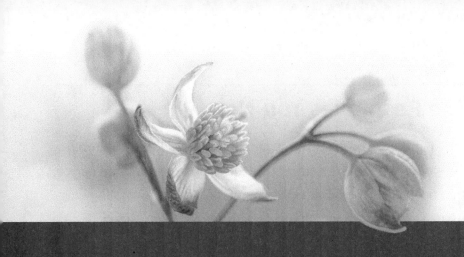

CHAPTER 3

Finding Resources

A MAJOR PART OF BEING A SELF-MANAGER is knowing how to find resources and get help when you need it. Asking for help is a strength. Finding and getting help makes you a good self-manager. In this chapter we offer some tools for finding resources and getting help to help yourself.

Don't assume because you can't do something alone that nothing can be done. This is seldom true. It is important to do the things you need and want to do. Finding a way to do them is worthwhile and rewarding.

Locating the Resources You Need

Most of us start looking for help by asking family or friends. This can be difficult for many different reasons. Sometimes we are afraid that people will not believe that our pain prevents us from doing what we want or need to do. Sometimes pride gets in the way. The truth is that most people want to be helpful but do not know how. Your job is to tell them what you need. Asking for help is discussed in Chapter 11, *Communicating with Family, Friends, and Health Care Providers*. Unfortunately, some people do not have family or close friends. Or sometimes, even if you have close people in your life, you cannot bring yourself to ask. And then sometimes family or friends are not able to give the needed help. Thankfully, there are many wonderful resources in our communities in addition to family and friends and on the internet we can use.

Finding resources can be a little like a treasure hunt. As in a treasure hunt, creative thinking can help you win the game. Finding what you need may be as simple as making a few phone calls or searching on the internet. Other times it may take sleuthing, like a detective. The successful community resource detective must find clues and follow leads. Sometimes this means starting over when a clue leads to a dead end.

Say you want to address a concern in your life. For example, suppose you find it difficult to prepare healthy meals every day. Standing for a long time is painful for you. After some thought, you decide that you want to continue cooking. Because standing is getting in the way, you think that you could continue cooking if you could cook while sitting. Someone else with the same problem might decide that they want food delivered. But your personal treasure hunt is figuring out how to cook without having to stand.

You look at kitchen stools and do not think they will work for you. So you decide that you need to redesign your kitchen. The hunt is on. Where can you find an architect or contractor who has experience in kitchen alterations for people with physical limitations? You need a starting point for your treasure hunt. You type the words "kitchen remodel" into a search engine. The internet has pages and pages of ads and listings for architects and contractors. It is overwhelming. Maybe you need to narrow your search.

Typing "kitchen design for physical disabilities" into the search box results in lots of tips from consumers and businesses, and there are also pictures to give you ideas. The first few contractors you contact are not experienced with solving your challenges. You finally find a company that seems to be just what you need, but it is located more than 200 miles (320 kilometers) away.

Now what? You have a couple of choices. You can contact every contractor that turned up in your search until you find what you need. This could be time-consuming. And even if you find someone suitable, you will still have to check references.

Where else could you find the information you need? Maybe someone who works with people with physical disabilities would know. This opens a long list of possibilities: occupational and physical therapists, the pain clinic, medical supply stores, the Center for Independent Living or Independent Living Canada, and organizations such as the Arthritis Foundation in the United States or the Arthritis Society in Canada. You decide to ask a friend who is a physical therapist.

Your friend does not have the answer but says, "Gosh, Dustin So-and-So just had his kitchen remodeled to accommodate his wheelchair." This seems like an excellent lead. You think that Dustin will almost certainly be able to give you the name of someone who does the kind of work you are seeking. He can also probably give you some ideas about the cost and hassle before you go any further. Unfortunately, Dustin turns out to be not much help. He didn't have a great experience, so he doesn't have much information that can help you. Now what?

Your next step might be trying to find a person in your community who is a "natural resource." These "naturals" or "connectors" seem to know everyone and everything about their community. There are people like this in every community. They tend to be folks who have lived a long time in the community. And they are very involved in it. They are also natural problem solvers. This is the person who other people turn to for advice. And they always seem to be helpful and have useful information.

The natural in your community could be a friend, a business associate, the mail carrier, your physician, your pet's veterinarian, the clerk at the corner grocery, the pharmacist, a bus or taxi driver, the school secretary, a real estate agent, the chamber of commerce receptionist, or a librarian. Think of this person as an information resource.

Sometimes the natural will taste the thrill of the hunt and, like a modern-day Sherlock Holmes, announce "the game is afoot!" and promptly join you in your search. For example, you ask your mail carrier, and she tells you about a contractor whose wife uses a wheelchair. She knows this because the guy just did a great job on a kitchen that is on her delivery route. You contact the contractor she names and find everything you need.

Let's review the lessons from this example. The steps in finding the resources you need are these:

1. **Evaluate your condition or situation and identify the problem.**

2. **Identify what you want or need.** Ask what you *can* do to improve your condition or situation and ask what you *want* to do to improve your condition or situation.

3. **Look for resources.**

4. **Ask friends, family, and neighbors for ideas.** (If you belong to online groups, ask members of those groups too.)

5. **Contact organizations that might deal with similar issues.**

6. **Identify and ask naturals in your community.**

One last note: The best sleuth follows several clues at the same time. This will save you lots of time and shorten the hunt. Watch out, though—once you get good at thinking about community resources creatively, you may become a natural yourself!

Resources for Resources

When you need to find goods or services, there are certain resources you can call on. One resource often leads to another. The natural is one of those resources, but your "detective's kit" needs a variety of useful tools. In this section we discuss both traditional and newer resources and how to find them. We begin with organization and referral services and finish with hints on how to make the most of the internet as a resource.

Organizations and Referral Services

Almost every community has one or more information and referral service. Sometimes these services cover a specific geographic area such as a city or county. Other times they are specific to a group, such as the Area Agency on Aging or the Government of Canada Programs and Services for Seniors. Sometimes they are specific to a condition such as a particular disability or disease. Several types of agencies operate these services. On an internet search engine or phone directory, search terms such as "United Way information and referral," "senior information and referral" (or "Area Agency on Aging" in the United States or "Council on Aging" in Canada), or "information and referral" or "211" in Canada. If you are using a telephone directory, be sure to check your county or city government or municipality or province listings.

Once you have the telephone number of a reliable information and referral service, your searches will become much easier. These services maintain huge files of referral addresses and telephone numbers. They can help you find information about just about any issue you

might have. Even if they don't have the answer you seek, they will almost always be able to refer you to another agency that can help.

Voluntary agencies such as the Arthritis Foundation and the American Chronic Pain Association in the US are rich resources. There are similar organizations in most other countries. For example, Canada has the Arthritis Society and the Chronic Pain Association of Canada. These agencies are funded by contributions from individuals and from corporate sponsors. They provide up-to-date information about health issues as well as support and direct services. You can usually subscribe to agency newsletters. Often, this puts you on the list to receive regular bulletins by mail or email. But you do not have to be a member or newsletter subscriber to qualify for their services. They are there to serve the public. Many of these organizations have wonderful websites. Websites can be accessed anywhere at any time if you have internet access. In cyberspace, you can live in rural North Dakota or the Canadian Arctic and get help on the web from Arthritis Australia in Sydney, Australia.

There are other organizations in your community offering information and referral services along with direct services. These include the local chapter of AARP (formerly known as the American Association of Retired Persons), CARP (formerly the Canadian Association for Retired Persons), senior centers, community centers, and religious social service agencies. These organizations offer information, classes, recreational opportunities, nutrition programs, legal and tax help, and social programs.

Don't overlook your local senior center. Most have social workers who may be very knowledgeable about resources. You do not need to be a senior to use this resource. There is probably a senior center or community center close to you. Your city government office or local librarian can tell you where such resources are, and the calendar section of your newspaper may lists current information about programs these organizations offer.

Most religious groups also offer information and social services to persons who need it. They provide services directly through the place of worship or through groups such as the Council of Churches, Jewish Family Service, or the Muslim Social Services Agency. To find out more about religious organizations, start with a local place of worship near you. People there can help you or refer you to someone who can help you. You usually do not need to be a member of the congregation or even of the religion to receive help.

Another option is to call your local hospital, clinic, or health insurance plan and ask for the social service department. Often, doctors are good resources and know about the physical and mental health services available through health care organizations.

Pain Clinics

If you have a pain clinic near you, health care providers there have a great deal of information and can also help you with your pain. Pain clinics focus on the diagnosis and management of all types of chronic pain, not just back pain or headaches. The providers there are experts on all aspects of chronic pain. In addition to medication and surgery, they also offer complementary treatments such as relaxation techniques, physical and occupational therapy, nutrition advice, and behavioral and psychological therapy. If you are dealing with reducing or eliminating opioid medications, the pain clinic is familiar with the tapering process. If they feel you need more than they can offer to reduce your opioid use, they can refer you to a rehab program. (For more on opioids and tapering, see Chapter 15, *Understanding Medications and Other Treatments for Chronic Pain*, page 329.)

Pain clinics can be a lifeline for someone with persistent chronic pain. Having all services available in one coordinated place (even if not physically in the same place) goes a long way to feeling hopeful. Ask your provider for a referral to a pain clinic, if you haven't already.

Libraries

Your public library is a particularly good resource if you are looking for information about your chronic condition. Libraries are not just collections of books. The resources your library can connect you to are vast and varied. Even if you are an experienced library detective, it's a good idea to ask the reference librarian to make sure you haven't overlooked a clue or two. Librarians see volumes of material cross their desks daily and are knowledgeable about the community (they may even be local naturals). If you cannot get to your local library, you can call or contact them online.

In addition to city or county libraries, in some communities there are other, more specialized health libraries. Ask any referral services you contact if there is a health library in your area. These libraries, such as the Government of Canada Health Library, specialize in health-related resources. They usually have a computerized database of useful information available in addition to the traditional print, audiotape, and videotape materials. Health libraries are typically maintained by nonprofit organizations and hospitals and sometimes charge a small fee for use. Even if there is no health library in your community, you can contact most health libraries online. They are used to getting questions from around the world.

Universities and colleges also have libraries. Most of the regional "government documents" sections of these libraries must be open to the public at no charge. US government publications exist on just about any subject, including a wide range of health-related subjects. You can find everything from information on organic gardening to detailed nutritional recipes, and these publications represent "your tax dollars at work." Public university and college librarians are usually very helpful locating what you need.

If you are fortunate enough to have a medical school in your community, you may be able to use its medical library. This is a place to go to for information rather than to look for help with tasks. Naturally, you can expect to find a great deal of information about disease and treatment at a medical library. Unless you have special knowledge about medicine, however, the detailed information you find in a medical library can be confusing and even frightening. Use medical libraries with care.

Most everyone knows about search engines like Google. But many don't know about Google Scholar, which lists peer-reviewed science articles. Peer-reviewed articles are checked for accuracy and trustworthiness by panels of professionals in the field. You can use Google Scholar just like Google to find the scientific literature on almost any topic. In your search results, you can always see the short abstracts for the articles. You can often read the entire articles as well.

Books

Books can be useful (indeed, you are reading a book now!). Many disease-related books contain reading and resource lists either at the ends of chapters or at the back of the book. These lists can be very helpful. We have a resource list that is updated regularly at www.bullpub.com/resources.

Newspapers and Magazines

Your local newspaper, especially if you live in a smaller community, can be an excellent resource. Most newspapers publish both paper and online versions. The online versions are often more thorough than the paper versions. Newspapers serving smaller communities or local sections of larger newspapers may include a local calendar of events page. This page can lead you to the organizations that are active in your community. Even if you are not interested in a featured event, calling the organization's contact telephone number may help you find something else you are interested in.

At a local bookstore or newsstand, there are a variety of general health magazines that can be useful. For example, some publications focus on specific health conditions such as arthritis, headaches, or fibromyalgia. You can also find many of these on the internet.

The Internet

Today most people have access to the internet. Even if you are not an internet user, you almost certainly know someone who is. Even if you do not have a computer, you can use one in your local library or one that belongs to a friend or family member. Internet search engines (Google, Bing, Yahoo, etc.) are the most frequently used tools. For most searches, this is where you will start.

The internet is the fastest-growing source of information today. New information is being added to it every second of every day. The internet not only offers information about health (or anything else you can imagine), it also provides several ways to interact with people all over the world. For example, someone who has interstitial cystitis, a painful and sometimes embarrassing condition, might find it difficult to find others with the same problem where she or he lives. The internet can put that person in touch with a whole group of such people whether they are across the street or on the other side of the world.

The good thing about the internet is that anyone can maintain a website, a Facebook page or other social network page, a blog, or a discussion group. That is also the bad thing about the internet. There are virtually no controls over who posts information or the accuracy or even safety of what is posted. So, although there is a lot of very useful information out there, you may also encounter incorrect or even dangerous information. Therefore, never assume that the information you find on the internet is trustworthy.

Rather, approach it with skepticism and caution. Ask yourself: Is the author or sponsor of the website clearly identified? Is the author or source reputable? Are credentials listed, and are they verifiable? Is the information contrary to what everyone else seems to be saying about the subject? Does common sense support the information? What is the purpose of the website? Is someone trying to sell you something or win you over to a particular point of view?

One way to analyze the purpose of the website is to examine its URL. The URL is the website's address on the internet. You find it in a bar in the upper-left corner of the computer screen. It starts with the letters http or www. The URL usually looks something like this:

www.selfmanagementresource.com

At the end of the main part of a US-based website's URL, you most commonly see .edu, .org, .gov, or .com. For non-US websites, the very last letters will represent the country of origin. Many Canadian-based websites end in .ca, so you have to determine whether a Canadian site that ends this way is affiliated with a school, nonprofit organization, government agency, or commercial enterprise. You may also see others, such as .biz or .info. This gives you a clue about the nature of the organization that owns the website. College or university website addresses end in .edu. Nonprofit organization website addresses end in .org. US governmental agency website addresses end in .gov. In Canada, the ending is .gc.ca for the federal government. Commercial organization website addresses end in .com.

As a rule of thumb, .edu, .org, and .gov websites are fairly trustworthy. However, be aware that a nonprofit organization (.org) can be formed to promote just about anything. A website address with a URL that ends with .com is usually a commercial organization trying to sell you a product or service. This doesn't mean that a commercial website can't be a good one. On the contrary, there are many outstanding commercial sites dedicated to providing high-quality, trustworthy information. These commercial sites may have advertising on them to cover the costs of providing this service by selling ads or by accepting grants from for-profit businesses such as pharmaceutical companies.

The URLs for some of our favorite reliable websites are listed at www.bullpub.com/resources. Please note that this is a commercial site owned and curated by the publisher of this book.

Social Networking Sites

Social networking sites and blogs are everywhere on the internet. Sites such as Facebook, Twitter, Instagram, TikTok, and Nextdoor are currently popular, but everything might change by the time this book is published. These sites enable the average person to communicate easily with others who want to listen (or read). Some sites, such as Facebook, require that users choose who is allowed to read their post. Others, such as Blogger, are more like personal journals that are open to anyone on the internet.

There are people living with chronic pain who are eager to share their experiences on social networking sites. Some sites have discussion forums where groups of people get together to share information and opinions. The information and support on these sites can be valuable, but again, be cautious: Some sites propose unproven and dangerous ideas.

Internet Discussion Groups

Google, Groups.io, and other internet providers offer discussion groups for just about anything you can imagine. To find discussion groups, go to the Google or Safari (or other) search engine home page and type "google groups" or "io groups" into the search box. You can narrow your search for a group specific to your situation by typing in something specific, such as "migraine" or "fibromyalgia" or "neck pain." Look for moderated groups. This means that a moderator enforces the rules of the group.

Anyone can start a discussion group about any subject. The people who start the groups run these groups. For any single health condition, there may be dozens of discussion groups. You can join them and the discussions if you wish, or you can just "lurk" (read without interacting). For people with complex regional pain syndrome, for example, a discussion group may allow them to connect to people who share their experiences. This may be their only opportunity to talk with someone else with their rare condition. These groups can also offer other benefits. For example, people with bipolar disorder might find it difficult to talk with someone face-to-face about their mental health concerns, but in an online group they may be able to give and receive information more freely.

Keep in mind that the internet changes by the second. Our guidelines reflect conditions at the time this book was written.

Becoming an effective resource detective is one of the jobs of a good self-manager. We hope

Apps and Tracking Devices

The internet is a valuable source for finding general information and it can also be useful for getting personalized information. There are many computer applications (apps) and tracking devices that can be very helpful with your self-management. For example, fitness trackers let you see your exercise patterns, and calorie trackers can help you with healthful eating. There are also apps and devices that promote relaxation and sleep techniques. More and more of these apps are coming on the market each day, and so anything we discuss here could be quickly outdated. But if you are considering using an app or tracking tool, here are some general things to think about:

1. Does it do what you want it to?

2. Will you use it?

3. Can you afford it? Some apps have a low monthly fee such as 4 or 5 dollars, but this adds up over time, and stopping the payments can sometimes be problematic if you decide you don't want to use it any longer.

4. Where does the data go, and do you care? Sure, you get access to data about your habits and lifestyle, but who else gets it? Your health care provider, your health plan, the company supplying the app? Are they keeping your data private?

that this chapter has given you some ideas about how to figure out what you need and how to find help in your community. Knowing how to search for resources will serve you better than being handed a list of resource agencies. If you find resources that you think we should add to our resource page, kindly send them to:

SMRC@selfmanagementresource.com

For a complete list of suggested further readings, useful websites, and other helpful resources, please see www.bullpub.com/resources.

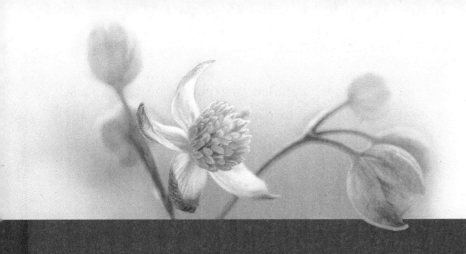

Understanding and Managing Common Symptoms and Problems

CHRONIC PAIN CONDITIONS ARE OFTEN ACCOMPANIED by other symptoms in addition to pain. These symptoms are signals from your body that something unusual is happening. Symptoms may include fatigue, poor sleep, depression, anger, stress, and memory problems and of course pain itself. Often symptoms cannot be seen by others, can be difficult to describe, and can occur at unexpected times. Although some symptoms are common, the ways in which they affect each person is very personal. What's more, these symptoms can interact with each other. This interaction may worsen existing symptoms and pain and even lead to new symptoms or problems.

Regardless of which symptoms you have or the causes of your symptoms, often the best strategies to deal with them are similar. Self-management tools are the key to success. In this chapter we discuss several common pain condition symptoms, their causes, and tools you can use to manage them. There is additional symptom management help in the next chapter too. Chapter 5, *Using Your Mind to Manage Pain and Other Symptoms*, provides detailed instruction on how to use your mind to calm your nervous system and deal with many of these symptoms.

Problem Solving with Common Symptoms

Learning to manage symptoms is very similar to problem solving, discussed in Chapter 2, *Becoming an Active Self-Manager*. To review these steps in detail, go to page 30. First, identify the symptom you are experiencing. Next, determine why you might have the symptom at this time. Consider possible options for self-management. Choose one and try it out and see what happens. This may sound like a straightforward process, but it is not always easy.

You may experience many different symptoms, and each symptom may have various causes. The ways in which these symptoms affect your life also differ. To make it less complicated, there are some practical things you can do to understand your symptoms and then manage them.

As you read this chapter, note that many of the symptoms we discuss have the same causes. Also, note how one symptom can lead to other symptoms. Understanding these patterns can make the management of pain less complex and confusing. For example, pain may cause you to tense your muscles in the area where you are hurting without even noticing that you are doing it. As a result, you change your posture. After a while, you are not standing straight and tall. Instead you are stooping a little. This change in posture may even change the way you walk. This new way of walking may change your balance, generate a new pain, or cause you to fall. As you gain a better understanding of this cycle of symptoms, you can identify better ways to address them. You may also find ways to prevent or reduce certain symptoms.

Observing Your Chronic Pain Patterns

One way to approach and manage symptoms is to keep a daily pain tracking diary or journal. This can be as simple as writing your symptoms on a calendar along with some notes about what you were doing before the symptom started or worsened. To learn even more about your pain, you might want to keep a behavioral worksheet. You can use the worksheet to help identify patterns related to chronic pain flare-ups.

Figure 4.1 on page 56 is a sample behavioral worksheet. Figure 4.2 on page 57 is a blank worksheet you can copy or write in. This worksheet has a column for writing down what happened immediately before the pain flare. It also has a column for things that happened earlier the day of the pain flare or even the day before the pain flare. To use a behavioral worksheet, you write down a few things that

Using Symptom-Management Tools

- Choose a tool to try, and be sure to give it a fair trial. We recommend that you practice using any new tool for at least two weeks before deciding whether it is going to be helpful. First, try using the tool in situations that are easier to manage. Once you experience success, try using it in more challenging situations.

- Try a variety of tools. Use each for a similar trial period. It is useful to try more than one tool because some tools may work better for certain symptoms than for others. You may find that you simply prefer some symptom-management techniques over others.

- Think about how and when you will use each tool. For example, some of these tools may require more lifestyle modification than others. The best symptom managers learn to be flexible. They learn to use a variety of techniques depending on their conditions and what they want and need to do each day.

- Place some cues in your environment to remind you to practice pain-management techniques. When mastering new skills, consistency is key. For example, place stickers or notes where you'll see them, such as on your mirror, near the phone, in your office, on your computer, or on your car's dashboard. Change the notes from time to time so you'll continue to notice them.

- Try linking each new tool with one of your established daily behaviors or activities. For example, practice relaxation before you go to bed, after you brush your teeth, or as part of your cool-down exercise.

- Ask a friend or family member to remind you to practice your pain-management tools each day. They may even wish to participate.

happened just before and just after a pain flare. The worksheet also includes a space for writing down the effects of the pain flare. That may be something short-term such as, "I decided not to meet my friends that afternoon." You might also include some longer-term effects of the pain flare, such as, "I notice that my friends call me less and less these days."

Completing a behavioral worksheet like this several times a week, over a number of weeks, can help you see patterns you did not notice before. Let's explore how you can learn more about your symptoms by completing a worksheet. For example, what patterns can you see in Figure 4.1? There are several. You may notice the following:

- Feelings early in the day (for example, frustration, guilt, or feeling really good) seem to set the stage for overdoing physical activities and spending a lot of time sitting, reaching, or standing.

- This physical activity is linked to, and might be triggering, pain flares.

Figure 4.1 **Sample Behavioral Worksheet**

Things that happen earlier in day or the day before the pain flare	Things that happen just before the pain flare	Problem	Things that happen after the pain flare	Things that happen later that day or the day after the pain flare
‣ Tired from not sleeping well ‣ Felt guilty I hadn't finished project I started last week	‣ Working at my computer for more than an hour	Pain flare 1	‣ Feeling really worried ‣ Stopped working and lay down when I couldn't stand the pain anymore ‣ Took extra pain medication ‣ Pain was not quite as bad after I rested and took meds	‣ Feeling more guilty about that project ‣ Thinking "I just can't get any work done" ‣ Thinking that medication helps pain, but I'd like not to take extra medication
‣ Frustrated about things I can't do ‣ Completed all my shopping for next two weeks	‣ Drove a long distance to get home ‣ Did a lot of reaching overhead to put all of the groceries away ‣ Did a lot of standing at counter and sink	Pain flare 2	‣ Lay down in bed for several hours with a heating pad ‣ Decided not to make the special meal I was planning ‣ Pain started to ease	‣ Feeling angry at myself that we had to order takeout again
‣ Woke up feeling really good	‣ Really enjoyed painting ‣ Stood for several hours at my art easel	Pain flare 3	‣ Spent afternoon in my recliner	‣ Resting helped with pain ‣ Feeling discouraged about not being able to do things that I enjoy

Figure 4.2 **Your Behavioral Worksheet**

Things that happen earlier in day or the day before the pain flare	Things that happen just before the pain flare	Problem	Things that happen after the pain flare	Things that happen later that day or the day after the pain flare

If this were your worksheet and you saw these patterns, you might think about:

- things you can do to deal when you feel these emotions. For example, you could use relaxation tools or calming self-talk.

- ways you can change the way you go about the activities you tend to overdo. For example, you could break long activities into more manageable steps or pace your activities better.

In Figure 4.1, note that lying down is common right after the pain. Although lying down did not get rid of the pain, it did reduce the pain. Being aware of this might make you think, "Can I schedule brief periods of lying down during the busy part of my day before my pain gets very bad to help keep my pain under control?" It would be interesting to see if doing this might also help reduce some of the feelings of guilt, frustration, and discouragement.

If you feel you cannot understand your pain, what causes it, or how it affects you, try using a behavioral worksheet. A behavioral worksheet can be a useful tool. In the worksheet, be sure to note whatever happens before and after an increase in your pain or other difficult or challenging events. When you do this for several days or weeks, you may spot common patterns. The patterns give you clues to how to manage your pain. For example, you may notice that on nights when you go out to dinner, you have trouble sleeping. Once you realize that, you become aware that when you go out, you tend to overeat and drink a couple cups of coffee after the meal. This is something you don't do at home in the evenings. Now you have ideas on how to adjust your behavior in the future to avoid experiencing sleep problems after a restaurant meal. Or you may notice that after you babysit the grandchildren you experience more pain than usual. This may cause you to consider what kinds of activities you are doing with the children. Can you modify those activities to include a nap for the kids and a rest break for you? Or is it one particular activity you do with them that is causing your pain flare-up? Recognizing patterns is the first step in symptom self-management for many people.

Figure 4.2 is a blank version of a behavioral worksheet for you to fill out for yourself. Once you learn more about your pain patterns, you can use other tools to try to address the patterns and reduce your pain.

Common Symptoms

The behavioral worksheets in Figures 4.1 and 4.2 are good tools to help you record and see the patterns in your symptoms. One benefit of observing these symptoms is that you can gain even more understanding of how one symptom (for example, pain itself) influences other symptoms (such as sleep, anger, or stress). You might find that a self-management tool that reduces your pain (for example, using relaxation methods or exercising) improves your sleep and reduces your stress level as well.

Read on to learn what you can do to manage some of the more common symptoms of chronic pain conditions. The following common symptoms are discussed in this chapter:

Pain

Pain can have many causes. We discussed reasons why chronic pain develops in Chapter 1, *Chronic Pain Self-Management: What It Is and How to Do It*, pages 9–11. You might want to review that material before reading this section. To read about specific pain conditions, see Chapter 16, *Managing Specific Chronic Pain Conditions*, pages 342–355. What follows is a brief description of some of the most common causes of pain.

- **Your pain condition or disease.** Pain can come from damage in or around joints and tissues, insufficient blood supply to muscles or organs, or an irritated nervous system, to name just a few sources. In a few conditions inflammation may cause pain, and in some cases there is no known cause. Whatever the initial cause, the ultimate result is disturbances at different levels of your nervous system—in your nerve cells, the spinal cord, and the brain. In other words, chronic pain.

- **Tense muscles.** When something hurts, the muscles in the area that hurts become tense. This is your body's natural reaction to pain. Your muscles tense to try to protect the area that hurts. Stress can also cause you to tense your muscles. Chronic muscle tension can lead to increased soreness or pain.

- **Muscle deconditioning.** When in pain, many people become less active. This inactivity leads to a weakening of the muscles, or muscle deconditioning. When your muscles are weak, they tend to complain anytime they are used. This is not because a muscle is damaged but because it has not been used in a while.

- **Lack of sleep or poor-quality sleep.** Pain often interferes with your ability to get either enough sleep or good-quality sleep. Poor sleep can also make pain worse, and it can make you less able to manage your pain.

- **Stress, anxiety, and emotions such as anger, fear, frustration, and depression.** These feelings are all normal responses to living with chronic pain. These feelings can amplify the experience of pain. This does not mean that the pain is not real. It is all too real. It just means that emotions such as stress and fear and other symptoms such as depression can make a painful situation worse.

- **Medication.** The medicines you are taking can sometimes cause pain, weakness, changes in your thinking, or abdominal or other physical or emotional discomfort. Ask your health care provider or pharmacist about the potential side effects of all your medication.

Controlling Your Pain

You are not helpless in the face of pain. How people self-manage pain—by changing the ways they act, think, and feel—can change the brain's response to pain. As a result, the brain itself can regulate the flow of pain messages by sending signals that open and close "pain gates" along nerve pathways in the spinal cord and in the brain itself (see the discussion of the gate control theory in Chapter 1, *Chronic Pain Self-Management: What It Is and How to Do It*, pages 3–4).

The brain can release natural and powerful chemicals such as endorphins (see page 5) that effectively block or reduce the pain you feel. For example, when people are seriously injured, they sometimes feel very little pain while they are focused on their injury. Your mood, how you focus your attention, and the way you view your situation—your thoughts and feelings— can open or close the pain gates.

Your day-to-day pain level is based on how your mind and body respond to pain. Here are four ways the mind and body interact when you have pain:

- **Inactivity.** You are not alone if, because of pain, you tend to avoid physical activity. This avoidance in turn causes you to lose strength and flexibility. The weaker and more out of shape physically you become, the more frustrated and depressed you feel. These negative emotions can open the gates and cause pain levels to rise.

- **Overdoing.** You may be determined to prove that you can still be active, so you overexert and push yourself to finish a task. At the same time, you ignore the signals your body sends about its need for rest. Pushing yourself only leads to more pain, which leads to more inactivity, more depression, and more pain.

- **Misunderstanding.** Your friends, family, boss, and coworkers may not understand that you are suffering and may dismiss your pain as "not that severe" or even as "not real." This can make you angry, guilty, or depressed.

- **Overprotection.** On the other hand, well-meaning friends, family, and coworkers might discourage you from doing things for fear that it will increase your pain. Sometimes, those around you can even take over things and prevent you from doing the things you like and want to do. This can also make you angry and frustrated. These feelings can increase your pain. Situations like this can also lead you to feel more discouraged, more dependent, and more disabled.

Fortunately, you can interrupt this downward spiral of negative mind-body and social interactions. If you've been told you have to live with pain, it doesn't mean you simply have to put up with it. You can have pain but still have a happy, fulfilling life. Learning to live with pain means learning to accept the idea that pain might be there much of the time but you can manage your pain and still have a meaningful life. When you are working on managing your pain, you have the opportunity to reevaluate your life values and goals. You can begin to pursue and focus on those things that give your life meaning. In a way, you can even think of this as a new beginning to manage the pain and get your life back on track. You can learn techniques that retrain the brain and calm your nervous system, such as:

■ Redirecting your attention to control pain

■ Challenging negative thoughts that support pain

■ Cultivating more positive emotions

■ Developing relaxation techniques

■ Slowly increasing your activity and reconditioning yourself

■ Learning pacing techniques to balance activity and rest

Consider this example of how one of these techniques might work. Imagine that you wake up in pain and think, "I'm going to be miserable all day; I won't get anything done." You can challenge this negative thinking or self-talk with more positive thoughts. Tell yourself instead, "I've got some pain this morning, so I'll start with some relaxation and stretching exercises.

Then I'll do some of the less-demanding things I want to get done this week."

This example shows how you can use your mind to reverse overly negative thinking. You can learn more about helpful thinking, relaxation, imagery, visualization, distraction, meditation, and other ways to use your mind in Chapter 5, *Using Your Mind to Manage Pain and Other Symptoms.*

Tools for Localized Pain Self-Management

Heat, cold, and massage are effective for managing localized pain (for example in the neck, back, or knees). These three tools work by stimulating the skin and other tissues surrounding the painful area. Heat and massage increase the blood flow to these areas, while cold makes the area feel numb. All three methods can close the gate and change the way the brain interprets body sensations.

Apply heat with a heating pad, a warm bath, or a shower (with the water flow directed at the painful area). You can improvise a heating pad by placing uncooked rice or dry beans in a sock. Knot the top of the sock and heat it in a microwave oven for 3 to 4 minutes. Before use, be sure to test the temperature so you don't burn yourself. Do not use popcorn!

Some people prefer cold for soothing pain, especially if the pain is accompanied by inflammation. A bag of frozen peas or corn makes an inexpensive, reusable cold pack. Whether using heat or cold, place a towel between the source and your skin. Also, limit the application to 15 or 20 minutes at a time (longer can burn or freeze the skin).

Massage is one of the oldest forms of pain management. Hippocrates (c. 460–380 BCE) said, "Physicians must be experienced in many things, but assuredly also in the rubbing that can bind a joint that is loose and loosen a joint that is too hard." Self-massage is a simple procedure that you can perform with little practice or preparation. Just gently rub or stretch the painful area with a little applied pressure. This stimulates the skin, underlying tissues, and muscles. Always use a nonirritating skin cream or oil for lubrication. If you prefer a cooling effect, use a mentholated cream.

There are three basic approaches to self-massage:

- **Stroking.** Place your hand on the muscle you want to massage. When you slightly cup the hand, the palm and fingers glide over the muscle as you massage. A slow, rhythmic movement repeated over the tense or sore area works best. Experiment with different pressures. If you have a condition such as complex regional pain syndrome, try putting your hand in warm water and then firmly stroking the painful area with your warmed hand.

- **Kneading.** If you have ever reached up and squeezed your own tense neck or shoulder muscles, you were kneading. Grasp the muscle between the palm and fingers or between the thumb and fingers as if you were kneading dough. Slightly lift and squeeze the muscle. Don't pinch the skin; work more deeply into the muscle. A slow, rhythmic squeeze and release works best. Don't knead one spot for more than 15 or 20 seconds.

- **Deep circular movement.** To create soothing heat (friction) that penetrates into muscle, make small circular movements with the tips of the fingers, the thumb, or the heel of the hand, depending on how large an area you are massaging. Keeping the fingers, thumb, or palm in one place, begin lightly making small circles and slowly increase the pressure. Don't overdo it. After 10 seconds, move to another spot and repeat.

Massage is not appropriate for all cases of pain. Do not use self-massage for a "hot" joint (one that is red, swollen, and warm to the touch) or an infected area. Avoid massage if you have phlebitis (inflammation of a vein), thrombophlebitis (a blood clot in a vein), or any kind of skin rash or irritation.

Medications and other treatments can also be useful for managing localized pain. You can read more about these in Chapter 14, *Managing Your Treatment Decisions and Medications* and Chapter 15, *Understanding Medications and Other Treatments for Chronic Pain*.

Tools for Chronic Pain Self-Management and Breaking the Pain Cycle

Managing chronic pain is a complex task. Like mastering all new tasks, it requires knowledge, practice, and patience. Sometimes you can't manage pain directly unless you use medications or other treatments your health care provider recommends. (These topics are discussed in detail in Chapter 14, *Managing Your Treatment Decisions and Medications*.) But often, without medication or medical intervention, you can self-manage other symptoms that are related to chronic pain, such as stress, poor sleep, and depression. If you can address even a couple of these symptoms, you will feel more in control of your pain. The rest of this chapter and Chapter 5, *Using Your Mind to Manage Pain and Other Symptoms*, are about self-managing common symptoms.

Many people experience pain in combination with several other common symptoms. Recall the discussion of the pain cycle in Chapter 1, *Chronic Pain Self-Management: What It Is and How to Do It*. (See Figure 1.2, page 10.) When you experience a number of symptoms at once, how do you decide which symptoms you should try managing? It is helpful to recognize how one symptom is linked to another symptom and also to think about what symptom comes first. Your behavioral worksheet (see Figure 4.2) might help you figure this out.

Figure 4.3 is a diagram based on information in a daily pain diary. The figure shows how symptoms are links in the pain cycle that lead to increased pain that interferes with daily activities. In this example, the trigger for the symptoms is the stress of caring for a very sick partner who requires around-the-clock help. This first link in the cycle is connected to waking in the night and not getting back to sleep. The sleep problems

result in fatigue, which in turn leads to the final link in the cycle: increased pain that makes it difficult to do most daily activities, including caregiving activities. This vicious pain cycle keeps repeating, with each link in the chain getting stronger and more difficult to change.

Recognizing the links in such a pain cycle helps identify the symptoms to target. To break the cycle in Figure 4.3, one strategy would be to focus on the first link in the chain: stress. Stress-management tools discussed later in this chapter (such as setting daily caregiving goals, getting and accepting help with caregiving, communicating concerns with your partner, and seeking support from friends) can be especially helpful. Self-managing stress can prevent the stress from linking with the other symptoms and behaviors to strengthen this chain and form this cycle.

Another strategy would be to focus on the link in the cycle that is the most difficult and challenging. For the situation illustrated in Figure 4.3, for example, a second strategy might be to self-manage fatigue and gain enough control over fatigue to prevent it from causing pain that interferes with daily activities. Pages 67–68 of this chapter introduce a number of tools for managing fatigue, including healthy eating, remaining physically active, and taking time to do things that you value and enjoy.

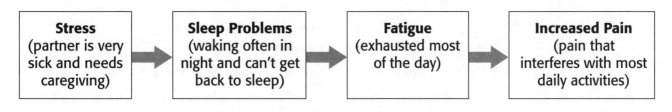

Figure 4.3 **Links in a Pain Cycle**

In addition to managing common symptoms, you can make lifestyle choices that positively influence your pain, your health, and your life. These include making physical activity and exercise a regular part of your week, healthy eating, managing your stress, improving your family and partner relationships, working with health care providers, and planning for the future. That's what the rest of this book is about. Taken together, these are all tools for you to use to manage chronic pain. Just as you cannot build a house with one tool, you often need many tools to manage chronic pain.

Breathing Problems

Shallow or labored breathing prevents your body from getting the oxygen it needs. Like other symptoms, breathing problems can have several causes.

Causes of Ineffective Breathing

Pain from weak, tense muscles can lead to ineffective breathing. When an area of the body hurts, the natural response is to tense the muscles in that area. This response is so automatic you are often unaware of how much tension you are carrying. Muscle tension can change how you move. You may move more slowly, or your posture may change so that your chest is not as open, leaving less room for your lungs to expand effectively.

Shallow breathing may result in muscles becoming weak and deconditioned (out of shape). This not only affects your breathing muscles, it can also affect the core muscles of your abdomen and the small muscles of your back. When muscles become deconditioned, they are less efficient at doing what they are supposed to do. They require more energy (and oxygen) to do their jobs.

Excess weight can also cause shortness of breath. Additional weight increases the amount of energy you use and therefore the amount of oxygen you need. Weight also increases the heart's workload. If you carry excess weight and you are inactive and have poor posture, your body must work harder to get the oxygen it needs.

Certain chronic pain conditions can directly impact posture and thereby reduce lung capacity. The list includes scoliosis, osteoporosis, and some severe forms of arthritis that attack the bones in the neck and back. Other causes of breathing problems include chronic lung diseases such as emphysema, chronic bronchitis, and asthma. These conditions usually require special medications and sometimes supplemental oxygen in addition to self-management techniques.

Shortness of breath can be frightening, and this fear can cause two additional problems. First, when you are afraid, you release hormones such as epinephrine. These hormones can cause more muscle tension and more shortness of breath. Second, you may stop activity altogether for fear exercise will hurt you. If this happens, you cannot build up the endurance necessary to help manage your chronic pain and breathing issues.

Tools for Breathing Self-Management

Just as there are many causes of ineffective breathing, there are many things you can do to manage this problem. When you feel short of breath, don't stop what you are doing or rush to finish your activity. Instead, slow down. If shortness of breath continues, stop for a few minutes. If your health care provider has prescribed medication for this problem, then take it.

The basic rule is to take things slowly and gradually. Increase your activity by not more than 25 percent each week. This means that increases in activity of 5 or 10 percent each week are just fine. For example, if you are currently able to garden comfortably for 20 minutes, next week increase your time in the garden by a maximum of 5 minutes. Once you can garden comfortably for 25 minutes, you can again add a few more minutes. To learn more about ways to increase your physical activity safely, read Chapter 6, *Organizing and Pacing Your Life for Pain Self-Management and Safety*, Chapter 7, *Exercising and Physical Activity for Every Body*, and Chapter 8, *Exercising to Feel Better*.

Finally, don't smoke. It might seem strange to think that smoking affects chronic pain, but it does. Recent studies have found a 20 percent increased risk of chronic musculoskeletal pain (such as back pain) in smokers.

Since we know that being exposed to secondhand smoke is also a health risk, you may want to avoid smokers as well. This can be difficult because smoking friends may not realize how they may be impacting your health. Your job is to tell them. Explain that you would appreciate it if they would not smoke when you are around. Also, make your house and your car "no smoking" zones. At home, ask people to smoke outside. In your car, tell them there is absolutely no smoking. They can smoke before they get in or after you reach your destination.

There are several tools that can help with better, more effective breathing. Here we describe two effective breathing self-management techniques:

Diaphragmatic Breathing

Ineffective breathing can be caused by a deconditioned diaphragm (a large muscle at the bottom of your rib cage) and deconditioned breathing muscles in the chest as well as by poor posture. In either case, the lungs are not able to function properly. The lungs do not fill well, nor do they get rid of old air effectively. Most people mainly use the upper lungs and chest for breathing. But you can breathe more deeply if you use diaphragmatic breathing, called "belly breathing." When you do this breathing technique properly, the diaphragm moves down into the abdomen and allows your lungs to expand fully with air. Diaphragmatic breathing strengthens your breathing muscles and makes them more efficient, so breathing is easier, and more oxygen is available to your body.

Interestingly, babies belly breathe instinctively with little effort. For adults, though, deep breathing requires a little practice. To learn to fully expand your lungs and practice diaphragmatic breathing, take these steps:

1. Lie on your back with pillows under your head and knees.

2. Place one hand on your stomach (at the base of your breastbone) and the other hand on your upper chest.

3. Breathe in slowly through your nose, allowing your stomach to expand outward. Fill your lungs with fresh air. The hand on your stomach should move upward, and the hand on your chest should not move or should move only slightly.

4. Breathe out slowly, through your mouth. At the same time, use the hand that is on your stomach to gently push inward and upward on your abdomen.

5. Practice this technique for 10 minutes, three or four times a day, until it becomes automatic. If you begin to feel a little dizzy, take a break or breathe out more slowly.

You can also practice diaphragmatic breathing while sitting in a chair.

1. Relax your shoulders, arms, hands, and chest. Do not grip the arms of the chair or your knees.

2. Think about your posture. Sit straight, gently slide your chin back, and feel your neck lengthen. Imagine the top of your head being gently tugged upward toward the ceiling. You may notice your abdominal muscles tightening just a little.

3. Put one hand on your stomach and the other on your chest.

4. Breathe in through your nose, filling the area around your waist with air. The hand on your chest should remain still and the hand on your stomach should move.

5. Breathe out through your mouth without force or effort.

Once you are comfortable with this technique, you can practice it almost anytime, while lying down, sitting, standing, or walking. Diaphragmatic breathing and good posture can help strengthen and improve the coordination and efficiency of the breathing muscles. This decreases the amount of energy you need to breathe and reduces overall muscle tension in your body. You can incorporate diaphragmatic breathing using any of the relaxation techniques in Chapter 5, *Using Your Mind to Manage Pain and Other Symptoms*.

Pursed-lip Breathing

A second breathing self-management technique, pursed-lip breathing, usually happens naturally for people who have problems emptying their lungs. Try this technique if you are short of breath or breathless.

1. Breathe in, and then purse your lips as if to blow across a flute or into a whistle.

2. Breathe out through pursed lips without any force.

3. Relax the upper chest, shoulders, arms, and hands while breathing out. Check for tension. Breathing out should take longer than breathing in.

Master one or both of these breathing self-management techniques and try them while doing daily activities. They will help you to better manage your shortness of breath. Breathing more easily can help you manage your pain.

Fatigue

Chronic pain can drain your energy, making fatigue a very real problem. Fatigue, not just pain, can keep you from doing things you'd like to do. Unfortunately, fatigue is often misunderstood by people who do not live with chronic pain. After all, others cannot usually see your fatigue. Spouses, family members, and friends sometimes do not understand the unpredictable ways that fatigue can affect you. They may think that you are just not interested in certain activities or that you just want to be alone. Sometimes you may not even understand why you feel so tired.

To manage fatigue, it helps to understand that your fatigue may be related to several factors, including the following:

■ **Chronic pain.** Chronic pain or other illness is a major strain on your body. People who are fatigued often use energy less efficiently. This is because the energy that could be consumed by everyday activities is being redirected to the parts of the body affected by the condition. When you are fatigued, your brain may release chemical signals that make your body conserve energy and require more rest. Also, some chronic conditions are associated with anemia (low blood hemoglobin), which can contribute to fatigue.

■ **Inactivity.** Muscles that are not used regularly become deconditioned, lose strength, and are less efficient. This can happen to all the muscles in our body, including the heart, which is made of muscle tissue. When the heart becomes deconditioned, its ability to pump blood is decreased.

Your blood carries necessary nutrients and oxygen to other parts of the body. When muscles do not receive these nutrients and oxygen, they cannot function properly. Deconditioned muscles tire more easily than muscles in good condition.

■ **Poor nutrition.** Food is our basic source of energy. When people are in chronic pain or experience pain flares, they often turn to eating foods that are high in fat and high in sugar (comfort foods). If you eat poor-quality food, eat too much food, or improperly digest food, fatigue can result. Chronic pain can cause a change in appetite. Some people overeat and gain weight. Extra weight causes fatigue by increasing the energy needed to perform daily activities. Other people lose their appetites. Eating too little, being underweight, or eating the wrong kinds of food can cause muscle tissue to break down. Less muscle means less strength and less energy. This leads to fatigue.

■ **Not enough rest.** Some people with chronic pain overdo activity and do not balance activity with rest. Others suffer from lack of sleep or poor-quality sleep. Either situation can result in fatigue. Managing sleep problems is discussed in more detail later in this chapter. You can find suggestions for balancing activity and rest in Chapter 6, *Organizing and Pacing Your Life for Pain Self-management and Safety*.

■ **Emotions.** Anxiety, fear, guilt, and depression can all cause fatigue. It can be exhausting to deal with the ongoing emotions that often accompany chronic pain. Being bored and not having enough to occupy your mind can also lead to fatigue. Most people are aware of the connection between stress and feeling tired, but fewer know that fatigue is a major symptom of depression. You can find more information later in this chapter about managing strong emotions, including depression (page 74), anger (page 81), fear (page 83), and guilt (page 85).

■ **Medication.** Some medications, including pain medications, can cause fatigue. If you think your fatigue is related to your medication, talk to your health care provider. Sometimes changing medications or dosages can lessen fatigue.

If fatigue is a problem for you, start by trying to understand the cause. Again, keeping track of your symptoms in a behavioral worksheet or pain diary (see Figures 4.1 and 4.2) may be helpful. Consider the possible causes of fatigue that are within your control to change. Are you eating healthy foods? Are you exercising? Are you pacing your activities with rest periods? Are you getting enough good-quality sleep? Are you effectively managing stress? If you answer no to any of these questions, you may have found one or more of the reasons for your fatigue.

Remember that your fatigue may be caused by things *other than your pain.* Therefore, to combat and prevent fatigue, you must consider and address other possible causes. This may mean trying a variety of self-management tools.

If your fatigue is the result of not eating well—if you eat too much junk food or drink too much alcohol for example—then the solution is to eat better-quality foods in the proper quantities or to drink less alcohol. For some, the problem may be a decreased interest in food, leading to decreased food consumption and weight loss. You can learn more about eating and weight and pain management in Chapter 9, *Healthy Eating and Pain Self-Management*, and Chapter 10, *Healthy Weight and Pain Self-Management*.

People often say they can't exercise because they feel fatigued. This misconception creates a vicious cycle: They are fatigued because of a lack of exercise, and they don't exercise because of the fatigue. Believe it or not, motivating yourself to exercise and being more active might be the answer. Walk around your house or try some gentle exercises like the Moving Easy Program in Chapter 8, *Exercising to Feel Better.*

You can learn more about starting an exercise program in Chapter 7, *Exercising and Physical Activity for Every Body,* and Chapter 8, *Exercising to Feel Better.* If you are having trouble getting started, try to just take a short walk each day for a few days in a row and see what happens. You may be surprised and learn a lot about the effects of even a brief amount of exercise!

If emotions are one of the causes of your fatigue, rest alone will probably not help. In fact, being inactive may make you feel worse, especially if your fatigue results from depression. We talk about how to deal with depression later in this chapter on pages 74–80. If you feel that your fatigue may be related to stress, read the section on managing stress on pages 86–91.

Sleep Problems

People with chronic pain often have sleep problems. In fact, two out of every three people with chronic pain, and almost everyone with fibromyalgia, report poor-quality sleep. You may have trouble falling asleep, wake too early and can't get back to sleep, wake up frequently in the night, or wake up feeling tired and achy. Sleep and pain experts think that the neurochemicals that are critical for regulating sleep and mood are low in people with chronic pain. That may be one of the reasons why chronic pain, poor sleep, and depression often go together. The problem of sleep and pain is even more complicated because some prescribed pain medicines (such as morphine or codeine) can cause sleep problems when they are taken for longer than a few weeks.

Sleep is a basic human need, like food and water. Good-quality sleep makes you feel refreshed, rested, and reenergized, ready to face the day. When you sleep, the body heals and repairs your muscles and tissues and provides energy to your vital organs, including the brain. Sleep may also play a role in regulating appetite. When you do not get enough good-quality sleep, you may feel fatigue, an inability to concentrate, irritability, increased pain, and weight gain. Of course, this does not mean that all these symptoms are always caused by a lack of sleep. Remember, the symptoms associated with chronic pain can have many causes. Nevertheless, improving the quality of your sleep can help you manage many of these symptoms, regardless of their cause. In fact, because sleep is so important, sleep and pain experts suggest that *improving sleep quality should be a major goal of all chronic pain treatment.*

How much sleep do you need? The amount varies from person to person. Many people think they do best with about 7½ hours each night. Yet research shows that some people feel refreshed with just 5 hours, while others need 8 to 10 hours to function well. If you are alert, feel rested, and function well during the day, chances are you're getting enough sleep. But if you get less good sleep than you require night after night, your mood and quality of life suffer.

Getting a Good Night's Sleep

Improving your sleep habits is one of the key steps you can take to help manage your pain. The self-management techniques discussed here are clinically proven to improve sleep quality for most people. They are not quick fixes like sleep medications, and they'll give you more effective (and safer) results in the long run. Allow yourself at least two to four weeks to work these into your routine, and do some problem solving around your personal sleep challenges. After four weeks you will likely see some positive results, and in 10 to 12 weeks you may enjoy long-term improvement.

Things to Do before You Get into Bed

- **Invest in a comfortable bed.** Your bed should allow for ease of movement and provide good body support. This usually means a good-quality, firm mattress that supports the spine and does not allow the body to sink in the middle of the bed. To increase firmness, place a bed board made of 1/2- to 3/4-inch (1 to 2 cm) plywood between the mattress and the box spring. Heated waterbeds, air beds, or memory foam mattresses are helpful for some people with chronic pain because they support weight evenly by conforming to the body's shape. If you are interested in these options, try them out at a friend's home or a hotel for a few nights to decide if one of them is right for you. An electric blanket or mattress pad, set on low heat, or a wool mattress pad are also effective at providing heat while you sleep. If you use electric bedding, follow the instructions carefully to prevent burns.

- **Keep your extremities warm.** Keep your hands and feet warm with gloves or socks. For painful knees, cut the toes off warm stockings and wear them as sleeves over your knees.

- **Find a comfortable sleeping position.** The best position depends on you and your condition. Sometimes small pillows placed in the right places can relieve pain and discomfort. Experiment with different positions and pillow placement. Also check with your health care provider for specific recommendations. One caution: Do not prop your head up on a mountain of pillows. This aggravates neck or back problems.

- **Elevate the head of the bed 4 to 6 inches (10 to 15 cm).** Do this if you have a problem with breathing, heartburn, or gastric reflux. You can prop sturdy wooden blocks under the bed legs or purchase an adjustable bed to raise your head during sleep.

- **Keep the room at a comfortable temperature.** This may be warm or cool. Each of us requires specific conditions to sleep better.

- **Use a vaporizer if you live where the air is dry.** Warm, moist air often makes breathing and sleeping easier. If you prefer cool air at night, use a humidifier.

- **Make your bedroom safe and comfortable.** Keep a lamp and telephone by your bed, within easy reach. Get rid of scatter rugs by your bed that may be a hazard and cause you to trip and fall. If you use a cane or walker, keep it by the bed where you can reach it easily and use it when you get up during the night.

- **Keep your eyeglasses by the bed.** This way if you need to get up in the middle of the night, you can easily put on your glasses and see where you are going!

Things That Negatively Affect Sleep to Avoid

- **Do not eat right before bedtime.** Many people feel sleepy after eating a big meal, but overeating is not a healthy way to fall asleep quickly. It will not result in a good night's sleep. Sleep is the time when your body can rest and recover. When it is busy digesting food, your body redirects valuable time and attention from the healing process. If you find that going to sleep feeling hungry keeps you awake, try drinking a glass of warm milk at bedtime.

- **Avoid alcohol.** You may think alcohol helps you sleep better because it makes you feel relaxed and sleepy, but in fact, alcohol disrupts the sleep cycle. Alcohol consumption in the evening can prevent you from getting deep sleep and lead to frequent wakings in the night.

- **Avoid or limit caffeine.** Caffeine is a stimulant that can keep you awake. Coffee, tea, colas and other sodas, and chocolate all contain caffeine. If you drink caffeinated beverages, drink them early in the day. If you have sleep problems, eliminate caffeine altogether to see if this has a positive effect on your sleep. But if you have been a regular caffeine user, don't stop caffeine suddenly. This can cause withdrawal symptoms such as headaches and the jitters. Instead, keep a log for a couple of days that tracks the number of caffeinated drinks you have each day. Gradually reduce the number of caffeinated drinks you have by one drink each day. There are noncaffeinated alternatives for almost every beverage.

- **Stop smoking and using e-cigarettes.** Aside from the fact that smoking can cause complications for your chronic pain, falling asleep with a lit cigarette can be a fire hazard. Furthermore, the nicotine contained in cigarettes is a stimulant. Like caffeine, nicotine impacts sleep. Quitting smoking may not be easy, but quitting is a huge step forward in managing your chronic pain condition. E-cigarettes are not an effective way to quit smoking. They are as addictive as regular cigarettes and cause the same health problems. For help with quitting nicotine, talk to your health care team or contact your local public health department or lung association.

- **Do not take diet pills.** Diet pills often contain stimulants, which may interfere with falling asleep and staying asleep.

- **Do not take sleeping medication.** Although sleeping pills may seem like the perfect solution for sleep problems, they are not a long-term answer. Sleeping medications tend to become less effective over time. Also, many sleeping pills have a rebound effect. That means that if you stop taking them, it becomes even more difficult for you to get to sleep or stay asleep than it was before you began taking them.

  Sometimes a doctor or other health care provider may recommend a short course of sleeping pills (a few weeks at most) and suggest you take them while improving your sleep practices overall. For example, your doctor may suggest you limit your time in bed and use your bedroom only for sleep and sex and nothing else. (See *Developing a Sleep-Friendly Routine* on page 72.) This combination of short-use medication and sleep-friendly practices may be helpful for people with chronic pain who have significant sleep problems. Sleep specialists agree that the techniques listed here offer the best long-term solution to poor sleep and are much more effective and safe than sleeping pills. Other types of medicines prescribed for your chronic pain may also improve sleep (see Chapter 15, *Understanding Medications and Other Treatments for Chronic Pain*).

- **Stop viewing blue-light emitting devices such as computers, TVs, tablets, cell phones, or some e-readers an hour before**

you go to bed. The light from these devices can disrupt your natural sleep rhythms.

- **Avoid diuretics (water pills) before bedtime.** If you are on diuretics, take them in the morning so your sleep is not interrupted by frequent trips to the bathroom. Unless your health care provider has recommended otherwise, don't reduce the overall amount of fluids you drink. Fluids are important for your health. However, you may want to limit the amount you drink right before you go to bed.

Developing a Sleep-Friendly Routine

In addition to preparing yourself and your bedroom for sleep and avoiding certain things that prevent sleep, take the following steps to set yourself up for sleep success.

- **Keep a regular rest and sleep schedule.** Go to bed at the same time every night and get up at the same time every morning. Even though you may feel tired on some mornings, getting up at the same time each day helps your body maintain its natural sleep cycle. If you wish to take a brief nap, take one in the afternoon and only lie down for 10 to 20 minutes, no more. Do not take a nap in the evening after dinner. Stay awake until you are ready to go to bed.

- **Reset your sleep clock when necessary.** If your sleep schedule gets off track (for example, you go to bed at 4:00 A.M. and sleep until noon one day), you need to reset your internal sleep clock. To do so, go to bed an hour earlier (or later) each day until you reach the hour you want to be your regular bedtime.

- **Exercise at regular times each day.** Not only does exercise help you sleep more soundly, it also helps establish a regular pattern for your day. Work out at the same time on the days you exercise. Avoid vigorous exercise in the evening before bedtime.

- **Get out in the sun every morning.** Exposure to sunlight is helpful, even if you are in the sun for only 15 or 20 minutes. A regular dose of morning sun helps sets your body clock.

- **Practice relaxation techniques at regular times each day.** The relaxation technique you practice doesn't have to be complicated. Even 10 minutes of daily deep belly breathing can help. Like regular exercise, this establishes a regular pattern to your day and quiets your nervous system. To learn more about techniques that can help you relax as you prepare for sleep, see Chapter 5, *Using Your Mind to Manage Pain and Other Symptoms*.

- **Develop a routine.** Do the same things every night before going to bed. This can be anything from listening to calm music on the radio to reading a chapter of a book to taking a warm bath. By developing and sticking to a "get ready for bed" routine, you are letting your body know that it's time to start winding down and relax.

- **Use your bedroom only for sleeping and sex.** If you have had pain for some time, you may have begun to use your bedroom for activities other than sleep. A number of these activities might lead you to feel more awake and alert. These activities might include watching TV, texting friends, or balancing your checkbook. When you do activities other than sleeping in bed, being in bed becomes a signal for your body to be alert. As a result, you cannot relax and fall asleep when it is time to do so. If you do these activities in bed because you are in pain and need to recline, move to another room where you can be comfortable and do all your reclining awake activities. Reserve your bedroom for sleep and sex only! If you find that you get into bed and you can't fall asleep, get out of bed after a few minutes and go into another room until you begin to feel sleepy again. Don't look at your cell phone or turn on any other blue-light emitting devices. Keep the lighting low when you are awake at night no matter what room you are in—bright lights signal to your body that it is time to be up and about.

What to Do When You Can't Get Back to Sleep

Many people can get to sleep without a problem, but then they wake up with the "early morning worries" and can't turn off their minds. Then they start to worry about not getting back to sleep This becomes a vicious circle.

To break this cycle, keep your mind occupied with pleasurable or interesting thoughts. Distract yourself instead of focusing on your worries. For example, try a distraction technique such as counting backward from 100 by threes or naming a flower or sports team for every letter of the alphabet. The relaxation techniques described in Chapter 5, *Using Your Mind to Manage Pain and Other Symptoms*, may also be helpful. If you still can't fall asleep, get up, leave your bedroom, and do something—read a book or play a game of solitaire (not on the computer; avoid blue-light emitting devices). After 15 or 20 minutes, go back to bed.

Does a racing mind often keep you awake? If it does, schedule a regular brief "worry time" each day well before bedtime. During worry time, write down your problems and concerns, and then make a to-do list. You can now relax and sleep well at night, knowing that you have some ideas to address your concerns. You may not solve your worries right away, but you will know that you have tomorrow's worry time to come up with new ideas.

Sleep Apnea and Snoring

If you are tired when you wake up in the morning, even after a full night's sleep, you may have a sleep disorder. People who have the most common sleep disorder, obstructive sleep apnea, often do not know it. When they are asked about their sleep, they respond, "I sleep just fine." Sometimes the only clue is that others complain about their loud snoring. Sleep specialists believe that obstructive sleep apnea is very common and alarmingly underdiagnosed.

When people have sleep apnea, the soft tissue in the throat or nose relaxes during sleep and blocks the airway. This makes breathing an extreme effort. The person struggles against the blockage for up to a minute, wakes just long enough to gasp for air, then falls back to sleep to start the cycle all over again. The person is rarely aware of being awakened dozens of times during the night. Sleep apnea leads to symptoms such as fatigue and pain, because the body does not get the deep sleep it needs to restore energy and heal.

Sleep apnea can be a serious or even life-threatening medical problem. It has been linked to heart disease and stroke. Sleep experts suggest that you be evaluated for sleep apnea or other sleep disorders if you are tired all the time in spite of a full night's sleep or you need more sleep now than when you were younger. It is especially urgent that you are checked if your spouse or partner reports that you snore.

Getting Professional Help for Sleep Problems

You can self-manage many sleep problems with the techniques discussed in this chapter, but there may be times when you need professional assistance. When should you get help?

- If your pain causes sleep problems two to three times a night and you are unable to fall back asleep reasonably quickly once you awaken

- If poor-quality sleep continues to seriously affect your daytime functioning (your job or your social relationships), after you have faithfully followed the sleep-management techniques described in this chapter

- If you have great difficulty staying awake during the day and your daytime sleepiness causes, or comes close to causing, an accident

- If your sleep is disturbed by breathing difficulties, including loud snoring with long pauses, chest pain, heartburn, leg twitching, or other related physical conditions

- If your sleep problems are accompanied by depression or problems with alcohol, sleeping medications, or addictive drugs

Don't put off asking for help. Discuss problems with your health care provider. Most sleep problems can be addressed. Once sleep is improved, many people find that there is an improvement in their chronic pain and their mood.

Depression

Most people with chronic pain sometimes feel depressed. Scientists think that an imbalance of certain chemicals in your brain (such as the neurotransmitters serotonin and norepinephrine) is involved in chronic pain, depression, and sleep disorders. Just as there are different degrees of pain, there are different degrees of depression. These range from feeling occasionally sad or blue to serious clinical depression. Clinical depression, which is also referred to as major depression, is characterized by a constant feeling of hopelessness and despair. Roughly a third of the people who experience chronic pain also experience clinical depression.

Sometimes people do not realize they are depressed. And often people do not want to admit to being depressed. Like other symptoms, depression can be treated with self-management techniques, with counseling, and with medication, The best treatment is specific to each person and is usually a combination of these.

What Is Depression?

Feeling sad sometimes is common. "Normal" sadness is a temporary feeling, often linked to a specific event or loss. People sometimes mistakenly use the word *depressed* to describe feeling sad or disappointed. A person might say, "I'm really depressed about missing out on visiting with my friends." In these circumstances people feel sad, but they can still relate to others and find joy in other areas of their lives.

Sometimes sadness affects people more deeply or lasts longer, as when you lose a loved one or are diagnosed with a serious illness. If, however, your sad feelings are especially severe, long-lasting, and recurrent, you may be experiencing clinical depression. Clinical depression drains the pleasure out of life, leaving you feeling hopeless, helpless, and worthless. If you are experiencing clinical depression, you may become numb, and even crying brings no relief.

Depression affects everything: the way you think, the way you behave, the way you interact with others, and even the way your body functions.

What Contributes to Depression?

Depression is not caused by personal weakness, laziness, or lack of willpower. Heredity, chronic pain conditions, medications, even the weather can all play a role in depression. The way you think, especially negative thoughts, can also produce and sustain a depressed mood. Negative thoughts associated with depression can be automatic, recur frequently, and often are not linked to any event or triggering cause.

Certain feelings and emotions also contribute to depression. They include:

- **Fear, anxiety, or uncertainty about the future.** Worries about finances, your family, or your pain or treatment can lead to depression. If you address these issues as soon as possible, both you and your family will spend less time worrying and have more time to enjoy life. This can have a healing effect. We talk more about these issues and how to deal with them in Chapter 17, *Planning for the Future: Fears and Reality*.

- **Frustration.** Frustration can have many causes. You may find yourself thinking, "I just can't do what I want," "I feel so helpless," "I used to be able to do this myself," or "Why doesn't anyone understand me?" The longer you entertain and accept these thoughts, the more alone and isolated you are likely to feel.

- **Loss of control over your life.** When you are living with chronic pain, many things can make you feel like you are losing control. These include having to rely on medications, having to see a health care provider on a regular basis, or having to count on others to help you do things you used to do yourself. Thinking you have lost control can make you lose faith in yourself and your abilities. Even though you may not be able to do everything yourself, you can still be in charge. Remember: as a self-manager, *you* are the manager for your own life.

A person may not even realize they are depressed, or they may feel it but attempt to hide

Am I Depressed?

Here is a quick test for depression: Ask yourself what you do to have fun. If you do not have a quick answer, consider your mood over the past two weeks. Have you had any of the following symptoms?

- **Little interest or pleasure in doing things.** An inability to enjoy life or other people may be a sign of depression. Symptoms include not wanting to talk to anyone, go out, or answer the phone or doorbell.

- **Feeling down, sad, or hopeless.** Feeling persistently blue can be a symptom of depression.

- **Trouble falling or staying asleep, or sleeping too much.** Awakening and being unable to return to sleep or sleeping too much and not wanting to get out of bed can signal a problem.

- **Feeling tired or having little energy.** Fatigue—feeling tired all the time—can be a symptom of depression.

- **Poor appetite or overeating.** This may range from a loss of interest in food to unusually erratic or excessive eating.

- **Feeling bad about yourself.** Have you felt that you are a failure or have let yourself or your family down? Do you doubt your self-worth or have a negative image of your body?

- **Trouble concentrating.** Have you found it hard to do such things as reading the newspaper, listening to a podcast, or watching television?

- **Sluggishness or restlessness.** Have you been moving or speaking so slowly that other people have noticed? Or the opposite—have you been much more fidgety or restless than usual? Either can be a sign of depression.

- **Wishing yourself harm or worse.** Thoughts that you would be better off dead or of hurting yourself in some way are often a strong sign of clinical depression.

Depressed people may also gain or lose weight, lose interest in sex or intimacy, lose interest in personal care and grooming, struggle to make decisions, and have more frequent accidents.

If several of these symptoms seem to apply to you, please seek help from someone you trust—your doctor, a member of the clergy, a psychologist, or a social worker. Do not wait for these feelings to pass. If you are thinking about harming yourself or others, get help now. Don't let a tragedy happen to you and your loved ones. In the United States, the national suicide prevention lifeline is 1-800-273-8255. In Canada, the number is 1-833-456-4566. In Quebec, the number is 1-866-APPELLE (1-866-277-3553).

Fortunately, treatments for depression, including antidepressant medications, counseling, and self-management techniques, are highly effective in decreasing its frequency, length, and severity. Depression, like other symptoms, can be managed.

it. Sometimes unrealistic cheeriness masks what a person is really feeling, and only the most sensitive observer recognizes the brittleness or phoniness of the mood. Refusal to accept offers of help, even in the face of obvious need for it, is a frequent symptom of unrecognized depression.

Depression can lead to withdrawal, isolation, and inactivity. These behaviors can cycle back to create more depressed feelings. One of the major problems of depression is that the more you isolate yourself, the more you drive away the people who can support and comfort you. Friends and family want to help you feel better, but often they don't know what to do. As you reject efforts to comfort and reassure you, they become frustrated and may eventually quit trying. The result is that a depressed person can end up saying, "See, I was right. Nobody cares."

Treating Depression

The most effective treatments for depression are antidepressant medications, counseling, and self-management techniques. We discuss each of these here.

Medication and Depression

Antidepressant medications help balance brain chemistry and are highly effective. You can learn more about them in Chapter 15, *Understanding Medications and Other Treatments for Chronic Pain*, on pages 333–334. They can also help relieve pain, lessen anxiety, and improve sleep. It can take several days to several weeks for most antidepressant medications to begin to work. Don't be discouraged if you don't feel better immediately. Stick with it. To get the maximum benefit you may need to take some medications for six months or more.

Most people experience side effects of antidepressant medication in the first few weeks. Side effects then lessen or go away. If the side effects you feel are not especially severe, continue to take your medication. As your body gets used to the medication, you will begin to feel better. Remember to take antidepressant medication every day. If you stop because you're feeling better (or worse), you may relapse. Antidepressant medications are not addictive. If you have significant side effects or if the medication is not helping, talk with your health care provider before stopping or changing your dose.

Counseling and Depression

Several types of psychotherapy, particularly cognitive behavioral therapy (CBT), can be highly effective in treating depression. Psychotherapy or counseling is often referred to as "talk therapy." CBT is a form of counseling that focuses on challenging and changing unhelpful thought patterns and helping people regulate their emotions and behaviors and learn coping strategies. CBT can help people think more realistically about their pain by encouraging them to change their thoughts, feelings, and behavior, including their stress responses. (Read more about CBT in the section on fear in this chapter on page 83 and in Chapter 15, *Understanding Medications and Other Treatments for Chronic Pain*, on page 338.)

As with medications, counseling rarely has an immediate effect. You may see a counselor for weeks (or longer) before you see improvement. The course of therapy can be brief, usually involving one to two sessions a week for several months. Counseling can be a good investment of your energy and time. By teaching you new skills and ways to think and relate, psychotherapy can help reduce your risk of recurrent depression.

Tools for Depression Self-Management

Depression self-management techniques can be surprisingly effective. You can learn many psychotherapy techniques on your own. For mild to moderate depression or just to lift your mood, the self-management strategies discussed here can be very productive. One study showed that reading and practicing self-help advice improved depression in nearly 70 percent of patients.

These skills and strategies can be used alone or added to medications and counseling.

- **Eliminate the negative.** Being alone and isolating yourself, crying a lot, getting angry and yelling, blaming your failure or bad mood on others, or using alcohol or other drugs usually leaves you feeling worse. Prescription tranquilizers or narcotic painkillers such as Valium®, Librium®, Restoril®, Vicodin®, codeine, sleeping medications, or other "downers" intensify depression or may cause depression as a side effect. However, if you have been prescribed one of these medicines, do not stop taking it before first talking with your health care provider. There may be reasons for continuing its use, or you may have withdrawal reactions.

Alcohol is also a depressant or downer. One of its key effects is that it makes you feel more discouraged. For most people, one or two drinks in the early evening are not a problem. However, if you can't stop thinking about alcohol during your day, or if alcohol is interfering in your life, you are having trouble with this drug. Talk about your alcohol use with your health care provider or seek help from a twelve-step program such as Alcoholics Anonymous.

- **Plan for pleasure.** When you are feeling blue or depressed, the tendency is to withdraw, isolate yourself, and restrict activities. That is the opposite of what you need to do. Maintaining or increasing activities is one of the best antidotes for depression. Go for a walk, call or video chat with a friend, look at a sunset, watch a funny movie, get a massage, learn another language, follow along to a yoga video, take a cooking class, or join a social club. Activities like these can help keep your spirits up and prevent or lessen depression.

Sometimes having fun isn't such an easy prescription. You may have to make an effort to plan pleasurable activities. Don't leave good things to chance. Consider making a list of what you'd like to do with your free time during the week and then schedule your fun each week. Even if you don't feel like doing it, try to stick to your activity schedule. That nature walk, cup of tea, or half hour of listening to music may improve your mood. You will never know if you do not try it.

If you don't feel much emotion and the world seems colorless, make an effort to put some living back into your life. Go to a bookstore and look through your favorite section. Listen or dance to some upbeat music. Exercise or schedule a massage so you can reconnect with your body. Eat your favorite spicy food. Treat yourself to a fragrant herbal bath, or try a cold shower. Go to a garden center and smell all the flowers. Even a walk around the block may bring a new adventure.

Make plans and carry them out. Look to the future. Plant some young trees. Look forward to your grandchildren's graduation from college even if your own kids are still in high school. If you know that one time of the year is especially difficult, such as Christmas or a birthday, make specific plans to be active during that period. Don't wait to see what happens. Be prepared.

■ **Take action.** Continue your daily activities. Get dressed every day and take pride in your appearance. Make your bed, get out of the house, go shopping, or walk your dog. Plan and cook meals. Force yourself to do these things even if you don't always feel like it.

Taking action to solve your most immediate problems provides the surest relief from negative feelings. You might decide to clean or organize a room or even just a desk drawer. Even a single simple action can boost your mood. Search websites you trust to learn more about a current events topic you are interested in. Call or write to an old friend or distant relative.

When you are feeling emotionally vulnerable, do not set major or difficult goals for yourself or take on a lot of responsibility. Break large tasks into small ones, set some priorities, and do what you can as best you can. (To review how to set priorities based on your values, read pages 31–32 in Chapter 2, *Becoming an Active Self-Manager.*) It is best not to make big life decisions when you are feeling depressed. For example, don't relocate without first visiting the new setting for a few weeks and learning about the community there. Moving can be a sign of withdrawal. Depression often intensifies when you are in a location away from friends and acquaintances. Besides, many troubles may move with you, and you may have left behind the support you may need to deal with your troubles.

■ **Socialize.** Don't isolate yourself. Seek out positive, optimistic people who can lighten your heavy feelings. Make an effort to see family and friends. Get involved in a church group, a book club, a community college class, a self-help class, or a nutrition program. If you can't get out, consider video chatting with friends, starting an online book club with people you know, or joining a group on the internet. If you join a public online group, be sure it is moderated—that is, that someone is in charge to enforce the rules of the group.

■ **Move your body to change your mood.** Physical activity lifts depression and negative moods. Depressed people often complain that they feel too tired to exercise. But the feelings of fatigue associated with depression are not due to physical exhaustion. Try to get 20 to 30 minutes of some type of exercise every day. It can be walking, yard work, chair dancing—anything. You may find that you have more energy. For more information on how to safely start moving and keep moving, see Chapter 7, *Exercising and Physical Activity for Every Body*, and Chapter 8 *Exercising to Feel Better*.

■ **Think positive.** Many people tend to be excessively critical of themselves, especially when they're depressed. You may find yourself thinking untrue things about yourself. Challenge automatic negative thoughts by changing the negative stories you tell yourself. For example, you may say to yourself, "Unless I do everything perfectly, I'm a failure." Try changing this belief to, "Success is doing the best that I can in any situation." Learn more about challenging negative self-talk and worst-case thinking on pages 102–104, in Chapter 5, *Using Your Mind to Manage Pain and Other Symptoms*. Also, when you are depressed, it's easy to forget that anything nice has happened at all. Make a list of some of the good or positive events in your life. You could even keep a gratitude diary and each day write one or two things that were positive. Learn more about expressing gratitude on page 114 in

Chapter 5, *Using Your Mind to Manage Pain and Other Symptoms*.

■ **Do something for someone else.** Lending a helping hand is a great way to change a bad mood. Arrange to babysit for a friend, read a story to someone who is ill or cannot see, or volunteer at a soup kitchen. If you can't get out, you can make calls to or write cards to folks in nursing homes. When you're depressed, you may greet this advice with thoughts like, "I've got enough troubles of my own. I don't need anyone else's." But if you bring yourself to help someone else, even in a small way, you'll feel better about yourself. When you help others, you are distracted from your own problems. Feeling useful is good for self-esteem. Helping others who are needier than yourself can help you appreciate your own abilities. Your problems may not seem as overwhelming. Sometimes helping others is the surest way to help yourself.

Don't be discouraged if it takes some time to feel better even once you start using these techniques. If, however, these self-management strategies are not turning things around for you and your depression becomes more severe, seek help from your health care provider or a mental health professional. Counseling or antidepressant medication (or both) can go a long way toward relieving depression. Seeking professional help and taking medications are not signs of weakness. They are signs of strength. Self-managers are strong.

Anger

Anger and frustration are common reactions to chronic pain. The uncertainty and unpredictability of living with pain may threaten your independence and control. You may find yourself asking, "Why me? It's so unfair." This is a normal response.

You may be angry with yourself, family, friends, health care providers, God or a higher power, or the world in general. For example, you may be angry at yourself for not taking better care of yourself. You may be angry at your family and friends because they don't do things the way you want. Or you might be angry at your doctor and other health care providers because they cannot fix your problems. Some people who are depressed or have anxiety disorders express their depression or anxiety with anger.

Chronic Pain and Anger

It is no wonder that people with chronic pain are sometimes upset. Anger and frustration, especially when poorly expressed, can stand in the way of good pain management. When you are angry you may lack motivation, be inactive, be hostile toward others, or "act out." Acting out may involve blowing up, shouting, or displaying other aggressive behavior. These behaviors can push away those who can most help you. The result is more isolation, anger, and frustration. The first step to self-managing your anger is recognizing and admitting that you are angry. The second step is identifying the reason for your anger. Managing anger also means finding acceptable ways to express your emotions.

Tools for Anger Self-Management

There are several things you can do to help manage your anger. Here we explain some of the more effective tools and techniques.

Reason with Yourself

How you interpret and explain a situation determines how you feel about it. You can make your anger less powerful by pausing and questioning your anger-producing thoughts. If you change your thoughts, you can change your response. Without either denying your feelings or giving in to the situation, choose how to react when you get upset. This sounds simple, but what gets in the way is that many people see anger as coming from outside—something over which they have little control. We see ourselves as helpless victims. We blame others and say, "You make me so angry!" We explode and then say, "I couldn't help it." We see spouses as selfish and insensitive, bosses as snobs or bullies, friends as unappreciative. So it seems that our only choice is an outburst of hostility. But with a little practice, even a seasoned hothead can master new and healthy responses. You can decide whether or not to get angry and then whether or not to act.

At the first sign of anger, count to three and ask yourself these three questions:

1. **Is this really important enough to get angry about?** Maybe this isn't serious enough to waste time and energy on. Will this make a big difference in your life? If not, it probably is not worth flying into a rage. Raise your anger threshold. Allow fewer things to trigger your anger in the first place. If you

can put up with more annoyances before you get angry, you can get angry less often.

2. **Am I justified in getting angry?** You may need to gather more information to really understand the situation. More information may prevent you from jumping to conclusions. More information can also help you understand why others act as they do. For example, you might fly into a rage when your friend is half an hour late for a concert before he tells you he was in a minor car accident on his way to the venue. If you wait to get all the information, you can avoid getting angry.

3. **Will getting angry make a difference?** More often than not, losing your cool does not work and may make you and others miserable. Exploding or venting increases your angry feelings, puts a strain on your relationships, and potentially damages your health.

Cool off

Any technique that relaxes or distracts you— such as meditating or taking a long walk—can help put out the anger fire. Slow, deep breathing is one of the quickest and simplest ways to cool off (see page 65). When you notice anger building, take ten slow, deep breaths before responding. Sometimes withdrawing and spending some time alone can cool down the situation. Physical exercise also provides a good natural outlet for stress and anger.

Talk without blaming

Learn how to communicate your anger with words, preferably without blaming or offending others. This can be done by using "I" (rather than "you") messages to express your feelings. (To learn how to use "I" messages, refer to pages 253–255 in Chapter 11, *Communicating with Family, Friends, and Health Care Providers*.) Know that, if you choose to express your anger verbally, people will not always be able to help you address the cause of your anger. Most of us are not very good at dealing with angry people. This is true even if the anger is justified.

If you really feel the need to vent, you may find it useful to seek counseling or join a support group. Nonprofit organizations, such as the various chronic pain, heart, diabetes, arthritis, and other health-related associations, may be useful resources that can help you find a group that is right for you.

Modify your expectations

Each of us has had to change what we expect from life along the way. For example, as a child you thought you could become anything—a fireman, a ballet dancer, a doctor, and so on. As you grew older, however, you evaluated these expectations, along with your talents and interests. Based on this evaluation, you modified your plans.

You can use this same adjustment process to deal with the frustration of having chronic pain. For example, it may be unrealistic to expect that you will ever be "all better." However, it is realistic to expect that you can still do many of the things you enjoy in life. Unfortunately, many people with chronic pain wait around until their problems improve. While they are waiting, they do nothing and become more inactive and frustrated. Changing your expectations can help you change your perspective. Instead of dwelling on the 10 percent of things you can no longer do, think about the 90 percent of things you can still do. Anger is normal when you have chronic pain. Part of learning to manage the condition involves acknowledging and accepting this anger and finding helpful ways to deal with it.

Falling out of fridge Dropping, Trouble opening

Fear

Pain and fear often go together. If you have pain for a long time, you might become fearful of things that are related to pain. For example, if you went on a long car trip and got a major headache, you might be afraid to go on other car trips. Situations that in the past caused a high level of pain can become big sources of anxiety.

Chronic Pain and Fear

If you had a lot of pain from a back injury that happened when you were picking something up off the floor, you might feel quite anxious about being told that doing this and other activities is necessary to your recovery. Attempts to do these activities can increase anxiety and also cause muscle tension and stress-related responses (such as increased heart rate) that make pain worse. You might see some activities as so much of a threat that you avoid doing them at all. Although avoiding activities works in the short run to prevent anxiety, in the long run, avoiding activities works against you.

There are several reasons why avoiding activities is a losing strategy. First, the tendency to avoid activity usually gets stronger over time. Although fear of pain might first lead you to avoid just one specific activity (such as going on a car trip or bending down to pick things up), over time fear increases the chances that you will avoid a whole range of activities that involve movement (including riding in the car to go anywhere, twisting, reaching, or getting up and down out of a chair). Second, avoiding activities leads to muscle weakness and a loss of physical fitness. Both of these make it more difficult and painful to do any activities— even the ones you used to enjoy. Third, as fear becomes stronger, much more of your attention and mental energy becomes focused on pain itself. Directing attention to pain may make it a lot harder to concentrate on other activities and things that are important to you (such as family events or work tasks). Finally, if fear of pain leads to avoidance of activities that are valued and meaningful, you are at risk of become more discouraged and depressed. As we noted in the section on depression (see page 74), depressed feelings make it harder to enjoy life. They also make it difficult to do things and lead to more inactivity, muscle disuse, and disability.

Counseling and Pain-Related Fear

Counseling for pain-related fear can be very effective. If you feel fearful often and your life is becoming more limited, consider cognitive-behavioral therapy (CBT). CBT has four basic parts. If you seek CBT therapy for pain-related fear, for example, your experience may involve these steps. First, the therapist works with you to determine your most important goals. Next, you learn about why exposure to feared situations can be helpful. Then the therapist works with you to identify a list of activities you are avoiding because of pain-related fear. To develop the list, the therapist might use a set of photographs of daily activities and ask you about how much concern/worry you have about each activity. The list you develop will include a range of activities, from those that are pretty easy for you (cause a low to moderate level of fear) to those that are the most difficult (cause the most fear). Finally, the therapist will help you to do behavioral experiments in which you will expose yourself several times to each of these activities. This will be done slowly, starting with the easiest activities. With repeated exposures to each activity, you will learn that many of the things you fear do not happen. You also will become more confident and less fearful. By doing activities you want to do, you get part of your life back and also gain tools to use in fearful situations in the future. You can learn more about this type of psychological therapy on page 338 in Chapter 15, *Understanding Medications and Other Treatments for Chronic Pain.*

Tools for Fear Self-Management

Self-management methods can be helpful if your pain-related fear and avoidance of activities is not too high.

■ **Reduce your overall level of anxiety.** Regularly practice the relaxation and meditation techniques you can learn about in Chapter 5, *Using Your Mind to Manage Pain and Other Symptoms*, on pages 97–104. Even 5 to 10 minutes of deep breathing two or three times a day is helpful.

■ **If your pain-related fear is not too high, you can be your own therapist.** Self-manage by following some of the principles of cognitive behavioral therapy. Make a plan to slowly try the things you fear. Make a list of five to ten things you avoid because you are afraid they will cause pain. The list should range from what you fear least to what you fear most. Expose yourself to each of these situations little by little. For example, if you fear driving in the car, you might start with driving just 5 or 10 minutes. For each thing you try, do it a number of times until your anxiety about it decreases and you feel more confident about managing fear. You might make some discoveries. For example, you may find that car rides on sunny days tend to trigger headaches more than on cloudy days. Maybe your problem is not the car rides but the light. Start with easier situations and progress to the more difficult ones. Go slow and easy. Keep at it until you feel you've mastered your fear and are no longer avoiding the situation.

Guilt ~~Failure Independence~~

People with chronic pain often feel guilty. This is common. The guilt might stem from different causes. You might feel guilty because you think that you have let down your family and friends. You might feel guilty that you cannot control the pain and think that you are weak. If you do not understand your pain, you are likely to feel more guilty because you might think that you are somehow causing your own pain.

People with pain who feel guilty are much more likely to report more severe pain and worry. They also report that pain interferes with (i.e., gets in the way of) their lives. This is especially true when people feel guilty much of the day. They also report spending much of their time trying to make sense of their pain. They might think a lot about who or what is to blame. They might wonder if the pain is due to something they have done or not done, or whether they have followed bad advice, or if they have used pain treatments that are not that helpful. If they are working, they report being a lot more tense at work and finding their work less satisfying.

If you are a person who is feeling guilty most of the time and the guilt is leading to depression, ask your health care team about depression counseling or medications. See page 74 in this chapter to learn more about depression self-management. If you feel guilty only some of the time and your guilt is not that severe, there are several self-management tools that might be helpful, including the following:

- **Know that you are not alone and reach out.** Guilty feelings are common in persons who have chronic pain. If you are avoiding family and friends and not communicating with them because of guilt, try to share your feelings and spend more time with others. This can reduce tension and worry and help you learn that people understand you and want to help you.

- **Seek out health professionals who can help you learn more about your pain.** This is especially useful if you don't understand the cause(s) of your pain or what the future of your pain is likely to be. People who can help include physicians, psychologists, nurse practitioners, physician associates, or physical therapists. Just as all health professionals are not surgeons, not all health professionals are pain experts. Ask around for a pain expert near you. Find someone who will spend the time to carefully review your history and medical records with you. Ask about your pain condition and your future. You may find that, as you learn more about your pain and its treatment, you can better self-manage your pain.

- **Relax your standards and give yourself some breaks.** There are several self-help tips you can try if you are a perfectionist and feel guilty when you don't live up to your own high standards. For example, you can set smaller and realistic daily action plans that you are pretty sure you can achieve. You can also keep a record of how many of these action plans you achieve so you can see your progress. Work on being easier on yourself using some of the self-compassion methods discussed on page 114. For example, try savoring pleasant experiences, keeping a list of things you are grateful for, etc.

Stress

Stress is a common problem. But what is stress? In the 1950s, the physiologist Hans Selye described stress as "the nonspecific response of the body to any demand made upon it." Others describe stress as the body's way of adapting to demands, whether pleasant or unpleasant. You may feel stress after experiencing negative events, such as the death of a loved one, or after joyful events, such as the marriage of a child.

How Does the Body Respond to Stress?

Your body is used to functioning at a certain level. When there is a need to change, your body adjusts. When your body needs to respond to stress, it reacts by preparing to take action. Your heart rate increases. Your blood pressure rises. Your neck and shoulder muscles tense. Your breathing becomes more rapid. Your digestion slows. Your mouth becomes dry. You may begin sweating. These are signals of what we call stress.

Why does this happen? To act, your muscles need a supply of oxygen and energy. Your breathing increases in an effort to inhale oxygen and to get rid of carbon dioxide. Your heart rate increases to deliver oxygen and nutrients to the muscles. At the same time, body functions that are not immediately necessary, such as the digestion of food and natural immune responses, slow down.

In general, these responses last only until the stressful event passes. Your body then returns to its normal level of functioning. Sometimes, though, your body does not return to its former comfortable level. If the stress continues for any length of time, your body continues to adapt to it. This chronic stress can lead to the onset of some chronic conditions and can make symptoms such as pain more difficult to manage.

How You Think about Stress Is Important

We've talked about how your body responds to stress and common situations that are stressful. One question you may have is: Why do some people respond to the same stressors in very different ways? Scientists have learned that the way you think about a situation is key to how you respond to a stressor. Consider two examples of how two different people might respond to the same stress event. In this example, the stress event is running low on gas, having to stop to refill the tank, and being late for an appointment with a new pain doctor.

In the first example, Fatima judges having to stop for gas as a real threat and has thoughts such as, "The doctor will think I forgot or don't care," "I've messed up the doctor's schedule and won't get in to see her," or "I'll never get another appointment." The more she focuses on these thoughts, the more tense and painful her neck and shoulder muscles become. She feels frustrated, anxious, embarrassed, and discouraged and has difficulty thinking clearly. After stopping to get gas, Fatima drives as fast as she can to get to her appointment. She arrives 25 minutes late and is too upset to go into the doctor's office.

Melanie, in contrast, judges the situation of running low on gas as more of a challenge. When she realizes she is going to have to stop, she feels herself tensing up a bit. She has some negative thoughts about herself ("I should have checked the gas last night or before I left") that lead her to feel annoyed or irritated at first. However, she also has thoughts that calm her down ("OK, I know some things I can do in this situation") and help her think more clearly. When Melanie stops for gas, she calls the doctor's office, tells them she will be late, and is told by the receptionist that they can fit her in later that afternoon. Melanie is relieved, drives to the doctor's clinic, and, because she now is early, decides to have lunch at a nearby café. She then goes to her rescheduled doctor's appointment and is pleased when it goes well.

These examples illustrate how the way you think about or judge an event can play a big role in how stressed out you become. If you focus on how much of a threat or how much harm an event will cause you, your body is much more likely to show stress responses (such as increased tension, higher blood pressure, rapid breathing rate, upset stomach, increased pain), and you are much more likely to feel emotionally upset (anxious, fearful, guilty). Becoming more aware of how you are thinking about small daily problems and common stressful events can be really helpful. It can also remind you to use self-management tools.

Most people cannot avoid some stress in their lives. Learning to live with stress and even adapt and grow from stress is an important self-management goal. something that makes them sick and should Although stress can be harmful, in other situations stress should be welcomed. Stress can help prepare you to take on both mental and physical challenges, motivate necessary lifestyle changes, and build resilience. The effect stress has on your health and well-being seems to be affected by your personal view or "mindset" about stress. Do you believe that stress is always bad and should be avoided? Or do you view stress as something that can sometimes enhance your health, growth, and performance? People with a "stress is enhancing" mindset do much better in stressful situations than people who see stress only as be avoided or reduced. Being open to viewing stressors as challenges rather than threats can help you learn and grow from stressful situations.

Techniques such as relaxation, meditation, and positive self-talk, which are discussed in Chapter 5, *Using Your Mind to Manage Pain and Other Symptoms*, help you adjust your response and lower your stress.

Common Stressors

Stressors are things that cause stress. There are many different kinds of stressors. They can be physical, emotional, or environmental. Regardless of what type of stressor you feel, the changes in your body are the same. Some sources of stress can be good, such as a job promotion, a wedding, a vacation, a new friendship, or a new baby. These stressors make you feel happy but still cause the changes in your body that we have discussed. Although there are different types of stressors, stressors are not independent of one another. In fact, one stressor can often lead to other stressors or increase the effects of existing stressors. Several stressors can also occur at the same time. For instance, fatigue can cause anxiety, frustration, inactivity, and loss of endurance. Let's examine some of the most common sources of stress.

Mental and Emotional Stressors

Mental and emotional stressors can also be either pleasant or uncomfortable. The joys you experience from meeting friends or seeing a child graduate may cause similar responses in your body as your feelings of frustration about your illness. Although this may seem surprising, the similarity comes from the way your brain perceives the stress.

Environmental Stressors

Environmental stressors can also be both good and bad. Environmental stressors may be as varied as a sunny day, a sandy beach, uneven sidewalks, loud noises, bad weather, a snoring spouse, or secondhand smoke. Each creates a positive or negative excitement that triggers the stress response.

Physical Stressors

Physical stressors include the physical symptoms of your chronic pain condition, but they also can be something as pleasant as picking up a new baby or going shopping. What do these physical stressors have in common? They increase your body's demand for energy. If your body is not prepared to deal with this demand, the results may be anything from sore muscles to fatigue or a worsening of other symptoms.

Exercise Is a Good Stressor

Remember that not all stressors are bad. For example, getting married, getting the job of your dreams, or having a baby are all positive stressors. Exercise is also a good physical stressor. When you exercise or do any type of physical activity, a demand is placed on your body. The heart works to deliver blood to the muscles. The lungs work harder, and you breathe more rapidly to keep up with your muscles' demand for oxygen. Your muscles are responding to the signals from your brain, which tells them to keep moving.

After you have exercised for several weeks, you will begin to notice a change. What once seemed really hard becomes easier. The same exercises put less strain on your heart, lungs, and other muscles because your muscles have become more efficient and you have become more fit. What has happened? Your body has adapted to stress. The same can happen with psychological stressors. Many people become more resilient and stronger emotionally after having emotional challenges and learning to adapt to them.

You can read more about exercise and stress and the positive benefits of being fit in Chapter

7, *Exercising and Physical Activity for Every Body*, and Chapter 8, *Exercising to Feel Better*.

Recognizing the Signs of Stress

Like most people, you can probably tolerate more stress on some days than on others. But sometimes you may be stressed beyond what seems to be your breaking point and feel that your life is out of control. Often it is difficult to recognize when you are under too much stress. The following are warning signs of excess stress:

- Nail biting, hair pulling, foot tapping, or other repetitive habits
- Teeth grinding or jaw clenching
- Tension in your head, neck, or shoulders
- Anxiety, nervousness, helplessness, or irritability
- Frequent accidents
- Forgetting things you usually don't forget
- Difficulty concentrating
- Fatigue and exhaustion

Some of these are also signs of chronic pain. That's why chronic pain is like a type of chronic stress.

Of course, there are many things that can make you feel stressed, not just your pain. Sometimes you may catch yourself behaving or feeling stressed. When you do, take a few minutes to think about what is making you feel tense. Take a few deep breaths and try to relax. Also, a quick body scan can help you recognize stress in your body. You will learn how to perform a body scan and other good ideas for coping with stress in Chapter 5, *Using Your Mind to Manage Pain and Other Symptoms*.

Know that nicotine, alcohol, and caffeine increase the stress response. Some people smoke a cigarette, drink a glass of wine or beer, eat sugary candy or starchy and salty junk foods, or drink a cup of coffee to soothe their tension, but this may actually increase stress. Eliminating or cutting down on these chemicals can help you feel less stressed.

Tools for Stress Self-Management

Dealing effectively with stress can start with a simple three-step process:

1. **Identify your stressors by making a list.** Consider every area of your life: family, relationships, health, financial security, living environment, and so on.

2. **Sort your stressors.** For each stressor, ask yourself two things: Is it important or unimportant? Is it changeable or unchangeable? Then place each of your stressors in one of four categories:

   - Important and changeable
   - Important and unchangeable
   - Unimportant and changeable
   - Unimportant and unchangeable

   For example, the need to quit smoking is changeable and important. Loss of a loved one is important and unchangeable. The bad record of your favorite sports team, a traffic jam, or bad weather is unchangeable and may or may not be important. What really counts is what you think about each stressor.

3. **Choose a strategy for each stressor.** Match your strategy to each stressor. Different strategies work for different stressors. In

the next sections, you will find some strategies to help manage the different types of stressors.

Managing Important and Changeable Stressors

Important and changeable stressors are best managed by taking action to change the situation and to reduce the stress. Useful self-management tools include problem solving, decision making, and action planning (see Chapter 2, *Becoming an Active Self-Manager*); relaxation techniques (see Chapter 5, *Using Your Mind to Manage Pain and Other Symptoms*); physical activity (see Chapter 7, *Exercising and Physical Activity for Every Body*, and Chapter 8, *Exercising to Feel Better*); and effective communication and seeking support from family and friends (see Chapter 11, *Communicating with Family, Friends, and Health Care Providers*).

Managing Important and Unchangeable Stressors

Important and unchangeable stressors are often the most difficult to manage. They can make you feel helpless and hopeless. No matter what you do, you cannot make another person change, bring someone back from the dead, or delete traumatic experiences from your life. Even though you may not be able to change the situation, you may be able to use one or more of the following tools to deal with it:

1. **Change the way you think about the problem.** For example, consider how much worse it could be, focus on the positive and practice gratitude (see page 114), distract yourself (see page 100), or simply accept what you can't change.

2. **Find some part of the problem that is changeable.** You can't stop a hurricane, but you can take steps to prepare for it, or you can rebuild if it's already struck. You can't make your brother quit tobacco, but you can make your car a nonsmoking and non-vaping zone.

3. **Reassess how important the problem is in light of your overall life and priorities.** Maybe your neighbor's criticism isn't so important after all.

4. **Change your emotional reactions to the situation.** You can't change what happened, but you can help yourself feel less distressed about it. Write your deepest thoughts and feelings in a journal (see page 115), seek support from family and friends, help others, practice relaxation techniques, use imagery, enjoy humor, or go for a walk.

Managing Unimportant and Changeable Stressors

If a stressor is unimportant, first try just letting it go. But if you can control it with relatively little effort, go ahead and deal with it. Solving small problems helps build your skills and confidence to tackle bigger ones. You can use the same strategies to address unimportant and changeable stressors that you use for important and changeable problems.

Managing Unimportant and Unchangeable Stressors

Unimportant and unchangeable problems are common hassles. Everybody has their share of these. The best solution is to ignore them. Starting now, you are given permission to let go of unimportant concerns. Don't let them bother you. Distract yourself with humor, relaxation, imagery, or focusing on more pleasurable things.

Stress Management and Problem Solving

Think about things you find stressful, such as being stuck in traffic, traveling, or grocery shopping and preparing a meal. First, look at what it is about the particular situation that is stressful. Do traffic jams bother you because you hate to be late? Are trips stressful because of uncertainty about your destination? Does meal planning and preparation involve too many steps and demand too much energy?

Once you have found the problem, begin looking for possible ways to reduce the stress. When you travel by car, can you leave earlier or let someone else drive or take public transit? Before a trip, can you contact someone at your destination and ask about wheelchair access, local mass transit, and other concerns? When you need to cook a meal, can you shop and cook on different days or can you shop and prepare food for the evening meal in the morning or take a short nap in the early afternoon on days you have to cook?

If you know that certain situations make you stressed, develop ways to deal with them before they happen. Rehearse, in your mind, what you will do when the situation arises so you will be ready. After you have identified some possible solutions, select one to try the next time you face the situation. Then evaluate the results. (This is the problem-solving approach that is discussed on pages 29–31 in Chapter 2, *Becoming an Active Self-Manager*.)

We have discussed how you can successfully manage some types of stress by planning for or changing the situation. But sometimes stress sneaks up on you when you don't expect it. Dealing with unexpected stress involves problem solving just as dealing with other stressful situations does. As noted earlier, tools for dealing with stress include getting enough sleep, exercising, and eating well. But sometimes stress is so overwhelming that these tools are not enough. These are times when good self-managers turn to consultants such as counselors, social workers, psychologists, or psychiatrists.

In summary, stress, like every other symptom, has many causes and can therefore be managed in many different ways. It is up to you to examine the problem and try to find solutions that meet your needs and suit your lifestyle.

Memory Problems

Many people worry about changes in their memory, particularly as they age. Although we all forget things, some people with chronic pain have memory problems that are not a normal part of aging. For people with chronic pain, memory problems may be caused by medications, other symptoms like depression, or other illnesses like dementia. But changes in memory and in thinking can also be a symptom of the pain condition itself. Scientists think this happens because the constant barrage of pain signals causes multiple changes in the brain. People with fibromyalgia seem especially

Self-Management Tips for Memory and Thinking Problems

- Talk to your family about your memory problems. If you do, they will better understand your behavior and support you.

- Give yourself enough time to finish a task. Try not to rush. Don't let others hurry you.

- Don't try to accomplish too many things at the same time. Do one task at a time. If a task is complex, break it down into smaller steps. See Chapter 6, *Organizing and Pacing Your Life for Pain Self-Management and Safety*, for other pacing suggestions. Avoid taking on more than you can handle comfortably.

- Be physically active. Exercise and movement increases the flow of blood and oxygen to the brain, which can help you think more clearly. To learn more, see Chapter 7, *Exercising and Physical Activity for Every Body*, and Chapter 8, *Exercising to Feel Better*.

- Practice relaxation techniques on a regular basis. Make relaxation part of your daily routine. Relaxation can quiet the nervous system, and, like physical activity, it can improve the quality of your thinking. Learn more in Chapter 5, *Using Your Mind to Manage Pain and Other Symptoms*.

- Reduce distractions. When you are trying to concentrate or pay attention to something, turn down the radio, shut off the TV, or find some place quiet.

- Reduce clutter in your home. Assign a place for things like your keys or cell phone and get in the habit of putting things back in their places after you use them. This will help keep you more organized.

- Use reminders to stay on track. Place sticky notes in different locations in the house, or make lists in a calendar or notebook. Set reminders on your computer or cell phone so that you remember appointments or tasks you want to do.

- Take a family member or friend with you to appointments. That way you won't miss out on information if you are having trouble paying attention or remembering new facts.

prone to memory and concentration concerns. This is commonly referred to as "fibro fog."

Fibro fog and memory problems related to other chronic pain conditions make it more difficult to complete everyday tasks. You might feel confused. It may be challenging to think clearly, pay attention, remember new information, or concentrate on new things. Although this can be upsetting and frustrating, there are things you can do to manage this symptom.

Recall that memory problems can be a sign of other disorders, such as depression or disease, or they may result from some of the medications you take for your pain. Be sure to talk with your health care providers openly about your problems with memory, concentration, or thinking. They will be able to assess your situation and help you manage your memory-related symptoms.

For a complete list of suggested further readings, useful websites, and other helpful resources, please see www.bullpub.com/resources.

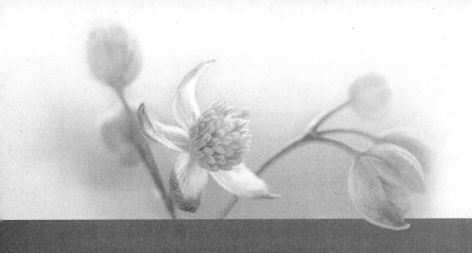

CHAPTER 5

Using Your Mind to Manage Pain and Other Symptoms

THERE IS A STRONG LINK BETWEEN thoughts, attitudes, and emotions and mental and physical health. As one of our self-managers said, "It's not always mind over matter, but mind matters." And in chronic pain, mind matters a lot. Brain-imaging studies have found that the emotional and thinking regions of the brain are connected not only to each other but to the part of the brain that detects body sensations. And all of these regions are connected to multiple pathways in the nervous system. What you think and feel can lessen or worsen your pain by opening or closing the pain gate in the spinal cord and influencing the complex network of nerve cells in the brain. (See pages 4–11 in Chapter 1, *Chronic Pain Self-Management: What It Is and How to Do It.*)

Although thoughts and emotions do not directly cause chronic pain, they can influence pain and many other symptoms. Research has shown that thoughts and emotions trigger certain hormones and other chemicals that send messages throughout the body. These messages affect how your body functions; they can, for example, alter your heart rate, blood pressure, breathing, blood sugar levels, muscle responses, immune response, concentration, fertility, and even your ability to fight off other illnesses. Both pleasant and unpleasant thoughts and emotions can make your heart rate and breathing increase or slow down.

When you feel a strong emotion, you often have a physical response. You may sweat, blush, tear up, and so on. All of us have experienced how the mind affects the body in this way. Sometimes just a memory or an image can trigger these responses. For example, try this simple exercise: Imagine you are holding a big, bright yellow lemon slice. You hold it close to your nose and smell its strong citrus aroma. Now you bite into the lemon. It's juicy! The juice fills your mouth and dribbles down your chin. You begin to suck on the lemon and its tart juice. What happens when you imagine this scenario? Your body responds! Your mouth puckers and starts to water. You may even smell the scent of the lemon. All of these reactions are triggered by the mind and its memory of your experience with a real lemon.

This example illustrates the power the mind has over the body. It also gives you a good reason to develop your mental abilities to help manage your symptoms. The mind can help relieve the unpleasantness caused by pain. With training and practice, you can learn to use the mind to relax your tense muscles, calm your nervous system, and improve your breathing. In this chapter, you will learn several ways to use your mind to manage pain and associated symptoms. These are sometimes referred to as "thinking" or "cognitive" techniques because they involve the use of our thinking abilities to make changes in the body. But before exploring the many cognitive and relaxation tools you can use to reduce your pain, it may help you to consider the bigger picture of your life. Figuring out what you value is a self-management tool that can help you prepare to use "thinking" techniques.

Thinking about Values: How It Can Help

Your thoughts, attitudes, and emotions are all rooted in your values. What are your values? To figure this out, you can ask yourself some questions: What is really important to you? What gives your life meaning? What are the principles that you want to guide your life? Try to write down your answers to these questions. Figuring out the answers can help you uncover your values. Many people find ongoing pain is so stressful that they end up just focusing on the immediate problems they face and simply trying to make it through the day. They give up thinking about "the big picture." Understanding and thinking about your values is very useful when coping with chronic pain.

Why are values important, and how can thinking about them help? Spending time focusing on what you value—what is most important to you as a person—can help you in many ways. Your values can help guide your actions. For example, if you realize that family relationships are what give your life meaning, then you are a lot more likely to make efforts to reach out to siblings, parents, and relatives. You may start to visit, phone, or email them more often, for example.

Knowing what your values are can also help you to step back from details of your day and see the broader landscape of your life. This can lead to a more positive and optimistic perspective. Instead of focusing on your daily pain, you can focus on your relationships or your role in your family and how you can become closer to people you care about. Thinking about your values can help you think about all the opportunities that are available for living in ways that really fit those values. It also can motivate you to pursue a path in life that fits with your deepest and true hopes and desires.

A focus on values can even make it easier to deal with daily stressors. If you are leading a values-focused life, you may be more likely to judge a daily stressor (like a pain flare or a delayed appointment) as a challenge to be dealt with rather than as something that is overwhelming that you can't handle. You may find your body is a lot less reactive to stress and that negative feelings are not as strong and/or don't last as long. In sum, being true to your values can help you become more resilient and more effective as a self-manager.

Goals and Values

We talk about setting goals in Chapter 2, *Becoming an Active Self-Manager*. Goals are things you want to accomplish. So what is the difference between a goal and a value? Your values are the things you think are valuable and important in life. Values are what really matters to you. Values give your life direction and purpose. Values include things such as being a good partner, being a good parent, growing as a person, caring for others, or taking care of your health. Values differ from goals in several ways. While a goal (for example, going out to dinner with your partner every week) can be accomplished, values are more like points on a compass. Values can't be reached, but they give your life direction.

If you focus only on goals and achievements, you may get caught up in the anxiety and uncertainty of achieving vs. not achieving them. If you fail to reach a goal, you may find that you get down on yourself or become a lot more critical of others in your life. You also might find, when you do reach a goal, that the satisfaction of achievement doesn't last that long. You don't really savor or enjoy the moment that much. Keeping the focus on values allows you to savor the joy of reaching a goal more fully because you can see a goal as part of a longer-term set of things you want to do to give your life meaning.

Identifying Your Values

Imagine you are asked, "When you look back on your life, what are the things that, over the years, mattered most to you and gave your life meaning?" What would your response be? Your answers to this question reveal a lot about your core values. Figure 5.1 on page 96 is an example of how someone might answer this question.

Figure 5.1 is a list of values provided by an art teacher who had to retire on disability because of chronic pain. Read this list and think about

These are one person's responses to the question, "What are the things that have mattered the most to you and have given your life meaning?"

Value
My relationship with my partner
My relationship with my children
My relationship with my friends
Making a difference in the lives of young people
Creating a warm and welcoming home space
Maintaining my health
Developing and nurturing my own spirituality
Visiting and supporting others who are sick and infirm

Figure 5.1 **Identifying Your Values**

what this teacher might have learned by making this list. Then write your own answers to the question at the start of this section ("When you look back on your life, what are the things that, over the years, mattered most to you and gave your life meaning?").

What can you learn from making a list of your values? First, it may help you understand who you really are. Sometimes, that sense of your true self gets lost in the shuffle. This is particularly true when you are dealing with an ongoing stressor, such as chronic pain. Reflecting on your true nature is a way of grounding yourself.

Second, listing your values can make you more aware of how you want to live your life. There are many potential paths you can follow, and you make choices every day about your life path. Third, focusing on values often causes people to think about how their current actions and goals fit with their true values. You might find that some of your actions (such as exercising daily) fit well with a core value (such as maintaining your health), while other actions that you do regularly (such as watching television for hours each day) take a lot of time and don't fit really well with any of your values.

Finally, making a list of core values can be the spark that helps you set and work on the actions and goals that fit with your values. Use your list of values as the basis for developing your action plans. (For more on action planning, see pages 34–37 in Chapter 2, *Becoming an Active Self-Manager*.) Focusing on your values is a great way to motivate yourself to follow your action plan. The goals you achieve through these action plans are even more meaningful when you do this because your goals and plans are strongly linked to how you want to live your life.

Tools for Relaxation Self-Management

Relaxation means different things to different people. If you think about it, you can probably identify the things you do that help you relax. The goal of relaxation self-management is to approach life with your mind and body in a a calmer state so that the mind and body are at rest. This allows you to reduce the tensions that can increase the intensity or severity of your symptoms.

You may have heard and read about using your mind to relax and how this can help you manage your pain. Like many of us, you may still be confused as to how to use your mind to relax and what the benefits of relaxation are. Relaxation involves using thinking or cognitive techniques to reduce tension from your body and mind. Relaxation can help you sleep better,

Quick and Easy Relaxation Tools

The relaxation tools in this chapter involve using your mind to help relax your body. However, before we get to these techniques, let's not forget about the quick and easy techniques that many of us use every day. Here is a short list of quick and easy relaxation tools:

- Take a nap or a warm, soothing bath.
- Curl up and read or listen to a good book.
- Watch a funny movie or a favorite TV show.
- Make a paper airplane and sail it across the room.
- Get a massage.
- Enjoy a glass of wine occasionally.
- Start a small garden or grow a beautiful plant indoors.
- Do crafts such as knitting, pottery, or woodworking.
- Read a poem or an inspirational saying.
- Go for a walk.
- Start a collection (coins, folk art, shells, etc.).
- Listen to your favorite music.
- Sing around the house.
- Crumble paper into a ball and use a wastebasket as a basketball hoop.
- Watch water move (ocean waves, a lake, or a fountain).
- Watch the clouds in the sky.
- Put your head down on your desk and close your eyes for 5 minutes.
- Rub your hands together until they're warm, and then cup them over your closed eyes.
- Vigorously shake your hands and arms for 10 seconds.
- Call a friend or family member to chat.
- Smile and introduce yourself to someone new.
- Do something nice and unexpected for someone else.
- Play with a pet.
- "Visit" a vacation spot in your mind.

breathe better, and feel less stress, anxiety, and pain. It can calm you and help you feel a sense of well-being. There are many different relaxation techniques. Some techniques help you relax your muscles, while others reduce anxiety and emotional stress or divert your attention from your symptoms. All of these help with pain and symptom management.

General Guidelines for Relaxation Self-Management

These general guidelines can help you successfully practice relaxation techniques.

- **Pick a quiet place and time.** Find a time and place where you will not be disturbed for at least 15 to 20 minutes. If this seems too long, start with 5 minutes. (By the way, in some homes the only quiet place is the bathroom. That is just fine.)

- **Try to practice the technique twice daily and not less than four times a week.** These are new techniques, and you need to repeat new techniques to master them.

- **Don't expect miracles or immediate results.** Sometimes it takes three to four weeks of consistent practice before you start to notice benefits.

- **Relaxation should be helpful.** At worst, you may find it boring, but if practicing any technique is an unpleasant experience or makes you more nervous or anxious, switch to a different symptom-management tool.

Relaxation Self-Management Tools That Take 5 to 20 Minutes

The two relaxation techniques we discuss next—body scan and relaxation response—take just a few minutes but are quite effective.

Body Scan

You will find a body scan script on page 99. You can record this script, have someone read it to you, or read it yourself and then try the scan. It is not difficult to remember what to do. To relax muscles, you need to know how to scan your body and recognize where you are tense. Once you know how to scan your body for tension, you can learn to release the tension. The first step is to become familiar with the difference between the feeling of tension and the feeling of relaxation. This exercise helps you to compare those feelings. With practice, you can spot and release tension anywhere in your body. Body scanning is best done lying on your back, but you can do it in any comfortable position.

Relaxation Response

In the early 1970s, physician Herbert Benson studied what he calls the "relaxation response." According to Benson, our bodies have several natural states. One example is the "fight or flight" response people experience when faced with danger. Another is the body's natural tendency to relax after feeling tense. This tendency is the relaxation response. As our lives become more and more hectic, our bodies stay tense for long periods of time. We lose our ability to relax. Achieving the relaxation response can help you change this.

To achieve the relaxation response, find a quiet place where there are few or no distractions. Get into a comfortable position. You should be comfortable enough to remain in the same position for 20 minutes.

Choose a pleasant word and a tranquil object or feeling. For example, repeat a word or sound

Body Scan Script

As you get into a comfortable position, allowing yourself to begin to sink comfortably into the surface below you, you may perhaps begin to allow your eyes gradually to close . . . From there, turn your attention to your breath . . . Breathing in, allowing the breath gradually to go all the way down to your belly, and then breathing out . . . And again, breathing in . . . and out . . . noticing the natural rhythm of your breathing . . .

Now allow your attention to focus on your feet. Starting with your toes, notice whatever sensations are there—warmth, coolness, whatever's there . . . simply feel it. Using your mind's eye, imagine that as you breathe in, the breath goes all the way down into your toes, bringing with it new refreshing air . . . And now notice the sensations elsewhere in your feet. Not judging or thinking about what you're feeling, but simply becoming aware of the experience of your feet as you allow yourself to be fully supported by the surface below you . . .

Next focus on your lower legs and knees. These muscles and joints do a lot of work for us, but often we don't give them the attention they deserve. So now breathe down into the knees, calves, and ankles, noticing whatever sensations appear . . . See if you can simply stay with the sensations . . . breathing in new fresh air, and as you exhale, releasing tension and stress and allowing the muscles to relax and soften . . .

Now move your attention to the muscles, bones, and joints of the thighs, buttocks, and hips . . . breathing down into the upper legs, noticing whatever sensations you experience. It may be warmth, coolness, a heaviness or lightness. You may become aware of the contact with the surface beneath you, or perhaps the pulsing of your blood. Whatever's there . . . what matters is that you are taking time to learn to relax . . . deeper and deeper, as you breathe . . . in . . . and out.

Move your attention now to your back and chest. Feeling the breath fill the abdomen and chest . . . noticing whatever sensations are there . . . not judging or thinking, but simply observing what is right here right now. Allowing the fresh air to nourish the muscles, bones, and joints as you breathe in, and then exhaling any tension and stress.

Now focus on the neck, shoulders, arms, and hands. Inhaling down through the neck and shoulders, all the way down to the fingertips. Not trying too hard to relax, but simply becoming aware of your experience of these parts of your body in the present moment . . .

Turning now to your face and head, notice the sensations beginning at the back of your head, up along your scalp, and down into your forehead . . . Then become aware of the sensations in and around your eyes and down into your cheeks and jaw . . . Continue to allow your muscles to release and soften as you breathe in nourishing fresh air, and allow tension and stress to leave as you breathe out . . .

As you drink in fresh air, allow it to spread throughout your body, from the soles of your feet all the way up through the top of your head . . . And then exhale any remaining stress and tension . . . and now take a few moments to enjoy the stillness as you breathe in . . . and out . . . Awake, relaxed, and still . . .

Now as the body scan comes to a close, come back into the room, bringing with you whatever sensations of relaxation . . . comfort . . . peace, whatever's there . . . knowing that you can repeat this exercise at any appropriate time and place of your choosing . . . And when you're ready, open your eyes.

(such as the word *one*) while gazing at a symbol (perhaps a flower) or concentrating on a feeling (such as peace).

Adopt a passive attitude. Empty all thoughts and distractions from your mind. You may become aware of thoughts, images, and feelings, but don't concentrate on them. Just allow them to pass.

To feel the relaxation response take the following steps:

- Sit quietly in a comfortable position.

- Close your eyes.

- Relax all your muscles, beginning at your feet and progressing up to your face. Keep your muscles relaxed.

- Breathe in through your nose. Become aware of your breathing. As you breathe out through your mouth, say the word you chose silently to yourself. Try to empty all thoughts from your mind; concentrate on your word, symbol, or feeling.

- Maintain a passive attitude, and let relaxation occur at its own pace. When distracting thoughts occur, ignore them by not dwelling on them, and return to repeating the word you chose. Do not worry about whether you are successful in achieving a deep level of relaxation.

- Continue this for 10 to 20 minutes. You may open your eyes to check the time, but do not use an alarm. When you finish, sit quietly for several minutes, at first with your eyes closed. Do not stand up for a few minutes.

- Practice this once or twice daily.

Distraction/Attention Refocusing

Our minds have trouble focusing on more than one thing at a time. We can reduce the intensity of symptoms by training our minds to focus attention on something other than our bodies and their sensations. This technique, called distraction refocusing or attention refocusing, is particularly helpful for people with chronic pain conditions.

Research shows that when a person focuses on pain, several areas of the brain show more intense pain-related activity than when the person is distracted from the pain. Many studies have found that people who constantly direct their attention to pain and think about it all the time are more likely to expect the worst from their pain problem and to feel helpless about controlling it. Consciously redirecting attention away from pain can help you feel better. With distraction/attention refocusing, you are not ignoring your pain or other symptoms. Instead, you are *choosing* not to dwell on them.

Sometimes it may be difficult to put pain or other anxious thoughts out of your mind. When you try to suppress any thought, you may end up thinking more about it. For example, try as hard as you can for the next few minutes to not think about a large tiger charging at you. Whatever you do, don't let the thought of that tiger enter your mind. Now work on this for a few minutes. After you are done, ask yourself, "What am I thinking about?" If you are like many people, you probably find that it is nearly impossible not to think about the tiger.

Although you can't easily stop thinking about something, you can distract yourself and redirect your attention elsewhere. For example, go ahead now and let yourself think about that large charging tiger. Now stand up, loudly slam your hand on the table, and shout, *"Stop!"* What happened to the tiger? Gone—at least for the moment.

Distraction is especially good for brief activities or times when you know you will have an increase in symptoms. For example, if you know climbing stairs will cause discomfort or that falling asleep at night is difficult, try one of the following distraction techniques:

- Make plans for exactly what you will do after the unpleasant activity passes. For example, if climbing stairs is uncomfortable or painful, think about what you will do once you get to the top. If you have trouble falling asleep, try making plans for some future event, being as detailed as possible.

- Think of a person's name, a bird, a make of car, or whatever, for every letter of the alphabet. If you get stuck on one letter, go on to the next

- Challenge yourself to count backward from 100 by threes (100, 97, 94 . . .).

- To get through unpleasant daily chores such as sweeping, mopping, or vacuuming, imagine your floor as a map of a country or continent. Try naming all the states, provinces, or countries, moving east to west or north to south as you work. If geography does not appeal to you, imagine your favorite store and where each department is located.

- Try to remember the exact words to favorite songs or the events in an old story.

- Try the *"Stop!"* technique. If you find yourself worrying or entrapped in frequently repeating negative thoughts, stand up suddenly, slap your hand on the table or your thigh, and shout *"Stop!"* With practice, you won't have to shout out loud. Just whispering *"Stop!"* or tightening your vocal cords and moving your tongue as if saying *"Stop!"* will often work. Some people imagine a large stop sign. Others put a rubber band on their wrist and snap it to break the chain of negative thought. Or pinch yourself. Do anything that redirects your attention.

- Redirect your attention to a pleasurable experience:
  - ▸ Think about something you find beautiful in nature.
  - ▸ Try to identify all the sounds around you.
  - ▸ Massage your hand.
  - ▸ Smell a sweet or pungent odor.

There are many variations to these examples, all of which can help you refocus attention away from your problem.

So far we have discussed short-term refocusing strategies that involve using only the mind for distraction, but long-term projects are also a good way to refocus your attention. In these cases, you focus on some type of activity. Find an activity that interests you and really focus on doing it. It can be almost anything, from gardening to cooking to reading or going to a movie or doing volunteer work. Think about what you find interesting about the project. Is it that you are accomplishing something, like helping others or learning something new? One of the marks of successful self-managers is that they have a variety of interests and always seem to be really involved in something valued or meaningful.

Challenging Negative Self-Talk and Worst-Case Thinking

We all talk to ourselves all the time. For example, when waking up in the morning, you might think, "I really don't want to get out of bed. I'm tired and don't want to go to work today." Or at the end of an enjoyable evening, you think, "Gee, that was fun. I should get out more often." What you think or say to yourself is your "self-talk." The way you talk to yourself is influenced by how you think about yourself, others, and the future. Self-talk can be a useful self-management tool when it's based on more positive thinking. Self-talk can also be a weapon that hurts or defeats you when it's habitually negative.

Negative self-talk and worst-case thinking damage your self-esteem, attitude, and mood. These thinking habits make your pain worse by opening the pain gate and making your other symptoms worse. What you say to yourself plays a major role in determining your success or failure in becoming a good self-manager. Negative thinking limits your abilities and actions. If you tell yourself "I'm not very smart" or "I can't" most of the time, you probably won't try to learn new skills because positive change just doesn't fit with how you think about yourself. Soon you you might think you are becoming a prisoner of your own negative beliefs.

Negative self-statements usually begin with something like, "I just can't do . . . ," "If only I could . . . ," "If only I didn't . . . ," or "I just don't have the energy." This type of negative thinking represents the doubts and fears you have about yourself in general. These statements also express your doubts and fears about your ability to deal with your pain condition and its symptoms.

A special kind of negative thinking is worst-case thinking. Worst-case thinking is especially common for people who have chronic pain. Worst-case thinking is when you think that the worst is going to happen. Imagine that after a week or so of having relatively little back pain, you suddenly have an increase in your back pain, a pain flare-up. If you are engaging in worst-case thinking, you might immediately begin to think you might become paralyzed or will have to live with excruciating pain for the rest of your life.

Worst-case thinking works against you in a number of ways. First, it makes it much harder to shift your attention away from pain. Second, it often leads you to feel helpless about managing your pain. Finally, because worst-case thinking makes you more emotionally upset, it makes whatever issue you are dealing with at the moment much more challenging. Worst-case thinking can cause such other problems as trouble sleeping, unhealthy eating, or angrily lashing out at family, friends, and coworkers.

Fortunately, you can change your self-talk and negative thinking. You can learn new, healthier ways to think about yourself so your self-talk can work for you instead of against you. By challenging the negative, self-defeating statements and replacing them with more positive, realistic ones, you can get your thinking working for you. You also can learn to manage symptoms more effectively.

Changing from negative self-talk to positive self-talk, like changing any habit, requires practice and includes the following steps:

1. **Listen carefully to what you say about yourself, both out loud and silently.** If you find yourself in a difficult situation and are feeling anxious, depressed, or angry, then try this. Write down what the situation is. For example, is it that you are getting up in the morning with pain, or are you struggling to do those exercises you don't really like, or are you having bad pain flares at the end of long days? Next, write down the unhelpful thoughts you are having about this situation. Unhelpful thoughts often come in three flavors: thoughts about yourself, thoughts about others, and thoughts about the future. Finally, write down the feelings that you have when you focus on these unhelpful thoughts. For example, the unhelpful thoughts might lead you to feel really anxious, depressed, or angry. Beginning to pay attention to the links between difficult situations, unhelpful thoughts, and difficult feelings is a first step in changing negative habits of thinking.

2. **Ask yourself if your negative thoughts are accurate.** Are you being too hard on yourself? Are you jumping to conclusions about what others are thinking? Are you assuming that the worst is going to happen in the future? Are you thinking about the situation in terms of black and white? Could things be gray?

3. **Challenge your negative thoughts.** Maybe you are making an unrealistic or unfair comparison, assuming too much responsibility, taking something too personally, or expecting perfection. Are you making assumptions about what other people think about you? What do you know for a fact? When you look at the evidence in this way, you will be better able to change these negative thoughts and statements. What would you tell a friend who is having such thoughts?

4. **Think about what has happened to you in the past in similar situations.** Often, we worry and fret for hours, days, or weeks about something that rarely or never happens. Do you usually experience a lot of pain when you socialize with others, or are you just afraid this might happen? We can use our past similar experiences to challenge our current negative thinking.

5. **Work on changing each negative statement to a more positive one.** For example, you might find yourself saying negative statements such as:

   ▶ "My pain is just terrible."

   ▶ "My pain will never get better."

   ▶ "Nothing will ever be the same."

   ▶ "I can't stand it anymore."

   ▶ "I'm good for nothing."

These negative statements work against you by increasing your distress and pain. You can challenge them by replacing them with more positive statements such as the following.

■ "My pain is really bad today, but I know it's only temporary."

- "By relaxing and taking a warm bath, I can make my pain more bearable. I just have to take things one day at a time."

- "Everything changes—I need to consider new ways of doing the things I enjoy."

- "I'm going to meet a friend for lunch to take my mind off the pain."

- "Other people need and depend on me; I'm worthwhile."

Notice that these comments do not suggest that everything is rosy and the pain will disappear. Instead they express a more realistic and positive outlook that can have a real effect on your pain experience.

6. **Write down and rehearse these positive statements, mentally or with another person.** Try writing down more positive, helpful statements on an index card and carry the card with you. Each time a negative thought occurs, take the card out and repeat the positive statement. With practice, this repetition of the more helpful self-talk can help you replace those old negative statements.

7. **Practice new statements in real situations.** This practice, along with time and patience, can help the new patterns of thinking become automatic.

8. **Rehearse success.** When you are unhappy with the way you handled a particular situation, try this exercise:
   - Write down three ways it could have gone better.
   - Write down three ways it could have gone worse.

   - If you can't think of alternatives to the way you handled it, imagine what someone whom you greatly respect would have done.

   - "Think about what advice you would give to someone else facing a similar situation.

At first, you may find it hard to change negative statements into more positive ones. With practice, you will start to see the benefits and it will get easier. Remember that mistakes aren't failures; they're opportunities to learn. Mistakes give you the chance to rehearse other ways of handling things. This is great practice for the future.

Allowing Yourself to Have Unwanted Thoughts and Feelings

Sometimes we struggle so hard not to have certain thoughts and feelings that the effort works against us. The struggle can become part of the problem, and trying to rid yourself of any and all unwanted thoughts and feelings about pain can actually work against you. An alternative way to manage this issue involves allowing unwanted thoughts and feelings to enter your mind. Let them come and go without working so hard to control them.

Why is allowing yourself to experience the full range of feelings helpful in managing pain? Struggling too hard to avoid negative thoughts can lead to your thinking more about them and feeling more upset. A part of pain self-management is accepting that sometimes we will experience difficult thoughts and feelings. Learning to observe and not overreact to unwanted responses can be helpful. Here are a couple of tips for

Getting Professional Help with Negative Thoughts

Sometimes negative self-talk is so automatic and intrusive that it seems like you cannot control it even when you really try. When this happens, you might feel stuck, unmotivated, or helpless to change these thoughts.

If you are focusing too much of your time on your pain, feel overwhelmed by negative thoughts about your pain, and cannot distract yourself, seek help from a professional such as a psychologist or therapist. If you don't have a therapist yet, discuss your concerns with your health care provider. Be open about how you are feeling. You may have an underlying depression that is stopping you from moving forward, which needs to be evaluated and treated. (See page 99 in Chapter 4, *Understanding and Managing Common Symptoms and Problems*.)

Getting help to understand and change your negative thought patterns could be a breakthrough for you and your pain management. Research has found that people with chronic pain who continually expect the worst are more disabled than those who have a more positive outlook. Changing thoughts and attitudes is very important.

---

learning how to accept unwanted thoughts rather than trying to avoid them:

Remind yourself: "My thoughts are just thoughts." If you find yourself getting caught up in a thought and unable to let go of it, it can help you to remember that thoughts are just temporary and that they come and go. Thoughts are not facts. When you have an unwanted thought, try just observing it rather than trying to control it. You may notice that the thought gets stronger and weaker. As you step back and simply observe the thought, you also might notice that it will fade a bit or go away altogether for a period of time. Observe how the thought affects your body. When the thought is present you may feel more tense and sick to your stomach, and your heart may pound or race. When the thought is absent or not as strong, the tension and other body responses may become less severe or go away. If you find you are struggling to control an unwanted thought, consider allowing yourself to experience the thought and observe what happens. You may find that you become much better at stepping back from the thought and related images and memories and end up feeling much better.

Consider this example. Christina had a pain flare the last time she went out shopping with her best friend, Joanne. Ever since then, she keeps thinking, "I'm such a terrible friend; Joanne will never want to go out with me again." The more Christina has the thought, the more upset she gets and the more convinced she becomes that she should cut off her relationship with Joanne. She concludes that this is an overly negative thought and that it is working against her. She decides the best thing to do is try to stop having it. So she tries to deal with the thought by ignoring it. When it pops into her mind, she does everything she can to distract herself. This simply doesn't work very well. The thought just keeps coming back, and she is getting more and more frustrated. Christina becomes convinced that she simply doesn't have enough willpower to overcome her negative ways of thinking.

What might happen if Christina took a different approach and simply paused and observed what happens when she starts thinking, "I'm such a terrible friend; Joanne will never want to go out with me again"? One thing is that she might notice that, after a while, the thought gets a bit weaker and after a little more time it comes up stronger again. She also might notice that other thoughts occur, such as, "Joanne is a true friend and always has been there for me even when I have not been able to go out with her." In other words, Christina may begin to see the thought as just a thought, something in her mind that comes and goes, but that it is not a fact. As a result she might learn that, when the thought comes up, she can let go of it rather than working so hard to control it. Christina may find that something interesting happens when she does this. She may find that she can have the thought without getting hooked by it or caught up in it. She can think about it without thinking that the thought is a true fact. Observing such thoughts also can take the emotional "sting" out of them. For example, after repeatedly pausing and observing the thought, Christina might find that it doesn't make her feel as discouraged or upset as it once did.

Ride the waves of your feelings. Your feelings are like waves in that they come and go. Rather than trying to control your feelings or avoid them, consider riding the waves of feelings. Keeping an image of waves in mind can be helpful when dealing with negative feelings. Like ocean waves, some feelings are strong and seem like they will last forever. However, if you watch waves you sometimes notice that as they approach the shore they change and may become weaker. When you ride the waves of emotion instead of ignoring them, you become aware of your feelings and how they change from moment to moment. In contrast, if you struggle so hard to control and fight off your negative feelings, you might miss the fact that they actually change in intensity and frequency.

Start by just noticing your feeling and putting a label on it (for example, sadness, fear, anger, guilt, etc.). Then focus on an image of yourself riding on the surface of the feeling like a surfer. Surfers don't fight the wave but instead go with it. If the feeling gets intense, stay with it. Notice what happens when you do focus on the feeling without judging it. Be curious about how you respond as the feeling gets stronger and weaker. Focus on how it feels in the moment and become more aware of how it changes from moment to moment. What sensations do you notice? Do you feel a sense of heaviness/lightness or warmth/cold? How is your body reacting? What changes in breathing and muscle tension do you notice? How do the changes in feelings affect how you might want to respond? How much are you tempted to try to fight or avoid the feeling? Notice how this urge changes when you stay with the wave and continue to ride it all the way into shore.

Riding the waves of feeling is one of the best ways to learn about yourself. Much of this learning comes from stepping back from the usual tendency to avoid, block, or push away difficult feelings. By riding the waves, you can learn that you don't have to control or act on a feeling. You can simply allow yourself to have the feeling and stay on the surface of it, noticing how it changes, and ride it out.

The mindfulness practices described on page 112 also address tools to manage thoughts and feelings by observing them come and go.

Exploring Imagery and Visualization

You may think that imagination is "all in your mind." But the thoughts, words, and images that flow from your imagination can have very real effects on your body. Your body often cannot distinguish whether you are imagining something or if it is really happening. Perhaps you've had a racing heartbeat, rapid breathing, or tension in your neck muscles while watching a movie thriller. These sensations were all produced by images and sounds on a film. During a dream, your body may have responded with fear, joy, anger, or sadness—all triggered by your imagination. If you close your eyes and vividly imagine yourself by a still, quiet pool or relaxing on a warm beach, your body responds to some degree as though you were actually there.

With guided imagery and visualization, you can use your imagination to relieve your symptoms. These techniques help you focus on healing images and suggestions.

Guided Imagery

Guided imagery allows you to refocus your mind away from your pain and other symptoms by transporting you to another time and place. It has the added benefit of helping you achieve deep relaxation by picturing yourself in a peaceful environment. This self-management tool is like a guided daydream.

In guided imagery, the images are suggested to you by a script like the ones included in this book on pages 110 and 111. With guided imagery, you focus your mind on a particular image. This usually begins with your sense of sight. For example, initially you focus on something visual. Involving your other senses—smells, tastes, and sounds—makes the guided imagery even more vivid and powerful.

Some people are highly visual and easily see images with their "mind's eye." However, if your images aren't as vivid as scenes from a great movie, don't worry. It's normal for the intensity of imagery to vary. To help you develop your ability to use images, start by focusing on a beautiful picture or a musical passage that you enjoy. Focus on as much detail as possible, and strengthen the images that come up by using all your senses.

With guided imagery, you are always completely in control. You're the movie director. You can project whatever thought or feeling you want onto your mental screen. If you don't like a particular image, thought, or feeling, redirect your mind to something more comfortable. You can use other images to get rid of unpleasant thoughts; for example, you might put unpleasant thoughts on a raft and watch them float away. Or sweep those thoughts away with a large broom or erase them with a giant eraser. You can even just open your eyes and stop the exercise.

The guided imagery scripts presented on pages 110 and 111 can help you take a "mental stroll." Here are some ways to use these scripts:

■ Read a script several times until it is familiar. Pause for about 10 seconds wherever there is a series of periods (. . .). Then sit or lie down in a quiet place and try to reconstruct the scene in your mind. Imagining the script should take 15 to 20 minutes to complete.

- Have a family member or friend slowly read the script to you. Remind them to pause for 10 seconds wherever there is a series of periods (. . .).

- Make a recording of the script and play it to yourself whenever convenient.

- Use a prerecorded tape, CD, or digital audio file that has a similar guided imagery script To find a script, see the link to our online resources at the end of this chapter.

Visualization

Visualization allows you to create your own images. Visualization is different from guided imagery, where the images are suggested to you. Visualization gives you a chance to use your imagination and create a picture of yourself doing the things you want to do.

All of us use a form of visualization every day—when we dream, worry, read a book, or listen to a story. In all these activities, the mind creates images for us to see. We also use visualization intentionally when making plans for the day, considering the possible outcomes of a decision we have to make, or rehearsing for an event or activity.

One way to use visualization to manage symptoms is to remember pleasant scenes from your past. Try to remember every detail of a special holiday or party that made you happy. Who was there? What happened? What did you do or talk about? Or you can remember a vacation or some other memorable and pleasant event.

Visualization also can be used to plan the details of some future event or to fill in the details of a fantasy. For example, how would you spend a million dollars? What would be your ideal romantic encounter? What would your ideal home or garden look like? Where would you go and what would you do on your dream vacation?

Another form of visualization involves thinking of symbols that represent the discomfort or pain you feel. For example, a painful joint might be red, or a tight chest might have a constricting band around it. After forming these images, you then change them in your mind. The red color might fade until there is no more color, or the constricting band stretches and stretches until it falls off. These new images can shift the way you think of the pain or discomfort.

Visualization is a useful tool to help you set and accomplish personal goals. After you write your weekly action plan, take a few minutes to imagine yourself doing the things you include on your action plan. Visualize yourself taking a walk, doing your exercises, or making a healthy meal. Visualization is a way to rehearse the steps you need to take in order to achieve your goals successfully. It helps you build confidence and skill.

Using Imagery for Self-Management of Specific Conditions

You have the ability to create special imagery to help ease (though not cure) your specific symptoms or illnesses. Use any image that is strong and vivid and meaningful to you. It works best if you use all your senses to create the image. The image does not have to be accurate for it to work. Just use your imagination and trust yourself.

These are examples of images that some people have found useful to help them deal with various situations:

For Tension and Stress

A tight, twisted rope slowly untwists.

Hard wax softens and melts.

Tension swirls out of your body and down the drain.

For Pain

You grasp the TV remote control and slowly turn down the pain volume until you can barely hear it; then it disappears entirely.

A cool, calm river flowing through your entire body washes away the pain.

A radiant white light finds the areas of pain and tension in your body and dissolves the pain and tension. As the light leaves your body, you feel warm and relaxed in its glow.

All of your pain is placed in a large, strong metal box that is closed, sealed tightly, and locked with a huge padlock. The box is placed on the deck of a ship that is heading out to sea.

For Depression

Your troubles and feelings of sadness are attached to big, colorful helium balloons and float off into a clear blue sky.

A strong, warm sun breaks through dark clouds.

You feel a sense of detachment and lightness, enabling you to float easily through your day.

For Cuts and Injuries

Plaster covers over a crack in a wall.

Cells and fibers stick together with very strong glue.

A shoe is laced up tight.

Jigsaw puzzle pieces come together.

For Arteries and Heart Disease

A miniature Roto-Rooter truck speeds through your arteries and cleans out the clogged pipes.

Water flows freely through a wide, open river.

A crew in a small boat rows in sync, easily and efficiently pulling the slender boat across the smooth surface of the water.

For a Weakened Immune System

Sluggish, sleepy white blood cells awaken, put on protective armor, and enter the fight against the virus.

White blood cells rapidly multiply like millions of seeds bursting from a single ripe seedpod.

For an Overactive Immune System (arthritis, psoriasis, etc.)

Overly alert immune cells in the fire station are reassured that the allergens have triggered a false alarm, and they go back to playing a game of poker.

The civil war ends with the warring sides agreeing not to attack their fellow citizens.

Use any of these images, or make up your own. Remember, the best ones are vivid and have meaning to you. Use the power of your personal imagination for health and healing.

Contemplating Prayer and Spirituality

There is strong evidence in the medical literature of the relationship between spirituality and health. According to the American Academy

Guided-Imagery Script: A Walk in the Country

You're giving yourself some time to quiet your mind and body. Allow yourself to settle comfortably, wherever you are right now. If you wish, you can close your eyes. Breathe in deeply, through your nose, expanding your abdomen and filling your lungs, and, pursing your lips, exhale through your mouth slowly and completely, allowing your body to sink heavily into the surface beneath you . . .

And once again breathe in through your nose and all the way down to your abdomen, and then breathe out slowly through pursed lips—letting go of tension, letting go of anything that's on your mind right now and just allowing yourself to be present in this moment . . .

Imagine yourself walking along a peaceful old country road. The sun is gently warming your back . . . the birds are singing . . . the air is calm and fragrant . . .

With no need to hurry, you notice your walking is relaxed and easy. As you walk along in this way, taking in your surroundings, you come across an old gate. It looks inviting and you decide to take the path through the gate. The gate creaks as you open it and go through.

You find yourself in an old, overgrown garden—flowers growing where they've seeded themselves, vines climbing over a fallen tree, soft green wild grasses, shade trees.

You notice yourself breathing deeply . . . smelling the flowers . . . listening to the birds and insects . . . feeling a gentle breeze cool against your skin. All of your senses are alive and responding with pleasure to this peaceful time and place . . .

When you're ready to move on, you leisurely follow the path out behind the garden, eventually coming to a more wooded area. As you enter this area, your eyes find the trees and plant life restful. The sunlight is filtered through the leaves. The air feels mild and a little cooler . . . You savor the fragrance of trees and earth . . . and gradually become aware of the sound of a nearby stream. Pausing, you allow yourself to take in the sights and sounds, breathing in the cool and fragrant air several times . . . And with each breath, you notice how refreshed you are feeling . . .

Continuing along the path for a while, you come to the stream. It's clear and clean as it flows and tumbles over the rocks and some fallen logs. You follow the path easily along the creek for a way, and after a while, you come out into a sunlit clearing, where you discover a small waterfall emptying into a quiet pool of water.

You find a comfortable place to sit for a while, a perfect niche where you can feel completely relaxed.

You feel good as you allow yourself to just enjoy the warmth and solitude of this peaceful place . . .

After a while, you become aware that it is time to return. You arise and walk back down the path in a relaxed and comfortable way, through the cool and fragrant trees, out into the sun-drenched overgrown garden . . . One last smell of the flowers, and out the creaky gate.

You leave this country retreat for now and return down the road. You notice you feel calm and rested. You feel grateful and remind yourself that you can visit this special place whenever you wish to take some time to refresh yourself and renew your energy.

And now, preparing to bring this period of relaxation to a close, you may want to take a moment to picture yourself carrying this experience of calm and refreshment with you into the ordinary activities of your life . . . And when you're ready, take a nice deep breath and open your eyes.

Guided-Imagery Script: A Walk on the Beach

Begin by getting into a comfortable position, whether you are seated or lying down. Loosen any tight clothing to allow yourself to be as comfortable as possible. Uncross your legs and allow your hands to fall by your sides or rest in your lap, and if you are at all uncomfortable, shift to a more comfortable position.

When you are ready, you may allow your eyes gradually to close and turn your attention to your breathing. Allow your belly to expand as you breathe in, bringing in fresh new air to nourish your body. And then breathing out. Notice the rhythm of your breathing—in . . . and out . . . without trying to control it in any way at all. Simply attend to the natural rhythm of your breath . . .

And now in your mind's eye, imagine yourself standing on a beautiful beach. The sky is a brilliant blue, and as some fluffy white clouds float slowly by, you drink in the beautiful colors . . . The temperature is not too hot and not too cold. The sun is shining, and you close your eyes, allowing the warmth of the sun to wash over you . . . You notice a gentle breeze caressing your face, the perfect complement to the sunshine.

Then you find yourself turning and looking out over the vastness of the ocean . . . You become aware of the sound of the waves gently washing up on shore . . . You notice the firmness of the wet sand beneath your feet, or if you decide to take off your shoes, you may enjoy the feeling of standing in the cool, wet sand . . . perhaps you allow the surf to roll up and gently wash across your feet, or perhaps you stay just out of its reach . . .

In the distance you hear some seagulls calling to one another and look out to see the birds gracefully gliding through the air. And as you stand there, notice how easy it is to be here, perhaps noticing some sensations of relaxation, comfort, or peace—whatever's there . . .

Now take a walk along the shore. Turn and begin to stroll casually along the beach, enjoying the sounds of the surf, the warmth of the sun, and the gentle massage of the breeze. As you move along, taking your time, your stride becomes lighter, easier . . . you notice the scent of the ocean . . . you pause to take in the freshness of the air . . . And then you continue on your way, enjoying the peacefulness of this place.

After a time, you decide to rest a while, and find a comfortable place to sit or lie down . . . and simply allow yourself to take some time to enjoy this, your special place . . .

And now, when you feel ready to return, you stand and begin walking back down the beach in a comfortable, leisurely way, taking with you any sensations of relaxation, comfort, peace, joy—whatever's there . . . Noticing how easy it is to be here. Continuing back until you reach the place where you began your walk . . .

And now pausing to take one last long look around. Enjoying the vibrant colors of the sky and the sea . . . The gentle sound of the waves washing up on the shore. The warmth of the sun, the cool of the breeze . . .

And as you prepare to leave this special place, taking with you any sensations of joy, relaxation, comfort, peace, whatever's there. Knowing that you may return at any appropriate time and place of your choosing.

And now bringing your awareness back into the room, focusing on your breathing . . . in and out . . . Taking a few more breaths . . . and when you're ready, opening your eyes.

of Family Physicians,* spirituality is a way to find meaning, hope, comfort, and inner peace in our lives. Many people find spirituality through religion. Some find it through music, art, or a connection with nature. Others find it in their values and principles.

Many people are religious and like to share their religion with others. Others do not practice a specific religion but do have spiritual beliefs. Our religion and beliefs can bring a sense of meaning and purpose to our lives. They can help us put things into perspective, set priorities, and find comfort during difficult times. Strong belief systems can help us with acceptance and motivate us to make difficult changes. Being part of a spiritual or religious community offers a source of support and the opportunity to help others.

Recent studies find that people who belong to a religious or spiritual community or who regularly engage in religious activities such as prayer or study have improved health. There are many types of prayer, any of which may contribute to improved health. Asking for help, direction, or forgiveness is one form of prayer. Offering words of gratitude, praise, and blessing is another. In addition, many religions have a tradition of contemplation or meditation. Prayer and meditation are probably the oldest self-management tools. Explore your own beliefs about what makes life meaningful and gives you hope. If you are religious, try engaging in prayer consistently. If you are not religious, consider adopting some form of reflection or meditative practice.

Also, if you are religious, consider telling your doctor or health care team. Although they won't ask, it is helpful for them to understand the importance of your beliefs in managing your health and life. Most hospitals have chaplains or pastoral counselors. Even if you are not in the hospital, these spiritual leaders will probably make time to talk with you. Choose someone you feel comfortable with. The advice and counsel of spiritual leaders can supplement your medical and psychological care.

---

*Adapted from the American Academy of Family Physicians: www.aafp.org/afp/2001/0101/p89.html and www.aafp.org/afp/2006/0415/p1336.html

Additional Ways You Can Use Your Mind to Manage Symptoms

These additional valuable techniques can help you to clear your mind, calm your nervous system, shift your emotional state, and reduce your tension and stress.

Practicing Mindfulness

Mindfulness involves keeping your attention in the present moment, without judging it as happy or sad, good or bad. When you are mindful, you try to live each moment—even painful ones—as fully and as mindfully as possible. Mindfulness is more than a relaxation technique; it is an attitude toward living. It is a way of calmly and consciously observing and accepting whatever is happening, moment to moment.

This may sound simple enough, but our restless, judging minds make it surprisingly difficult. Just like a restless monkey jumps from branch to branch, our mind jumps from thought to thought.

To practice mindfulness, focus on the present moment. The "goal" of mindfulness is simply to observe—with no intention of changing or improving anything. Even though the practice is not about "improving" your thoughts, people are positively changed by the practice. According to new scientific studies, the practice of mindfulness is linked to positive changes in areas of the brain associated with memory, learning, and emotion. Considerable research has demonstrated the benefits of mindfulness practice in relieving stress, easing pain, improving concentration, and relieving a variety of other symptoms. Observing and accepting life just as it is, with all its pleasures, pains, frustrations, disappointments, and insecurities, enables you to become calmer, more confident, and better able to manage whatever comes along.

To develop your capacity for mindfulness, follow these guidelines:

■ Sit comfortably on the floor or on a chair with your back, neck, and head straight but not stiff.

■ Concentrate on a single object, such as your breath. Focus your attention on the feeling of the air as it passes in and out of your nostrils. Don't try to control your breathing by speeding it up or slowing it down. Just observe it as it is.

■ Even when you resolve to keep your attention on your breathing, your mind will quickly wander off. When this occurs, observe where your mind went (for example, to a memory, a worry about the future, a bodily ache, or a feeling of impatience). Then gently return your attention to your breathing.

■ Use your breath as an anchor. Each time a thought or feeling arises, momentarily acknowledge it. Don't analyze it or judge it. Just observe it and return to your breathing.

■ Let go of all thoughts of getting somewhere or having anything special happen. Just keep stringing moments of mindfulness together, breath by breath.

■ At first, do this practice for just 5 minutes, or even 1 minute at a time. Eventually, you may wish to gradually extend the time to 10, 20, or 30 minutes.

Because the practice of mindfulness is simply the practice of moment-to-moment awareness, you can apply it to anything: eating, showering, working, talking, running errands, or playing with your children or grandchildren. Mindfulness takes no extra time.

Activating Your Quieting Reflex

The quieting reflex technique was developed by a physician named Charles Stroebel. It will help you deal with short-term stress such as the urge to eat or smoke, succumb to road rage, or react to other annoyances. By activating what's called the sympathetic nervous system, this technique relieves muscle tightening and jaw clenching and stops you from holding your breath. It should be practiced frequently throughout the day, whenever you start to feel stressed. It can be done with your eyes opened or closed.

To engage in the quieting reflex exercise, follow the steps outlined below:

1. Become aware of what is annoying you: a ringing phone, an angry comment, the urge to smoke, a worrisome thought—whatever.

2. Repeat the phrase "alert mind, calm body" to yourself.

3. Smile inwardly with your eyes and your mouth. This stops facial muscles from making a fearful or angry expression. The inward smile is a feeling. It cannot be seen by others.

4. Inhale slowly to the count of three, imagining that the breath comes in through the bottom of your feet. Then exhale slowly. Feel your breath move back down your legs and out through your feet. Let your jaw, tongue, and shoulder muscles go limp.

With several months' practice, the quieting reflex becomes an automatic skill.

Enjoying Nature Therapy

Many people suffer from what has been called "nature deficit disorder." Thankfully, this disorder can be cured with regular doses of the outdoors. For thousands of years, exposure to natural environments has been recommended for healing. Taking a break from artificial lighting, excessive computer and TV screen time, and indoor environments can be restorative. A brief walk in a park or a longer visit to a beautiful outdoor environment can restore the mind and body. When the weather is poor, visit a garden nursery to inhale the fragrance of the flowers and see the color and beauty. Or bring nature indoors with plants, pets, and nature photography. Even a few minutes of playing with or stroking a pet can lower blood pressure and calm a restless mind.

Expressing Gratitude

One of the most effective ways to improve your mood and overall happiness is by focusing your attention on what's going well in your life. For what are you grateful? Research demonstrates that people can increase their happiness by practicing gratitude exercises. We encourage you to try these three:

■ **Write a letter of thanks.** Write and then deliver a letter of gratitude to someone who has been especially kind to you but that you have never properly thanked. Perhaps it's a teacher, a mentor, a friend, or a family member. In the letter, express your appreciation for the person's kindness. Include some specific examples of what the recipient has done for you. Describe how the actions made you feel. Ideally, read your letter to the person, face-to-face if possible. Be aware of how you feel, and watch the other person's reaction.

■ **Acknowledge at least three good things every day.** Each night before bed, write down at least three things that went well today. No event or feeling is too small to note. By putting your gratitude into words, you can better appreciate and remember your blessings. Knowing that you will need to write each night changes your mental filters during the whole day. You will tend to seek out, look for, and specially note the good things that happen. If doing this daily is too much or begins to seem like a routine chore, do it once a week.

■ **Make a list of the good things in your life that you take for granted.** For example, if your chronic pain has affected your knees, you can still be grateful that your elbows and hands are unaffected. Celebrate a day that you don't have a headache or back-ache. Counting your blessings can add up to a better mood and more happiness.

Listing Your Strengths

Write a list of your talents, skills, achievements, and positive qualities, big and small. Celebrate your accomplishments. When something goes wrong, consult this list of positives to put your problem in perspective. It then becomes just one specific experience, not something that defines your whole life.

Putting Kindness into Practice

This world is plagued by violence and suffering. When something bad happens, it's front-page news. As an antidote to this misery, despair, and cynicism, practice acts of kindness. Look for opportunities to give without expecting anything in return. Here are some examples of kind actions:

■ Hold the door open for the person behind you.

■ Give an unexpected gift of movie or concert tickets.

■ Send an anonymous gift to a friend who needs cheering up.

■ Help someone with a heavy load.

■ Relate positive stories about helping and kindness.

■ Cultivate an attitude of gratefulness for kindness you receive.

■ Plant a tree.

■ Smile and let people cut ahead of you in line or on the freeway.

■ Pick up litter.

■ Give another driver your parking space.

Be creative. Acts of kindness are contagious and have a ripple effect. In one study, people who were given an unexpected treat (cookies) were later more likely to help others.

Writing Away Stress

It's hard work to keep deep negative feelings hidden. Over time, this cumulative stress undermines your body's defenses and may even weaken your immunity. Confiding feelings to others or writing them down puts them into words and helps to sort them out. Words help people understand and absorb a traumatic event and eventually put it to rest. Sharing feelings gives a sense of release and control.

In his book *Opening Up*, the psychologist James Pennebaker described a series of studies about the healing effects of confiding or writing. One group was asked to express their deepest thoughts and feelings about something bad that had happened to them. Another group wrote about less personal and emotional topics such as their plans for the day. Both groups wrote for 15 to 20 minutes a day for three to five days in a row. No one read what either group had written.

The results were surprisingly powerful. When compared with the people who wrote about ordinary events, the ones who wrote about their bad experiences reported fewer symptoms, fewer visits to the doctor, fewer days off from work, improved mood, and a more positive outlook. Their immune function was enhanced for at least six weeks after the writing exercise. This was especially true for those who expressed previously undisclosed painful feelings.

Try doing the "write thing" when a problem or a memory is bothering you. It could be when you find yourself thinking (or dreaming) too much about an experience or when you avoid thinking about something because it is too upsetting. It may be when there's something you would like to tell others but don't for fear of embarrassment or punishment.

The following guidelines can help you use writing as a way to deal with negative experiences:

- Set a specific schedule for writing. For example, you might write 15 minutes a day for four consecutive days, or one day a week for four weeks.

- Write in a place where you won't be interrupted or distracted.

- Don't plan to share your writing—that could stop your honest expression. Save what you write or destroy it, whichever you prefer.

- Explore your very deepest thoughts and feelings and analyze why you feel the way you do. Write about your negative feelings such as sadness, hurt, hate, anger, fear, guilt, or resentment.

- Write continuously. Don't worry about grammar, spelling, or making sense. If clarity and coherence come as you continue to write, so much the better. If you run out of things to say, just repeat what you have already written in different words.

- Even if you find the writing awkward at first, keep going. It gets easier. If you just cannot write, try talking into a tape recorder for 15 minutes about your deepest thoughts and feelings.

- Don't expect to feel better immediately. You may feel sad or depressed when your deepest feelings begin to surface. This usually fades within an hour or two or a day or two. The overwhelming majority of people report feelings of relief, happiness, and contentment soon after writing for a few consecutive days.

- Writing may help you clarify what actions you need to take. But don't use writing as a substitute for taking action or as a way to avoid things.

Mental Strength and Resilience

Having chronic pain means facing many life difficulties and daily hassles. Chronic pain can strain your relationships with others, make it difficult or impossible to work, lead to financial problems, and contribute to other health problems (such as weight gain, sleep problems, etc.). Becoming an effective self-manager does not mean that you will never experience these

Building Mental Strength

Here are some of the tips for building mental strength you can learn more about in this book:

1. **Use relaxation techniques.** Practice muscle relaxation or engage in activities that you find relax you naturally. For example, take a warm bath or listen to your favorite music. (See page 97.)

2. **Refocus your attention.** Direct your attention away from pain to something pleasant that you can get absorbed in (like watching a beautiful sunset) or takes a lot of mental energy (like counting backwards or memorizing the words to a new song). (See page 100.)

3. **Engage in positive and realistic thinking and self-talk.** Pay attention to what you say to yourself. Revise overly negative statements about yourself, others, and the future to more realistic and positive statements. (See page 102.)

4. **Practice using guided imagery.** Review the guided imagery scripts on pages 110 and 111. Or focus on a special image that is meaningful to you (for example, your favorite vacation spot) and try to remember every detail. (See page 108.)

5. **Consider prayer or explore your spirituality.** Draw on spiritual tools that are meaningful to you. These might include readings, meditation or contemplation exercises, or music that enhances your spirituality. (See page 109.)

6. **Practice mindfulness.** Focus on the present moment, for example by paying attention to your breathing. Simply observe what happens without judging anything that comes up. (See page 112.)

7. **Engage your quieting reflex.** To strengthen your ability to relax in challenging situations, practice the quieting reflex exercise frequently. (See page 113.)

8. **Enjoy pets, plants, and nature.** Get out of the house and put yourself in outdoor settings where you can focus on the sights, sounds, smells, and other physical sensations of natural environments. (See page 114.)

9. **Schedule worry time.** Set aside a specific time to focus on your worries. During that time, don't do anything other than think about your worries and develop action plans for addressing them. If a worry comes up at another time of the day, jot it down and forget about it as best you can. Then revisit it during your worry time. (See page 73.)

10. **Practice gratitude.** Focus your attention on what is going well for you by making a list of good things that happened to you each day or writing a letter of thanks to another person. (See page 114.)

11. **Write about your stress.** Keep a journal and write about the things that are stressing you. Be sure to write about the feelings and thoughts that you are having, particularly those that you have not shared with others. (See page 115.)

problems. What self-management does is enable you to increase your mental strength to deal better with these challenges.

Mental strength, also called mental resilience, is the ability to deal with and recover from tough events. As you become stronger and more resilient, you will still react to both minor hassles and major life events. However, as you become more resilient, the level of distress you feel will be lower and will not last as long. Basically, you will be able to bounce back from these life difficulties.

How do people build physical strength? Chapter 7, *Exercising and Physical Activity for Every Body*, and Chapter 8, *Exercising to Feel Better*, are full of exercise tips for building physical endurance, flexibility, and strength. These tips may involve doing exercises and activities that you might have avoided doing in the past because of pain or other reasons. If you follow these tips, you are likely to find that the exercises are difficult at first but get easier as your strength and physical endurance increase.

You can build mental strength and resilience in much the same way. Don't avoid activities or situations that are emotionally difficult because they might cause fear, anxiety, or other strong negative emotions. Instead, make a commitment to work on putting yourself in these situations. Start with situations that are easier for you and, as your mental resilience gets stronger, gradually work on the more challenging situations.

This chapter (and other chapters in this book) provide many exercise tips for building mental strength. These tips have several things in common. All of them ask you to take actions to build mental strength rather than avoid situations, thoughts, and feelings that might be difficult. All of them also provide opportunities for learning and growth. Each exercise is like a behavioral experiment in which you can learn about self-management strategies. You might find something about a strategy that worked well for you, as well as something about the strategy that you need to change the next time you do the experiment.

Relaxation, imagery, and positive, more realistic thinking can be some of the most powerful tools you can add to your self-management toolbox. They can help you manage pain and other symptoms as well as master the other skills discussed in this book. As with exercise and other acquired skills, using your mind to manage your health condition requires both practice and time before you begin to notice the benefits. If you feel you are not accomplishing anything, don't give up. Be patient and keep on trying. However, if your symptoms get worse, see your health care provider as soon as you can. Let your caregiver know about the techniques you are trying. Give a full picture of what you do to manage your pain condition and your health. This will help ensure safe, coordinated care.

For a complete list of suggested further readings, useful websites, and other helpful resources, please see

www.bullpub.com/resources.

"How we spend our days is, of course, how we spend our lives."
— Annie Dillard, *The Writing Life*

CHAPTER 6

Organizing and Pacing Your Life for Pain Self-Management and Safety

Andrea retired from her job early. She was looking forward to spending more time with her young grandchildren and joining the YMCA's social club. A few months after retirement she developed chronic knee and back pain. She tried to attend social events but came home in severe pain. If she played with her grandchildren one day, she ended up spending the next day in bed. Andrea became depressed and often stayed in bed all day. She became weak and tired. Friends and family tried to help, but she turned them away or discouraged them. She showered only once a week. It seemed that no matter what she did, the pain got worse.

A friend suggested to Andrea that she limit her activity to just 10 minutes at a time. She was surprised that this seemed to work, but 10 minutes was not enough. She wanted her life back. She talked with her health care provider, who suggested she keep a record of what she could do, how long she could do it, and what seemed to set off pain. (See Figure 4.1, page 56). She learned that every day was not the same and that

119

she needed to pay attention to how her pain changed activity by activity, day by day. She also learned that small things sometimes set off her pain.

With the help of a worksheet like the one in Figure 4.2 (page 57), Andrea noticed that exercises like those in the Moving Easy Program increased her pain-free time while she straightened up her kitchen. A guided imagery technique recommended by another friend calmed her and enabled her to do more (see pages 110 and 111). She worked with her health care team to find medications that were more effective. She saw an occupational therapist, who had many helpful ideas.

Now, Andrea rests the day before and the day after her grandchildren visit, and they are able to play and enjoy games together. Recently she enjoyed a short outing with her local YMCA social group. Even though Andrea still struggles at times, she is relieved that she has gotten her life back.

This chapter is about organizing your living space and pacing your activities. The self-management tools in this chapter may be useful to you and help you reduce your pain. After you figure out what is causing pain that you can avoid, you can take steps to use good body mechanics, organize your space, modify your activities, and pace yourself. All of these are self-management tools that can help you live a safer and more independent life. Throughout this chapter, we share several tools to help you prevent injury, pace your activity, and increase your safety. Pick and choose the tools that you think will work best for you. The aim is for you to be able to do the things you need and want to do.

Monitoring and Understanding Your Pain

To gain a better understanding of your pain, use a pain diary or a behavioral worksheet. (See Figures 4.1 and 4.2, pages 56 and 57, in Chapter 4, *Understanding and Managing Common Symptoms and Problems*.) If you fill out a series of worksheets like these over time, you will see patterns that you did not know about. These patterns can offer insight into changes you can make to your activities that might help you feel better over time. You can also use your worksheet to test new approaches in real time by noticing what works and what causes early signs of pain.

After filling out and reading her behavioral worksheets, Andrea (who we introduced in the story that opens this chapter) noticed that her fatigue and pain were beginning much earlier than she thought, and she learned to identify early signs of pain flares. Her observations led her to add planned rest breaks and activity breaks to her days. This allowed her to spend less time in bed and more time doing what she wanted to do.

One thing to be aware of when monitoring your pain with a worksheet: Some people overfocus on their pain when keeping a record of it, and researchers have found this overfocusing makes things worse. Try to stay neutral in your observations. Be open to learning from your record and finding new approaches to managing your pain without becoming negatively fixated on the record of your pain.

Using Good Body Mechanics

Body mechanics is the way people move during daily activities. Good movement starts with good posture. Proper body mechanics and proper posture during daily activities contribute to effective pain management. Consider what some people who live with chronic pain have to say about body mechanics:

- "I suffered with severe headaches for years and consulted many specialists and tried many medications, but none worked well for me. I bought special prescription glasses for using the computer, which helped some but not enough. Then one day I changed my desk setup. I added a screen, keyboard, and mouse to my laptop. I got a new chair with armrests and a footrest so my feet touched the ground. I use this setup daily. Most of my headaches are gone."

- "I started limping. I moved less, I was not sleeping well, and my back started hurting. Eventually I went to a physical therapist. She showed me how to walk slower with good body alignment and encouraged me to use a cane. Wow, did that all help! I have strengthened both my knees, and I can keep doing the things I love."

- "I pay attention to my posture and the way I move when I am cooking, washing dishes, and doing laundry. I used to strain my back by twisting and bending, and now I complete these tasks without an increase in pain."

Practicing Good Standing and Sitting Posture

Your spine has three natural curves: the neck, the upper back, and the lower back. These natural curves reduce strain. They protect your back by helping your body absorb the "shock of movement," and they offer support when you hold positions (i.e., while sitting, standing, etc.). Good posture maintains these curves. You have good posture when all your body parts are in alignment. This prevents strain on muscles, ligaments, tendons, and joints.

Figures 6.1 and 6.2 on page 122 illustrate good sitting and standing posture. To practice good posture, pull in and lift your stomach muscles to support your trunk when standing, sitting, or changing positions. Lifting your stomach muscles helps you align your body and takes strain off your back. Try it and you will notice a difference.

Use the following checklist to achieve good posture, as shown in Figure 6.1. If ideal posture increases your pain, consult a physical therapist or occupational therapist.

- ears over shoulders
- shoulders over hips (shoulders even and relaxed)

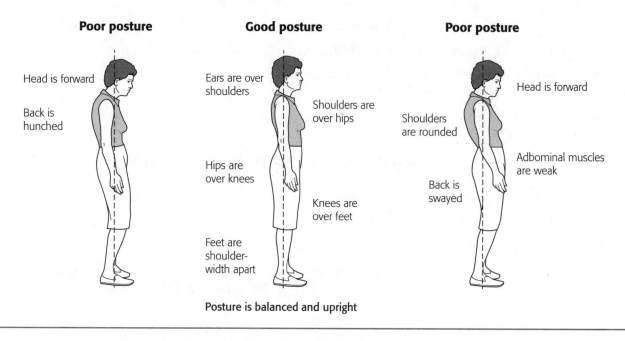

Poor posture   **Good posture**   **Poor posture**

Head is forward

Back is hunched

Ears are over shoulders

Shoulders are over hips

Hips are over knees

Knees are over feet

Feet are shoulder-width apart

Posture is balanced and upright

Head is forward

Shoulders are rounded

Adbominal muscles are weak

Back is swayed

Figure 6.1 **Standing Posture**

- stomach muscles gently tightened and lifted

- hips over knees

- knees over feet (knees straight but not locked)

- feet shoulder-width apart (even weight on both feet)

For exercises to improve posture, see pages 159–163.

Good sitting posture, which is shown in Figure 6.2, looks like this:

- ears over shoulders

- shoulders relaxed and not elevated

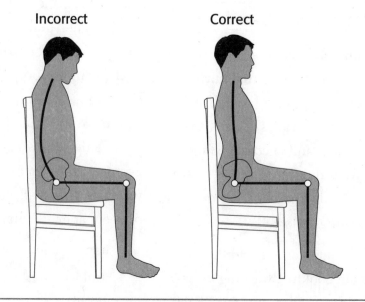

Incorrect   Correct

Figure 6.2 **Sitting Posture**

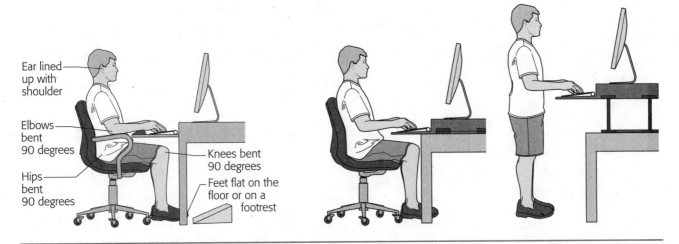

Figure 6.3 **Proper Sitting and Standing Posture for Computer Use**

- upper back relaxed and over hips
- stomach muscles gently tightened and lifted
- hips bent 90 degrees
- knees bent 90 degrees
- buttocks flat on seat with even weight on both hips
- feet flat on floor or footrest

Tips for Good Posture and Computer Use

Posture is also important when using computers and electronic devices (for example phone, laptop, tablet). Figure 6.3 demonstrates proper posture at the computer when using a regular desk and a standing desk.

Use good posture when using a laptop. Long periods of laptop use in improper positions can cause pain. If you prefer a laptop at home or in the office, consider getting a separate keyboard and a separate monitor. This allows you to set up your laptop as shown in Figure 6.3.

Standing desks (also known as sit-to-stand desks; see Figure 6.3) allow people to be more active and sit less. There is limited research on their use for pain management. If you purchase one, make sure you can keep good posture when you are using it, whether you are sitting or standing. Position your keyboard so that when typing, your elbows are bent at 90 degrees. There should be a wrist rest so that you can take the strain off your shoulders. The top of the monitor should be at or slightly below eye level. If you wear bifocals, consider lowering the monitor 1 to 2 inches for more comfortable viewing.

Tightness in your forearm muscles, tension in shoulders, or pain in hands is often the result of long hours working on a computer. Here are some additional tips to combat problems with computer use:

- An adjustable screen is a big help in maintaining good posture.
- Computer features such as screen magnifiers and text-to-speech software can conserve your energy and reduce eye and hand strain.

Body Mechanics for Daily Activities

Using good posture for daily activities such as getting dressed, taking a shower, or simply changing position protects your back and limbs. Here are some tips to reduce pain and enhance safety:

- Bend your knees and bend at the hips if you need to lean forward to pick something up. Do not bend at the waist, as it strains your spine.

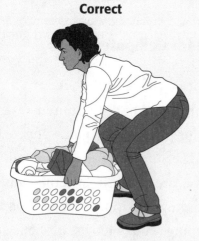

Correct

Protect your back by bending your knees and bending at your hips.

Incorrect

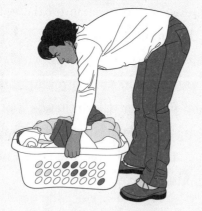

Do not bend at the waist.

- Use assistive devices (see pages 128–130) or change your position to avoid awkward body posture. For example, consider putting your feet on a low stool to put on socks, or use a sock aid. Use a long-handled sponge to reduce bending and twisting to wash your back or feet in the shower.

- Reduce twisting, especially while bending forward. One helpful trick is to imagine you are wearing a belt buckle. Make sure to keep your imaginary belt buckle and your feet pointing in the same direction.

- Take time to feel steady before you move. To avoid getting dizzy when moving from a seated or lying position, stand up slowly and remain in one place a moment before you start to move. This is very important when you are getting out of bed.

- Take three deep breaths or use breathing exercises to stay calm during challenging movements, and use the exhale part of the process to reduce muscle tightening.

Gently tighten and lift your stomach muscles to support your spine while sitting or standing, and when changing positions.

- Warm-up and pain-relief exercises can increase your productivity and reduce pain. Warm-up exercises such as taking a short walk or doing the Moving Easy Program introduced in Chapter 8, *Exercising to Feel Better* (page 173), can warm the muscles and increase circulation. Stretch breaks help lengthen and relax tight muscles and prevent pain flares. The neck, shoulders, wrists, and back are areas that become tight when working at a computer. Curve and Arch, Wrist Stretch Up and Down, Raise It Up and Ear to Shoulder are some Moving Easy Program stretches that address these areas (see pages 161, 170, and 175). If you have tightness in another area such as the ankle, consider Ankle Rotation (see page 184).

Changing Positions Safely

Posture and body mechanics are important when you change positions. This is when you are likely to twist, rush, or get into awkward positions. All of these are likely to increase pain.

This section illustrates step-by-step instructions for a few common daily activities that require changes in position. Carefully review the instructions and the figures and try to follow the steps. Ask a friend or family member to watch you the first time you practice to make sure you are doing things correctly. The key thing is to feel safe and steady. If these instructions do not work for you, consult an occupational or physical therapist. If you have been given different instructions by a health care provider, follow the recommendations your caregiver has given you.

Moving from Sitting in an Armchair to Standing

1. Take two deep breaths to relax your muscles, and make sure not to hold your breath

2. Slide your hips forward to sit near the front half of the chair.

3. Make sure your feet are flat on the floor, making a 90-degree angle with your knees.

4. Lean forward until your nose is over your toes.

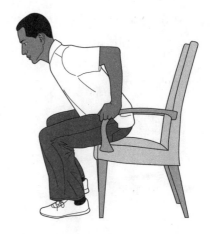

5. Tighten your stomach muscles and gently push from the arms of the chair and your hips to come to a standing position.

For additional tips, see the Sit-to-Stand exercise in Chapter 8, *Exercising to Feel Better* (page 165).

Getting into Bed

1. Sit on the bed about a foot from the pillow.

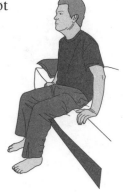

2. Scoot back so that you are not on the edge of the bed. The back of your knees should be touching the mattress.

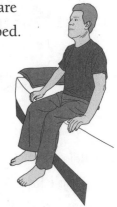

3. Lower your body slowly onto your arm that is closest to the pillow.

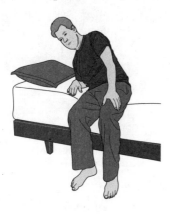

4. Bend your knees and pull your body onto the bed. You may need assistance from a friend, caregiver, or family member. You can also use a leg lifter (see Figure 6.6) on page 130, which is a very simple tool that can mean the difference between getting in bed by yourself or needing help.

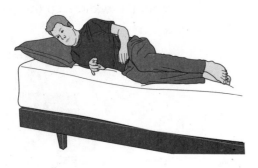

5. Roll onto your back.

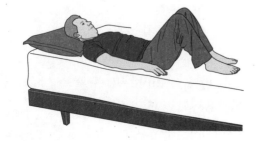

6. Relax your legs and get comfortable. Some people have less pain if their joints are supported. Ask a physical therapist or occupational therapist for specific recommendations for pillows, wedges, or other supports.

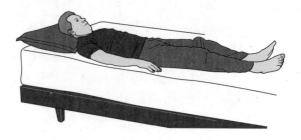

Using a Cane

Many people refuse to use a cane, only use one occasionally, or do not use one properly. They may think that a cane makes them look old or disabled. They do not want to appear weak. Some even believe that using a cane weakens muscles or should only be used if one side is weaker than the other. Most of these assumptions are incorrect. Have you noticed that serious hikers often use walking sticks for added safety, balance, and stability? Like walking sticks, a cane can increase balance and stability and prevent falls. A cane can help you go farther and do more things with less pain. Although making the decision to use a cane regularly can be a difficult step, it may help to think of it as not giving up independence or giving in to pain but instead gaining a tool to increase independence, reduce pain, and prevent injury.

A single-point cane (Figure 6.4) increases safety and balance. It provides added stability while walking and allows walking on uneven ground or going up and down curbs with greater ease. When pain or weakness is greater on one side, a cane allows walking with less pain. Many people find that using a cane increases their confidence, makes them feel steadier, and decreases their pain. Canes come in many colors and designs

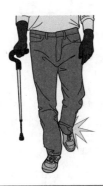

Figure 6.4 **A Single-Point Cane**

and can be stylish. For centuries they were even valued as accessories like jewelry or hats.

Here are tips for selecting and using a cane:

Grip. If you have hand or arm pain, a handle about 1½ to 2 inches (4 to 5 cm) in diameter is best. Test the handle and make sure it allows for a comfortable grip without having to squeeze too tight or is not so large that it strains your hand.

Tip. The rubber tip on the end of a cane grips the floor and gives you traction. If you are given a cane or have had yours for a long time, make sure the tip and especially the tread on the bottom of the tip are in good shape. If the tip looks worn, buy a replacement at a pharmacy or medical supply store.

Fit. If you are given a cane, make sure it fits you properly. You can adjust most canes.

- **Position:** With the cane in your hand, bend your elbow at a comfortable angle of about 15 degrees. You might bend your elbow slightly more if you are using the cane mainly for balance.

- **Height:** Cane height matters. If your cane is too long, you will have to work harder to pick it up and put it down. If it is too short, you will lean to one side and lose your balance. In both cases, unbalanced posture can

increase pain. To make sure your cane is the right height, hang your arm at your side straight down. The top of your cane should line up with the crease in your wrist.

Proper form. These are general instructions for using a single-point cane.

- Stand up straight. Lift and tighten your stomach muscles for more support.

- Keep the cane close to your body.

- Hold the cane in a vertical position.

- To maintain a normal walking pattern, step forward with the cane and the leg on the opposite side at the same time. If you are weaker on one side or have a more painful side, hold the cane in the hand of your stronger side. If you do not have more pain on one side, hold the cane in the hand that feels more comfortable to you.

- When you are ready to walk, step out with the leg on the opposite side of the hand holding the cane. In other words, if you are holding the cane in your right hand, step out with your left leg.

- Make sure to step out with your leg and the cane at the same time. When you step forward with the other leg (the leg on the side where you are not holding the cane), keep the cane in place.

- Make sure to touch the cane to the ground. If you don't touch your cane to the ground, it provides no support and may increase the risk of injury.

- Do not drag your cane.

If you feel unsteady or continue to have pain, you may need a different type of cane or assistive device. Ask to see a physical therapist. This is a time to call in a self-management consultant.

Using Assistive Technology to Make Activities Easier and Safer

Like all technology, the purpose of assistive technology is to make life easier. Assistive technology can help you have less pain and fatigue. All of us have used assistive technology. For example, a step stool that helps you reach high shelves is a kind of assistive technology. There is a device to help you do almost everything. Your job as a self-manager is to find the ones you need to do your daily activities safely. The questions to ask are: "What devices are available?" "How do I use the device properly?" and "Does this device help my pain and/or fatigue?"

Think about your daily life. What causes your pain and pain flares? What wears you out? You may want to review your pain or symptoms journal to answer these questions. Next, ask yourself, "Are there any devices that might help?" This section lists and describes assistive technology that many people find helpful, so this is a good place to start if you are thinking about buying something new.

The bathroom is a place where accidents are common. Use the following assistive devices to be safer when you are in the bathroom:

- Raised toilet seats, shower chairs, and grab bars (Figure 6.5) reduce strain on your knees, hips, and back. They can be helpful if you cannot stand for long periods of time or have difficulty moving from sitting to standing.

- For bathing, a long-handled sponge can reduce bending and twisting.

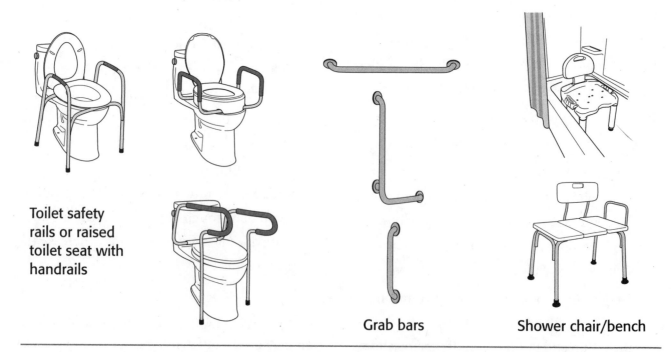

Toilet safety rails or raised toilet seat with handrails

Grab bars

Shower chair/bench

Figure 6.5 **Raised Toilet Seats, Shower Chairs, and Grab Bars**

■ Install a handheld showerhead and use a pump dispenser for shampoo or body wash to make bathing easier. (The showerhead makes it easier to reach all parts of your body with water, and the pump dispenser is easier to handle than a slippery bar of soap.) A bath glove can also be used to lessen the amount of time and energy spent pinching or holding a washcloth.

■ There are devices to help with wiping after using the toilet. These can also reduce twisting if you have movement restrictions. Look for self-wiping toilet aids when searching online or at a medical supply store. You can also consider a bidet, which uses water to clean yourself after going to the bathroom.

If you struggle to dress, consider buying new clothing items that are a size larger. Look for clothes with a looser fit and a larger neck opening. You can add Velcro closures to clothing if buttons or zippers are a problem for you. Use elastic shoelaces to reduce pinching—with elastic shoelaces, you simply slip your foot into the shoe with a shoehorn and don't have to tie or untie the laces. If bending results in lower back pain, use a long-handled shoehorn. Sitting to put on your shoes is a good strategy as well. A leg lifter can also help you in the bedroom, especially if it is a challenge to get into bed safely (see page 125). A reacher can help you reach your shoes and socks to put them on and take them off. It can also be useful to pick up items from the floor (see page 130).

There are also many assistive devices available for the kitchen. Some of these are shown in Figure 6.6 on page 130. Helpful kitchen devices include the following:

■ A food processor, a mandoline for slicing, and easy-grip utensils (also known as built-up utensils) make cooking and eating easier. Many kitchen home stores carry these, or you can shop for them on the internet. You can also create your own easy-grip utensils by sliding utensil foam tubing (1½ to 2 inches, or 4 to 5 cm, in diameter) on the handle to hold the utensil.

■ Lightweight dishes, silverware, pots, and pans reduce strain on shoulders, wrists, and hands.

■ Nonslip table mats and scooped plates can make food preparation and eating easier.

■ Use a rolling cart to transport multiple items at once rather than carrying or making repeated trips. Consider sliding heavy items along the counter rather than lifting them.

To find assistive technology devices, check a local medical supply store, drugstore, or online. Online purchase is often easiest. Do an online search using search terms such as "assistive equipment" or "assistive devices" plus the room where they will be used (for example, "bedroom," "bathroom," "kitchen"). You can also look for a "lending closet," senior center, or community organization that rents or loans out equipment such as mobility aids and bathroom safety equipment. Some community organizations give away used equipment. If you have equipment you no longer use, you can donate it.

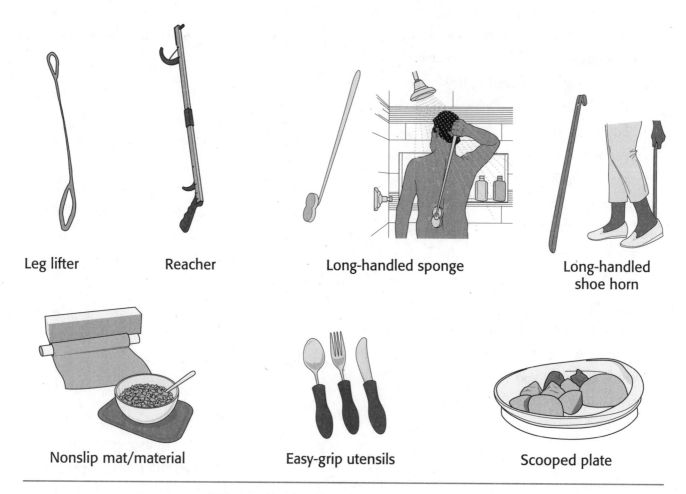

Leg lifter   Reacher   Long-handled sponge   Long-handled shoe horn

Nonslip mat/material   Easy-grip utensils   Scooped plate

Figure 6.6 **More Assistive Technology to Make Tasks Easier**

Organizing Your Home for Safety

Just as simple devices can help you, small changes in your home can make daily activities easier and contribute to successful pain self-management.

Arranging Your Space

These are some proven strategies that can make your living space safer and easier to live in independently.

- **Remove clutter.** Keep pathways clear. Keep cables and cords off the floor, and consider wireless options. Get rid of any scatter rugs, which can be easy to slip on.

- **Rearrange furniture.** Place furniture to support rest breaks. For example, you might position a sturdy chair with arms in your bedroom to use for dressing. Perhaps you can use another sturdy chair in the kitchen. You can rest in this chair while waiting for food to cook or water to boil. If you have good balance but want to cook in a seated position, look for a high stool that supports good posture.

- **Reorganize items in your cabinets.** Put the items you use most often in the front of the cabinet in easy reach. This prevents bending over and reaching for items every time you use them. Store regularly used items between shoulder and hip height.

■ **Keep frequently used items in each room or, if you live in a multistory home, on each floor.** Keep canes, phones, reading glasses, and other useful items in the areas where you often use and need them. It is OK to have more than one of these items. Rushing to find and answer the phone can result in increased pain and fall risks. If you place a phone in every room or keep a cell phone in your pocket, you never have to rush and risk a fall to answer a ringing phone.

Choosing Furniture to Reduce Strain and Pain

The right furniture can also help keep you safe and reduce pain flares.

■ **Choose sturdy, firm chairs with arms.** Make sure they support good posture rather than have a rounded back, which does not. It is easier to get up from a kitchen chair with arms than from a recliner or sofa, reducing the risk of falls or twists.

■ **Use beds and chairs at the right height.** Chairs or beds that are too low can be difficult to get out of without straining. Chairs that are high and do not have backs, such as stools, do not provide back support. A high bed is easier to get out of, but it is harder to get into. Consider purchasing a bed that is height adjustable. If you are having difficulty getting out of a bed or a chair, consult

with a rehabilitation professional, such as an occupational therapist or physical therapist.

Modifying Activities

After normal daily activities such as paying bills, doing laundry, or preparing breakfast, you may have pain. But it may be difficult to figure out exactly which actions are causing pain flares. Breaking down painful activities into steps makes it easier to simplify or modify them. For example, consider all the steps for making a salad:

1. Stoop, bend, and reach to gather ingredients from refrigerator and bowls and utensils from cabinets.

2. Lift or carry ingredients and tools to work surface.

3. Chop or tear salad ingredients. Open jars or cans for olives or other ingredients.

4. Make or add salad dressing.

5. Toss ingredients.

6. Clean counters, tools, and utensils.

7. Put supplies away.

Some people make a salad without thinking. For others it is a painful task. In Figure 6.7 on page 132, you can see some ways to make tasks less painful and less tiring. On the right are specific ways to modify the salad-making task. To try these modifications for yourself, start by guessing what might help and testing out that modification to see if it does. You may find it helpful to use one modification or several. Fill out the blanks in Figure 6.8 on page 132 to try to modify a task that you find difficult.

Figure 6.7 **Modifications for Making a Salad**

Goal	Modification
Reduce carrying or lifting.	Use a cart on wheels to gather supplies.
Reduce steps/simplify.	Buy a bag of already prepared salad greens to avoid chopping.
Change positions/improve body mechanics.	Sit to make the salad (or take seated rest breaks).
Use assistive equipment.	Use salad tongs with large handles that do not require gripping; use an easy-to-use (or automatic) can opener and knives with easy-grip handles.
Rearrange storage for easier access.	Store supplies you use often between hip and shoulder level.

Figure 6.8 **Modifications for Making a Task Easier**

Take a minute and think about a task that you find painful. Write it down here:

_____

Consider the steps involved and list them here:

1. _____

2. _____

3. _____

4. _____

5. _____

6. _____

Now list potential ways to make this task easier

1. _____

2. _____

3. _____

4. _____

5. _____

6. _____

Principle	Modification to Test
Reduce carrying or lifting.	
Reduce steps/simplify/divide task into smaller steps.	
Change positions/improve body mechanics.	
Use assistive equipment.	
Rearrange storage for easier access.	
Other:	

When you come up with your list, try the modifications that you think will be the most helpful. Avoid testing all ideas at one time.

Limiting Time on Tasks

Another way to modify daily activities (such as washing or putting away dishes) is to limit how much time you spend on them. Do this by timing yourself to see how long you can do the task without pain or other symptoms. If you find that after 15 minutes you have pain, do the activity for 10 minutes. Do not power through tasks. You do not have to complete a task in one push. You can come back and finish later. This works for dusting, cleaning, cooking, and other routine chores. Try doing just one room at a time or even just one side of a room. Prep your vegetables in a separate step from preparing and serving your meal. Empty one shelf of your dishwasher at a time and do the other shelf later. Fold a few items of laundry at a time. This strategy can also work for tasks like bill payment. Especially if you create a bill-paying station with all the supplies ready to go, it can be easy to work in shorter bursts.

If you tend to get lost in a task and feel the pain later after your task is completed, consider setting a timer for rest breaks. Or make a playlist of favorite songs that will finish when you need to stop. You can also break a task into steps. Then make a schedule to do just one step a day and complete the entire task over several days. This way you can complete the task without increased pain. For example, each day just dust one room or sort one cabinet in the garage.

Activity Pacing

If pain has made it difficult to do the thing you need and want to do, activity pacing is one of the most useful self-management tools that can help you enjoy a more active lifestyle again. It involves adding rest breaks and doing activities at a slow pace. Using the activity pacing tools in this chapter, you can design a schedule that allows you more control over your routine of activities.

Research has shown that activity pacing increases time on tasks, reduces joint stiffness, and reduces fatigue. It allows people with chronic pain to avoid too much or too little activity. Everyone is different, so apply the information as it fits your personal situation. Whether you are new to chronic pain management or a seasoned veteran, think of right now as a fresh start. Life changes. Your body changes. Your activities change.

Balancing Activity and Rest

When you deal with chronic pain, it can be difficult to strike the right balance between activity and rest. Common sense may tell you to stop an activity if it hurts. Acute pain is nature's way of telling us to pay attention, to rest, and to heal. But chronic pain requires a different approach. Stopping all activity can make your condition worse. Being inactive can cause new pain from stiffness and weak muscles. The trick is to find the balance between different types of activity and rest. Do as much as you can without increasing your pain.

It is common for people with chronic pain to go to extremes of either avoiding an activity or overdoing it. Here are some examples.

Avoiding Activity

Five years ago at age 70, Francisco developed chronic hip and back pain. He stopped walking and moving and let his family do everything for him. Francisco thought resting would help. Instead, it made things much worse. He became weak, and when he wanted to stand up from his favorite chair, it took two or three tries. When he finally stood up, he was short of breath. His pain got worse, he became depressed, and he felt helpless. He felt fortunate that his wife helped him use the bathroom and get dressed, but he found he had stopped doing almost everything he used to do.

Francisco's story is not unique. Fear of pain leads people to avoid activity, but avoiding activity can lead to more pain and often more fatigue. It is a vicious cycle, as shown in Figure 6.9. Resting too much has many negative effects. It can lead to further disability, additional depression, and more pain. If you have ever been in bed for several days, you will likely recall how weak and wobbly you felt the first few times you were up and about. This weakened state is called disuse

syndrome. Being inactive affects strength, pain, fatigue, and your mental state in just a few days.

Overdoing Activity

Nikita has chronic back pain. She works from her home office. In the morning she gets up early to clean the kitchen and make breakfast for her family before starting work on the computer at 9:00 A.M. Nikita works straight until noon. She is very focused and ignores any pain when she is working. For the past few months, she has been working even harder. At the same time, she started walking a half hour five days a week. Her pain has gradually gotten worse. She is limping by the end of her day. She has been told that exercise is helpful. She does not want to get weak and keeps on walking. But recently she had to stay in bed for several days and increase her pain medications. She is beginning to wonder if there is a better way to manage her pain.

Like those who rest too much, those who push themselves, ignore pain, and overdo their activities are also in a vicious cycle (Figure 6.10). The longer this cycle continues, the longer the recovery time. It can be very discouraging to be trying to do more and more and in fact be doing less and less.

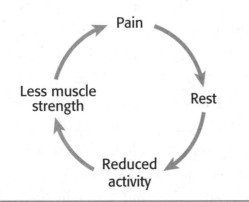

Figure 6.9 **Vicious Cycle of Inactivity**

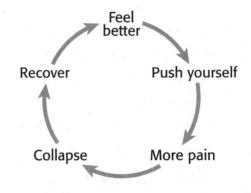

Figure 6.10 **Vicious Cycle of Overdoing Activity**

Exercise Can Help Reduce Pain

Margaret has lived with rheumatoid arthritis for many years. Her back and hands hurt; she felt tired and needed to rest often. She started with the Moving Easy Program and soon graduated to an exercise program designed for people with arthritis. She took the program, and after a few weeks she felt less stiff and had more energy. The program leaders told people to slow down or stop briefly if they were tired or noticed an increase in pain. They encouraged Margaret to substitute an exercise that did not cause pain when the class did one that she found painful. When the class ended, she started walking 5 minutes every day around her neighborhood. Just like in the class, she started slow. She paid attention to her body and eventually increased to a 10-minute walk once or twice a day. During the rest of her day, Margaret added rest breaks and changed position when tired. She paid more attention to her posture. Margaret reports now that the exercise class started a chain of positive changes.

Creating an Activity Pacing Schedule

So far in this chapter, we have talked about body mechanics, assistive technology, reorganizing your home, and modifying tasks. We hope you have also looked at your daily activities to see if you are doing too much or too little or maybe some of each. Here are some tips to help you create an activity pacing schedule:

1. **Make a list of the things you do each day in an average week.** Start by looking at a typical day. When you make the list, note which activities cause pain and which do not. Notice your tendency to do too much or too little. Figure out what you *need* to do each day and *want* to do each day.

2. **Prioritize.** Think about what you need to get done. If you don't have time in your day to be very active, think about little things you can do to become more active. Avoid squeezing too much in a day. This leads to rushing, exhaustion, and more pain. If you are too busy, identify your priorities. What things can you skip or do less frequently? Can you get help with your responsibilities so you can spend time in healthier activities?

3. **Make modifications to balance rest and activity.** Working without a break, ignoring pain, and hurrying to finish a task can cause pain or make existing pain worse. Read through the list below and identify a few modifications you think will help you balance rest and activity. Think about a way to fit a modification into your schedule, try it, and decide if it is helpful. Consider the following modifications:

   ■ Rest before you are tired even if it means not completing something in one attempt.

   ■ Stop and stretch or rest at the earliest sign of pain or fatigue. For example, take scheduled stretch breaks every 20 to 30 minutes while working on your computer.

- Plan daily breaks or a break during the toughest time of your day. Take a few minutes to do a relaxation exercise or read an article in your favorite section of the paper.

- If you need to do a tiring activity, limit other activities that day.

- Rest before or after a special but tiring event, such as an outing with grandchildren or a holiday shopping trip.

- If you want to keep doing one task longer, change positions. For example, while attending a weekly phone conference meeting, sit for a while and then stand. There is special equipment to make working and standing and sitting easier (see the standing desk in Figure 6.3).

- Break an activity into parts. Change an activity so it is less complex or less time consuming.

- Alternate easy and difficult activities each day.

- Build in warm-ups such as walking, stretches, and relaxation before activities that require movement such as housecleaning, yard work, or gardening.

- Schedule regular activities for pleasure or recreation that work with your ability level. These can range from less physical activities such as a book club meeting or a phone call with a friend to more physical activities such as a walk around a small local park.

4. **Listen to your body and adjust your schedule.** You may have planned to do an activity for an hour but you end up feeling pain after 20 minutes. The schedule you create is an experiment, so listen to your body and adjust if the schedule is not working. Try a different position or a rest break. Perhaps you can modify this activity or fit it into your schedule on another day.

5. **Consider your stress, nutrition, and sleep.** If activities that typically don't make you tired or cause pain begin to wear you out, maybe something else is contributing. Think about what you are eating, what is going on in your life, and whether you are sleeping well. You may need to adjust your schedule during times of high stress or when you are not eating or sleeping well. Consider this story from a person with chronic pain:

> "I went to my exercise class one day, and doing the exercises raised my pain level to a 10. This had not happened before. The instructor asked, 'What did you eat today?' I said, 'Nothing, just black coffee.' She followed up by asking, 'How did you sleep last night?' I responded, 'Not well.' I then began to notice how sleep and what I eat affects my pain."

For more on how sleep, stress, and nutrition can affect pain, read Chapter 4, *Understanding and Managing Common Symptoms and Problems*, Chapter 5, *Using Your Mind to Manage Pain and Other Symptoms*, Chapter 9, *Healthy Eating and Pain Self-Management*, and Chapter 10, *Healthy Weight and Pain Self-Management*.

In the next part of this chapter, we revisit Francisco and Nikita to review their typical days. We then explore how they can revise their schedules for better activity pacing.

Figure 6.11 **Typical Day for Francisco**

Time	Actual Activity
7 A.M.	Woke up
8:45 A.M.	Got out of bed
9 A.M.	Morning self-care and dressing with help from his wife
10 A.M.	Breakfast
11 A.M.	TV
12 noon	TV
1 P.M.	Lunch
2 P.M.	TV
3 P.M.	Nap
4 P.M.	TV
5 P.M.	Nap
6 P.M.	Dinner
7 P.M.	TV
8 P.M.	TV
9 P.M.	TV
10 P.M.	TV

When he reviewed his schedule (Figure 6.11), Francisco noticed that he was watching TV or napping in his favorite chair most of the day. His family encouraged him to do more, and he agreed. He started with dressing himself almost every day. At first he could put on his shirt, but he still needed help with his pants and socks. After a couple of weeks, even putting on socks was easier. Francisco thought about what else he could do, such as walking or visiting with his grandchildren. He started with two minutes of walking around the house during commercials five or six times a day. If he had any pain, he stopped and rested for a minute and only walked a minute the next few times. Once or twice a day he did a few exercises from the Moving Easy Program during commercial breaks. (See Chapter 8, *Exercising to Feel Better*, pages 173–189.)

Within a month, Francisco had more energy and noticed he was awake in the late afternoon and was able to spend more time with his grandchildren who lived next door. He also began walking around the block with his wife 10 minutes every day after breakfast. They increased this a few minutes at a time. They got up to half an hour, but then Francisco had to back off because he was feeling more pain after the walks. He learned that gradual change works. After he had a difficult day, he did less the next day. After a couple of months, Francisco could stand up on the first try and he was not short of breath. He was realizing he missed playing cards with his friends and was thinking about how he could start doing that again.

Francisco was successful because he wanted to feel better. He made changes slowly and paid attention to his pain. He did his exercises carefully and with good posture. He changed his position every hour when he sat in his chair. His wife and family encouraged him and gave him control to make the changes he wanted. They encouraged him to restart past activities he enjoyed. Because he was not napping and sitting all day, he slept better at night and had more energy to socialize. He slowed down but did not stop when he had setbacks.

Looking at her schedule (Figure 6.12 on the next page), Nikita realized she was busy without a break from morning to night. Her priority was to work her eight-hour work shift. To do this she needed to simplify her work around

Figure 6.12 **Typical Day for Nikita**

Time	Actual Activity
7 A.M.	Clean kitchen
8 A.M.	Make breakfast
9 A.M.	Work on laptop
10 A.M.	Work on laptop
11 A.M.	Work on laptop
12 noon	Lunch
1 P.M.	Work on laptop
2 P.M.	Work on laptop
3 P.M.	Work on laptop
4 P.M.	Fast walk
5 P.M.	Prepare dinner
6 P.M.	Dinner
7 P.M.	Clean up
8 P.M.	Shower; prepare for next day
9 P.M.	Read in bed
10 P.M.	Go to sleep

the house. She talked with her husband and two teenage children about helping with cooking and kitchen cleanup. The family decided on easy breakfast and lunch items each person could manage themselves. They made a schedule so that a different person was responsible for dinner each evening. Nikita wanted to cook dinner two days a week and one on the weekend. These changes lightened her daily workload around the house.

Nikita tried this new schedule and felt less rushed. After a week or two, she added a short relaxation activity before work. She began to notice she felt less muscle tension and less

pain. Nikita looked at the modifications to balance rest and activity on page 133 to get some rest break ideas. She decided to change positions every 30 minutes and take a 5- to 10-minute rest every hour. During her rest break she did a few exercises from the Moving Easy Program. At first, she moved too fast. This made her pain worse. She slowed down and watched her posture and positioning. The exercise gave her some pain relief.

Nikita also reduced her long post-work walk to a shorter walk and added stretch breaks that did not increase her pain in the afternoon. After her workday, she relaxed and talked with her family at dinner. She wanted to find a fun family activity like a board game to do in the evenings at least once a week.

As a result of these changes, Nikita now feels less rushed and better able to manage her schedule most days. She is still trying out new modifications that can help her during a full workweek with frequent deadlines.

Nikita and Francisco both realized they could learn a lot from reviewing the schedules for their typical days. Success came with trying new activities and modifications gradually and evaluating if they helped. Both benefited from family support. They used many of the ideas in this chapter to modify their day step by step to create a more satisfying and rhythmic schedule. Both were able to add healthy activities to their schedules and felt better as a result. As they continue to feel better, they are looking into doing more fun activities.

Returning to Activities You Let Go

Marta has chronic lower back and knee pain. She took a leave from her career after a long, difficult pain flare. During her time off she made many changes, including taking regular rest breaks and short exercise breaks and doing a regular relaxation practice. She hired help for cleaning, cooking, and laundry for a short period when her pain was at its worst. She returned to work and spoke to her supervisors about accommodations. They agreed on assistive technology and schedule modifications to support her success at meeting work demands.

Marta was feeling better and started to think about activities she enjoyed in the past and might want to do again. Playing the piano and gardening were activities that came to mind. She decided gardening was what she really wanted to be doing again. She knew it might be challenging and realized she would have to do it differently. She asked friends and looked online for resources about gardening with chronic pain. She was surprised by how many ideas and resources she found.

Marta listed the steps in a typical day of gardening and came up with several modifications. These included planting in a raised garden bed on legs (Figure 6.13), using lightweight tools,

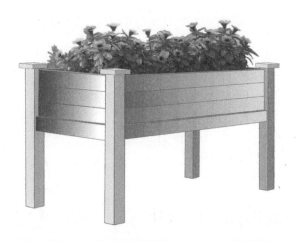

Figure 6.13 **A Raised Garden Bed**

and keeping gardening materials in a tool chest outside near the bed. She listed tasks she needed help with such as purchasing soil for filling the raised bed. She paid her neighbor's son to buy soil and fill the bed. She selected plants that were easier to grow and did not need daily care. When gardening, she took rest breaks before she was tired and paid attention to her body to limit twisting and bending. Martha grew flowers in her box and felt very happy watching her flowers grow. She had figured out a way to resume an activity she had let go.

Managing Pain Flares

A pain flare is extra pain that often is linked to overdoing your activities, fatigue, stress, rushing, an overly packed day, or something else that affects your schedule. Some pain conditions have more flares than others. To limit your pain flares, do not ignore pain. Maintain good sleep, eating, relaxation, and exercise habits. Add warm-up activities into your routine. It is valuable to learn the difference between a flare and something that requires a medical visit. This is something to discuss with your health care provider.

When you have a pain flare, the impulse is to stop everything and just rest. Instead, try pausing or modifying the activity that increases pain. At the same time, increase health-promoting activities, such as practicing good sleep hygiene and relaxation techniques, and take more rest breaks. If possible, avoid stopping everything and putting your whole schedule on hold.

Managing chronic pain requires noticing what makes your pain worse, making changes slowly, and recognizing what works and what does not.

It requires patience. Activity pacing helps you create a routine that meets your needs. Starting with one small change can make a difference. Be kind to yourself, and slowly fill your tool kit of pain self-management tools and techniques. The bottom line is to feel in control of your life and to do the things you need and want to do.

For a complete list of suggested further readings, useful websites, and other helpful resources, please see

www.bullpub.com/resources.

"Activity and rest are two vital aspects of life. To find a balance in them is a skill in itself. Wisdom is knowing when to have rest, when to have activity, and how much of each to have. Finding them in each other—activity in rest and rest in activity—is the ultimate freedom."

— Sri Ravi Shankar, *Celebrating Silence: Excerpts from Five Years of Weekly Knowledge*

Exercising and Physical Activity for Every Body

ACTIVE PEOPLE ARE HEALTHIER AND HAPPIER than people who are not active. This is true for people of all ages and conditions, including people with chronic pain. Inactivity can cause or worsen pain, disability, and other illness. In order to better manage your chronic pain, you need to learn how to balance activity and rest. Chapter 6, *Organizing and Pacing Your Life for Pain Self-Management and Safety*, explains the importance of planning for appropriate rest periods throughout the day. Equally important is planning for regular activity and exercise.

Physical activity keeps you fit so you have the strength, stamina, and energy to do the things you want to do in life. Being fit helps you manage your chronic pain over the long run. Scientific research shows that regular exercise helps chronic pain, improves functioning, and boosts overall health and well-being. Research also shows that people who participate in flexibility, strengthening, and endurance exercise, as well as programs including tai chi, yoga, and qigong, have improvements in pain and daily activity.

141

You probably know that physical activity and regular exercise are important, but when you have chronic pain it can be difficult to know what you can do and how to do it. The good news is that there is plenty of information to help you get started and be successful. For example, there are government guidelines that explain the importance of physical activity and offer programs to get you started. These guidelines spell out what kinds of exercise or physical activities are best and how much you need. In this chapter and the next chapter (Chapter 8, *Exercising to Feel Better*), you will learn about these guidelines and about how to make wise exercise choices.

Of course, learning what to do is not enough. You also must do it! It is up to you to make your life more enjoyable, more comfortable, and healthier through physical activity. As is the case in every chapter, the information about exercise in this book is not intended to take the place of medical or other health professional advice. If you already have a prescribed exercise plan that differs from the suggestions here, be sure to share this book with your health care provider or therapist before changing your program.

Why Exercise?

Decades of research confirm that regular exercise is key to a healthier life. It improves levels of strength, energy, and self-confidence and lessens feelings of stress, anxiety, and depression. It can help you sleep better and feel more relaxed and happier. In addition to reducing chronic pain, exercise can prevent and help in the management of heart disease and diabetes. It improves blood pressure, blood sugar, and blood fat levels. Exercise can help you maintain a good weight, which takes stress off your weight-bearing joints.

Exercise is often the largest part of pain rehabilitation programs. A recent review of nondrug treatments for chronic pain found that exercise is the best and most long-lasting way to reduce pain and improve function for people with chronic lower back pain, hip and knee osteoarthritis, fibromyalgia, and tension headaches. In people with various types of widespread pain, exercise improves the ability to do normal activities; reduces pain, tenderness, and fatigue; and increases muscle strength. Strengthening and stretching exercises improve chronic neck pain and some types of headaches. Many people with leg pain from poor circulation or other causes can learn to walk farther and more comfortably with a regular exercise program. Strong muscles help people with arthritis protect their joints by improving stability and absorbing shock. Regular exercise also helps nourish joints and keeps cartilage and bone healthy. There is evidence that regular exercise can help prevent blood clots, which is one of the reasons it can be of particular benefit to people with heart and vascular diseases.

When you are physically active and exercise, you improve strength, flexibility, and endurance and you can participate in more meaningful activities. You also reduce your risk of falls and other injuries from strained muscles, over-stressed joints, fatigue, and poor balance.

That is all good news. The better news is that it doesn't take hours of painful, sweaty exercise to achieve health benefits. Studies show that even short periods of moderate physical activity can improve health and fitness, lessen pain and improve everyday functioning, reduce disease risks, and boost mood. Being active also helps you feel more in control of your life and less at the mercy of your chronic pain. The bottom line: *keep moving!*

Kinds of Exercise

Just as different foods (such as carbohydrates, protein, fats, and fiber) provide different benefits, different kinds of exercise have different effects on your body. There are four major types of exercise. We list and explain each one here:

- **Endurance (aerobic).** Your endurance depends on the fitness of your heart, lungs, and muscles. The heart and lungs must work efficiently to send enough oxygen-rich blood to your muscles. Your muscles must be fit enough to use the oxygen. Aerobic ("with oxygen") exercise uses the large muscles of your body in continuous activity. Walking, swimming, dancing, mowing the lawn, or riding a bike are all aerobic forms of exercise. Many studies show that aerobic exercise lessens pain and fatigue, promotes a sense of well-being, eases depression and anxiety, promotes restful sleep, and improves mood and energy levels.

- **Flexibility.** Being flexible helps you move comfortably and safely. Limited flexibility can cause pain, lead to injury, and make muscles work harder and tire more quickly. You lose flexibility when you are inactive or your daily movement is limited. Certain illnesses and diseases can also result in a loss of flexibility. The good news is that even if you have chronic pain, you can improve flexibility and manage pain by doing gentle stretching exercises.

- **Strength.** You must use your muscles to make and keep your muscles strong. Inactive muscles weaken and atrophy (shrink). When your muscles get weak, you feel weak and tire quickly. For many people, disability and lack of mobility is due to muscle weakness. Exercises strengthen muscles when they require your muscles to do more work than those muscles are used to doing.

- **Balance.** For good balance, you need strong and coordinated muscles in your trunk and legs, flexibility, and good posture. Though there are many causes of falls (such as poor vision, poor lighting, obstacles such as rugs on the floor, dizziness, and being tired or distracted), being strong and coordinated is very important and can help prevent falls and injury.

Physical Activity Guidelines

Many countries and some institutions, including the World Health Organization (WHO), have guidelines for the type and amount of physical activity you need to do to be healthy. The guidelines are pretty much the same all over the world and apply to adults with and without chronic illness and disability. When you read the guidelines, it is important to remember that they are goals to work toward; they are not the starting point. On average, only about 25 percent of people exercise enough to meet these guidelines. Don't worry that everyone else can meet these goals and only you can't.

Your goal is to gradually and safely increase your physical activity to a level that is right for you. You may be able to exercise as much as the guidelines indicate, but maybe you won't. The important point is to use the information to be more active and healthier in a way that is right for you. Start doing what you can do now. Even a few minutes of activity several times a day is a good beginning. The important thing is to do some activity that works for you, make it a habit, and gradually increase the time or number of days a week that you do it.

The following guidelines are from the US Department of Health and Human Services. Remember, they are a guide to where you could go, not a requirement for where you should be right now.

- Adults should do moderate endurance (aerobic) exercise for at least 150 minutes (2½ hours) each week or vigorous-intensity activity for at least 75 minutes each week.

- Aerobic activity should be performed at least 10 minutes at a time, spread out through the week. Being active at a moderate intensity in 10-minute sessions throughout the day provides the same health benefits of longer sessions.

- Moderate-intensity muscle-strengthening exercise of all major muscle groups should be done at least two days a week.

- If people cannot meet the guidelines, they should be as active as they can and avoid inactivity. The newest guidelines emphasize that moving for 10 minutes at a time is important and useful.

In Canada, the Canadian Society for Exercise Physiology (CSEP) publishes the Canadian Physical Activity Guidelines for people 18 to 64 years old and 65 years and older. You can find these guidelines at www.csep.ca/guidelines. The Canadian guidelines also emphasize the following two points:

- More physical activity provides greater health benefits.

- Those with poor mobility should perform physical activities to enhance balance and prevent falls.

Endurance Exercise

Endurance exercise helps you be more energetic and more active. There are many kinds of endurance exercise. Any physical activity involving your arms and legs that you can keep up for at least 10 minutes can be an endurance exercise and qualifies as physical activity. Most of the time we think of activities such as walking, swimming, biking, dancing, or exercise classes as endurance activities. However, doing household chores or working in the yard can be endurance exercises too. Some regular activity is better than none. Remember that the activity you choose should be comfortable enough that you can eventually keep it up for at least 10 minutes.

How often you exercise (frequency), how long you are active each time (time), and how hard you work (intensity) all work together. You can choose the frequency, time, and intensity to adjust your exercise effort. It is better to begin by underdoing rather than overdoing.

Frequency

Frequency is how often you exercise. Every other day is a good way to start. Guidelines suggest that you exercise three to five days a week. If possible, do not go more than two days in a row without exercising.

Time

Time is the length of each exercise session. The guidelines suggest you exercise at least 10 minutes at a time. As you build your endurance, you can increase the time of each session and do several 10-minute sessions in a day.

Intensity

Intensity describes your exercise effort—how hard you are working. Low to moderate intensity is safe and effective. When you exercise at moderate intensity, you can tell that your body is working but you feel that you can continue for a while and you can talk normally. High-intensity exercise is not necessary to get benefits, and it increases chances for injuries. You are exercising at a high intensity if you feel breathless, can't talk while you are exercising, or feel you can only continue for a few seconds. How hard you work to exercise depends on how fit you are now. For example, a 10-minute brisk walk is low intensity for an athlete but is high intensity for someone who hasn't been active for a while. When you begin endurance exercise, you may want to begin at a low intensity until you have a good idea of how you are feeling.

Figure out what is moderate intensity for you so that you don't work too hard. There are several ways to do this, including the following:

- **Talk Test.** When exercising, talk to another person or yourself, or recite poems or song lyrics out loud. If you are doing moderate-intensity exercise, you can speak comfortably. If you can't carry on a conversation because you are breathing too hard or are short of breath, you're exercising at a high intensity. Slow down. The talk test is an easy and quick way to recognize your effort. If you have lung disease, the talk test might not work for you. If that is the case, try the perceived-exertion scale.

Table 7.1 **Moderate-Intensity Exercise Heart Rate, by Age (CDC guidelines at cdc.gov)**

Age	Exercise Pulse (beats per minute)	Exercise Pulse (15-second count)
30s	122–144	30–36
40s	115–137	29–34
50s	109–129	27–32
60s	102–122	25–31
70s	96–114	24–29
80s	90–106	23–27
90 and above	83–99	21–25

- **Perceived Exertion.** Rate how hard you're working on a scale of 1 to 10. One, at the low end of the scale, is sitting down, doing no work at all. Ten is working as hard as possible—in other words, very hard work that you couldn't do for more than a few seconds. A good level for moderate aerobic exercise is between 3 and 5 on the 1-to-10 scale. When you are exercising, ask yourself where you are on the scale. Work a little harder if your exertion is too low, or ease up if your exertion is too high.

- **Heart Rate.** Unless you're taking heart-regulating medicine (such as beta-blockers), checking your heart rate is another way to measure exercise intensity. The faster your heart beats, the harder you're working. (Your heart also beats fast when you are frightened or nervous, but here we're talking about how your heart responds to physical activity.) Endurance exercise at moderate intensity raises your heart rate to a range between 65 and 76 percent of your safe maximum heart rate based on your age. The safe maximum heart rate gets lower with age. That means your safe exercise heart rate decreases as you get older. There are a number of ways to find your heart rate. Some types of gym equipment have hand grips that take your pulse. Cell phone apps, smart watches, and monitors you wear on your wrist or belt can also measure your heart rate. It is your job to know what exercise heart rate is best for you. Table 7.1 lists general guidelines for you to follow.

Putting Together Your Own Endurance Program

You can build your endurance exercise program by varying frequency, time, and activities. We recommend that you start slowly with low- to moderate-intensity exercise and increase frequency and time as you work toward the recommended guideline of 150 minutes each week. A good way to meet the guideline goals for physical activity is to accumulate 30 minutes of moderate physical activity on most days of the week. This is just 10 minutes three times each day or 30 minutes all at once. It is your choice. This can be a combination of walking, stationary bicycling, dancing, swimming, or chores that require moderate-intensity activity. It is important to remember that 150 minutes is a goal, not your starting point.

Example Exercise Programs

If you begin exercising just 2 minutes each time you are active, you will likely be able to build up to meet the recommended goal of 10 minutes, three times a day. Not everyone can reach the guideline goal, but almost everyone can learn to be active enough to achieve important health benefits. Being physically active regularly will bring health benefits. Moderate intensity is a goal. If you do not currently exercise and are inactive in general, starting off at low intensity is a good idea.

These moderate-intensity programs will allow you to reach 150 minutes of aerobic exercise each week:

- a 10-minute walk at moderate intensity three times a day, five days a week

- a 30-minute bike ride at moderate intensity (on mostly level ground) three days a week plus a 30-minute walk twice a week

- a 45-minute aerobic dance class at moderate intensity twice a week plus two 30-minute walks each week

- gardening and yard work (digging, raking, lifting) 30 minutes a day, five days a week

If you are just starting, try beginning with:

- a five-minute walk around the house three times a day, five days a week (total 75 minutes)

- a water exercise class that lasts 40 minutes twice a week and two 10-minute walks on two other days a week (total 120 minutes)

- low-impact aerobics class once a week (50 minutes) and a 15-minute walk on two other days a week (total 110 minutes)

Warming Up and Cooling Down

When you exercise at moderate intensity, it is important to warm up first and cool down afterward. To warm up, do several minutes of a low-intensity activity to allow your muscles, heart, lungs, and circulation to gradually get ready to work harder. Warming up reduces the risk of injuries, soreness, and irregular heartbeat. Cooling down helps your body return to its normal resting state. Repeat your warm-up activity or take a slow walk to cool down. Doing gentle flexibility exercises during your cool-down can be relaxing and help reduce muscle soreness and stiffness.

Choosing Your Endurance Exercise

In this section, we discuss a few common endurance exercises. All of these exercises strengthen your heart, lungs, and muscles as well as relieve tension and help you manage your weight. Most of these exercises also strengthen your bones (water exercise is the exception).

Walking

Walking is easy, inexpensive, safe, and can be done almost anywhere. You can walk by yourself or with companions. Walking is safer than jogging or running and puts less stress on the body. It is an especially good choice if you have been sedentary or have joint or balance problems. If you walk to shop, visit friends, and do household chores, then you can probably walk for exercise. A cane or walker doesn't need to stop you from getting into a walking routine. If you haven't been walking for a while, 5 or 10 minutes may be enough to begin. As you get more comfortable, alternate brisk walks and slow walks and build up your total time. Each week increase your brisk walking interval by no more than 5 minutes. Try to build to a total of 20 or 30 minutes of brisk walking. Remember that your goal is to walk most days of the week, at moderate intensity, for sessions that are at least 10 minutes long.

Before starting your walking program, consider these tips:

- Walk on a flat, level surface. Fitness trails, shopping malls, school tracks, streets with sidewalks, and quiet neighborhoods are good places.

- Warm up and cool down with a stroll.

- Set your own pace. Better to start off slowly than try to go too fast and tire out too quickly.

Be sure your shoes fit comfortably and are in good repair. Shoes with laces or Velcro let you adjust width as needed so you get more support than slip-ons. If you have problems tying laces, consider Velcro closures or elastic shoelaces that don't require tying and untying. Many people buy shoes with removable insoles and replace them with more shock-absorbing insoles. You can find insoles in sporting goods stores, drugstores, and shoe stores. When you shop for insoles, take your walking shoes with you. Try on the shoe with the insole inserted to make sure there's enough room for your foot. Insoles come in different sizes and can be trimmed with scissors for a custom fit. If your toes take up extra room, try the three-quarter insoles that stop just short of your toes. If you have prescribed inserts in your shoes already, ask your therapist about insoles for walking shoes.

If you have pain in your shins when you walk, you may not be warming up long enough. Try some ankle exercises from the Exercises for Hands and Feet section (pages 184–186) in Chapter 8, *Exercising to Feel Better*, before you start walking. Start your walk at a slow pace for at least 5 minutes. Keep your feet and toes relaxed.

Sore knees are another common problem for walkers. Fast walking puts more stress on knee joints. Slow down at first or walk for shorter distances or shorter intervals. Do the Knee Strengthener and Ready-Go exercises (pages 164 and 165) in Chapter 8, *Exercising to Feel Better*, as part of your warm-up.

You can reduce cramps in the calf and pain in the heel by walking slowly to warm up. If you have circulation problems in your legs and get cramps or pain in your calves while walking, alternate between comfortably brisk and slow walking. Slow down and give your circulation a chance to catch up before the pain is so intense that you must stop. Exercise may help you gradually walk farther with less cramping or pain. If these suggestions don't help, check with your health care provider or therapist for suggestions.

Swimming

For most people with chronic pain, swimming is excellent exercise. Swimming uses your whole body. If you haven't been swimming for a while, consider a refresher course. To make swimming an aerobic exercise, you eventually need to swim continuously for 10 minutes. Try different strokes, changing strokes after each lap or two. This lets you exercise all joints and muscles without overtiring any one area.

Swimming is an excellent aerobic exercise, but it does not improve balance or strengthen bones. Because swimming involves the arms, it can lead to excessive shortness of breath. This is especially true for people with lung disease. However, for people with asthma, swimming may be the preferred exercise, as the moisture helps reduce shortness of breath. People with heart disease who have severely irregular heartbeats and have had an implantable defibrillator (AICD) should avoid swimming.

Before starting your swimming program, consider these tips:

- The breaststroke and freestyle (crawl) normally require a lot of neck motion and may be uncomfortable. To solve this problem, use a mask and snorkel so that you can keep your face in the water and breathe without twisting your neck.

- Wear goggles. The chemicals in the pool may irritate your eyes.

- A hot shower or soak in a hot tub after your workout helps reduce stiffness and muscle soreness.

- Always swim where there are qualified lifeguards, if possible, or with a friend. Never swim alone.

Water Exercise

The buoyancy of water allows you to move and strengthen your muscles and cardiovascular system more easily and with less stress than exercise on land. If you don't like to swim or are uncomfortable learning strokes, you can walk laps around a pool or join water exercise classes. Most community centers that have a pool offer classes. The deeper the water you stand in, the less stress there is on joints. However, water above the chest can make it hard to keep your balance. Let the water cover more of your body just by spreading your legs apart or bending your knees a bit. If you have access to a pool and want to make your own routine, there are many water exercise books available. You can also find water exercise videos online. Suggestions for water temperature from US and Canadian national arthritis organizations range from 84 to 92 degrees F (29 to 33 degrees C).

Before starting your water exercise program, consider these tips:

- Wear footgear designed for water. Some styles have Velcro straps to make them easier to put on.

- If you are sensitive to cold or have Raynaud's syndrome, wear water gloves, a wet suit or tights, and a shirt made for use in the water.

- Wearing a flotation belt or life vest adds extra buoyancy and comfort by taking weight off your hips, knees, and feet.

- As on land, moving more slowly makes exercise easier. In the water, regulate exercise intensity by how much water you push when you move. For example, when you move your arms back and forth in front of you underwater, it is hard work if you hold your palms facing each other. It is easier if you turn your palms down and slice your arms back and forth with only the narrow edge of your hands pushing against the water.

- Be aware that additional buoyancy allows for greater joint motion than you may be used to, especially if you are exercising in a warm pool. Start slowly, and do not exercise too vigorously even if it feels good. Wait until you know how your body will react and feel the next day.

- If you have asthma, exercising in water can help you avoid the worsening of asthma symptoms that occurs during other types of exercise. This is probably due to the beneficial effect of water vapor on the lungs. Remember, though, that for many people with lung disease, arm exercises can cause more shortness of breath than leg exercises.

- If you have had a stroke or have another condition that may affect your strength and balance, make sure that you have someone help you in and out of the pool. You can add to your safety and security by finding a position close to the wall or staying close to a buddy who can lend a hand if needed.

- If the pool does not have steps and it is difficult for you to climb up and down a ladder, suggest that pool staff position a three-step kitchen stool in the pool by the ladder rails. This is an inexpensive way to provide steps for easier entry and exit. The steps are easy to remove and store when not needed.

Stationary Bicycling

Stationary bicycles offer the fitness benefits of bicycling without the outdoor hazards. Stationary cycling doesn't put excess strain on your hips, knees, and feet; you can easily adjust how hard you work; and weather doesn't matter. Some people with paralysis of one leg or arm can exercise on stationary bicycles with special attachments for their paralyzed limbs. The stationary bicycle is a particularly good alternative exercise—use the bicycle on days when you don't want to walk or do more vigorous exercise or when you can't exercise outside.

Before starting your stationary bicycling program, consider these tips:

- Make it interesting. Watch a video or listen to an audiobook or music as you pedal along. Some people take a "bike trip" and keep track of their miles and chart their route on a map. Keep a record of the times and distances of your bike trips. You will be amazed at how far you can go.

- Stationary bicycling uses different muscles than walking. Until your leg muscles get used to pedaling, you may be able to ride for only a few minutes. Start with no resistance. Increase resistance slightly as riding gets easier. When you increase resistance, it has the same effect as bicycling up hills. If there is too much resistance, your knees may get sore or you will tire out and stop before you get the benefit of endurance.

- Pedal at a comfortable speed. For most people, 50 to 70 revolutions per minute (rpm) is a good place to start. Some bicycles have an rpm rate readout. If not, you can add up the number of times your right foot reaches its

Stationary Bicycle Checklist

A safe stationary bike has the following features:

- The bicycle is steady when you get on and off.
- The resistance is easy to set and can be set to zero.
- The seat is comfortable and can be adjusted so your knee is almost straight when the pedal is at its lowest point.
- The pedals are large, and the pedal straps are loose to allow the feet to move slightly while pedaling.
- There is enough space between the bike frame so that your knees and ankles do not touch when you pedal.
- The handlebars allow good posture and comfortable arm positions.

lowest point in a minute to calculate rpm. As you get used to bicycling, you can increase your speed. However, faster is not necessarily better. Listening to music at the right tempo makes it easier to pedal at a consistent speed. Experience will tell you the best combination of speed and resistance.

- Set a goal of 20 to 30 minutes of pedaling at a comfortable speed. Build up your time by alternating intervals of brisk pedaling or more resistance with less exertion. Use your heart rate, the perceived-exertion scale, or talk test (see page 145) to make sure you aren't working too hard.

- On days when you're not feeling your best, maintain your exercise habit by pedaling with no resistance, at a lower rpm, or for a shorter period of time.

Exercising on Other Exercise Equipment

If you have trouble getting on or off a stationary bicycle or don't have room for a bicycle where you live, you might try a restorator. A restorator is a small piece of equipment with foot pedals that you can attach to the foot of a bed or put on the floor in front of a chair. To find a restorator, ask your therapist or health care provider or call a pharmacy that carries exercise equipment.

A restorator allows you to exercise by pedaling. You can vary the resistance and adjust for leg length and knee bend. This is a good alternative to an exercise bicycle for people who have problems with balance, weakness, or paralysis. People with other chronic illnesses, such as lung disease, may also find the restorator to be an enjoyable way to start an exercise program.

Arm cranks or arm ergometers are bicycles for the arms. People who are unable to use their legs for active exercise can improve their cardiovascular fitness and upper body strength by using an arm crank. It's important to work closely with a knowledgeable therapist or instructor to set up your program, because using only your arms for endurance exercise requires different intensity monitoring than using larger leg muscles. Many people with lung disease may find arm exercises to be less enjoyable than leg exercises because they may experience shortness of breath.

There are many other types of exercise equipment. These include treadmills, rowing machines, cross-country skiing machines, mini trampolines, stair climbers, and elliptical machines. Most are available for use at gyms and recreation centers. They are also sold in both commercial and home models.

If you're thinking about starting to use exercise equipment, know what you want to achieve. For cardiovascular fitness and endurance, choose equipment that will help you exercise as many parts of your body at one time as possible. The motion should be rhythmic, repetitive, and smooth. The equipment should be comfortable and safe, and using it should not put stress on your joints. If you're interested in purchasing a new piece of equipment, try it out for a week or two before buying.

Land-Based Exercise Classes

Exercise classes at a local gym, senior center, or recreation center can be fun and safe. You can get aerobic exercise in classes that include dancing, such as Zumba or Jazzercise. More traditional dancing such as salsa, ballroom, and square dancing also provides good aerobic exercise. Classes in tai chi, qigong, and some other martial arts are popular and help with endurance, strength, balance, and relaxation. Yoga is helpful for flexibility, strength, balance, and relaxation, but for the most part yoga classes are not aerobic exercise. You can learn more about tai chi and yoga in Chapter 8, *Exercising to Feel Better*.

When you are new to classes, introduce yourself to the instructors. Let them know who you are, that you may need to modify some movements, and that you will ask for advice. If you don't know other people in a class, try to get acquainted. Be open about why you may do things a little differently. You'll be more comfortable, and you may find others who also have special needs. Ask the instructor to show you how you can modify the routines to better suit you, whether it is to go more slowly, reduce arm work, take breaks, or shorten a routine.

Being different from the group in a room walled with mirrors takes courage, conviction, and a sense of humor. The most important thing you can do for yourself is to choose an instructor who encourages everyone to exercise at their own pace and a class where people are friendly and having fun. Observe classes, speak with instructors, and participate in at least one class session before committing to and paying for a class.

Before starting an exercise class, consider these tips:

- Wear comfortable, well-fitting shoes with nonslip soles.

- Protect your knees. Keep your knees relaxed (aerobics instructors call this "soft knees").

- Don't overstretch. The beginning (warm-up) and end (cool-down) of the session will include stretching and strengthening exercises. Remember to stretch only as far as you comfortably can. Hold the position, and don't bounce. If needed, ask your instructor for an alternative exercise.

- Alternate the kinds of exercise you do. Many exercise facilities have a variety of exercise opportunities, including equipment rooms with cardiovascular machines, pools, and aerobics studios. If you have trouble with an hour-long aerobics class, see if you can join the class for the warm-up and cool-down and use a stationary bicycle or treadmill during the aerobics portion. Many people have found that this routine gives them the benefits of both an individualized program and the social enjoyment of group exercise.

■ There are many excellent exercise YouTube videos, DVDs, and videotapes for use at home. These vary in intensity, from very gentle chair exercises to more strenuous aerobic exercise. Review the videos and ask your health care provider, therapist, or exercise professional for suggestions.

Self-Tests for Endurance: Checking Your Progress

For some people, feeling more energetic and healthier is enough to indicate progress. Others may need proof that their endurance exercise program is making a measurable difference. To measure your success, use one or both of the endurance fitness tests described in this section. Pick the one that works best for you. Record your results before you start. After two to four weeks of exercise, repeat the test and check your improvement. Talk to your health care providers or exercise professionals to set reasonable and safe goals for yourself.

■ **Measure by distance.** For walking and bicycling, note how far you go in a set time. See how far you travel in 5 or 10 minutes, for example. Measure distance by counting how many blocks you go or keep track of your steps with a step monitor. If you are swimming, count the lengths of the pool. Your goal is to cover more distance in less time or the same distance with less exertion.

■ **Measure by time.** Measure a given distance to walk, bike, swim, or water-walk. You can pick a few blocks, measure an actual distance, or determine lengths in a pool. Start timing and move at a moderate pace. At the end of the distance, record how long it took you to cover your course and your perceived exertion (on a scale from 1 to 10). Your goal is to complete the distance in less time or with less exertion.

Exercise Opportunities in Your Community

Many people who exercise regularly do so with at least one other person. Two or more people can keep each other motivated. A whole class can become a circle of friends. On the other hand, exercising alone gives you the most freedom. You may feel that there are no classes that would work for you, or you don't have a buddy to accompany you. If so, use the suggestions in this chapter and Chapter 8, *Exercising to Feel Better*, to design your own program. As you progress, you may find that these feelings change.

Most communities offer a variety of exercise classes, including special programs for people over 50, adaptive exercises, mall walking, fitness trails, tai chi, and yoga. The following are good places to look for classes:

■ **Check with the local Y, community and senior centers, parks and recreation programs, adult education classes,** organizations for specific conditions (e.g., arthritis, diabetes, cancer, heart disease), and community colleges. These programs vary widely in terms of what they offer and in the training of the exercise staff. The classes usually are inexpensive, and the staff is responsive to people's needs.

■ **There are several exercise programs that research has shown to be helpful to older people as well as people with arthritis and other specific conditions.** To find one of these programs, visit the Evidence-Based Leadership Collaborative's website at www.eblcprograms.org/evidence-based/map -of-programs/.

■ **Public health offices often sponsor classes that are appropriate for a wide range of ages and needs.**

■ **Hospitals often have medically supervised classes for people with heart or lung disease (cardiac or pulmonary rehabilitation classes).** These programs tend to be more expensive than other community classes, but they may include medical supervision.

■ **Health and fitness clubs usually offer aerobics or aerobic fitness classes, weight training, cardiovascular equipment, and sometimes a heated pool.** They charge membership fees.

Your Exercise Program: Solving Possible Problems

Table 7.2 lists a number of problems that may occur during exercise and possible solutions. Note that some concerns are serious enough that you should stop your exercise, seek help, and talk to a health care provider before resuming.

Table 7.2 **If Exercise Problems Occur**

Problem	Advice
Irregular or rapid heartbeat; pain, tightness, or pressure in the chest, jaw, arms, or neck	Stop exercising. Ask for help immediately. Contact your doctor. Don't exercise again until your doctor has cleared you.
Shortness of breath lasting past the exercise period	Tell your doctor right away. Don't exercise again until your doctor has cleared you.
Light-headedness, dizziness, fainting, cold sweat, or confusion	Lie down with your feet up or sit down with your head between your knees. Seek help and get medical advice immediately. Don't exercise again until your doctor has cleared you.
Shortness of breath or calf pain from circulation or breathing problems	Warm up by going slowly at first. Take short rests to recover, and keep going if you can. Contact your doctor. Don't exercise again until your doctor has cleared you.
Excessive tiredness after exercise, especially that continues into the next day	Exercise less hard next time. If tiredness lasts, check with your doctor.

Finding the Right Program for You

Ask about these things when you explore community programs:

- **Classes with moderate- and low-intensity exercise designed for beginners.** You should be able to observe classes and participate in at least one class before signing up and paying.

- **Qualified instructors who are experienced working with people who have similar abilities as you.** Knowledgeable and experienced instructors are more likely to understand special needs and be willing and able to work with you.

- **Membership policies that allow you to pay by the class or for a short series of classes or let you freeze your membership at times when you can't participate.** Some fitness facilities offer different rates depending on how many services you use.

- **Facilities that are easy to get to, park near, and enter.** Parking lots, dressing rooms, and exercise sites should be accessible, safe, and professionally staffed.

- **Staff and members who are friendly and easy to talk to.**

- **An emergency management protocol and instructors certified in CPR and first aid.**

■ ■ ■

This chapter has been about physical activity and endurance exercise. The next chapter, Chapter 8, *Exercising to Feel Better*, addresses posture, flexibility, strength, and balance. It discusses exercises you can choose to meet your needs and provides more information about community classes such as tai chi and yoga. It includes a full introduction to the Moving Easy Program (MEP), which is a comprehensive and gentle set of range-of-motion exercises, as well as self-tests to check your progress.

**For a complete list of suggested further readings,
useful websites, and other helpful resources, please see**

www.bullpub.com/resources.

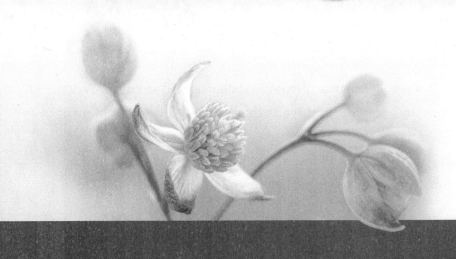

"The miracle is not that I finished, the miracle is that I had the courage to start."

—John Bingham,
Penguin Chronicles #1,
March 1995

CHAPTER 8

Exercising to Feel Better

A common problem with chronic pain is that if you have chronic pain, you often start using your body in different ways to try to lessen your pain. Perhaps you aren't as active and don't exercise as much. If this is happening to you and you recognize the changes, you are on the right track. There is an old adage: use it or lose it. If you don't use your body—by moving your muscles and joints and being active—you will start to lose stamina, strength, and flexibility. If you experience chronic pain and become less active and limit your usual activities, you may become depressed or anxious, feel tense, and experience more pain. As this happens, being active becomes harder and more painful. Often it seems easier to just stay still than to try to move and maybe hurt more.

In Chapter 7, *Exercising and Physical Activity for Every Body*, you learned about the different types of exercise you can do. That chapter discussed the importance of keeping physically active when you have chronic pain and how to fit at least 30 minutes of endurance exercise and physical activity into your day. This chapter contains illustrations and descriptions of specific exercises and exercise programs that you can safely do to feel more comfortable and relaxed and to improve your posture, flexibility, balance, and strength. When you improve these abilities, your daily life will be easier, more comfortable, and safer. Activity will be easier, less painful, and more rewarding. You will be healthier and feel better.

How to Use This Chapter

This chapter contains four sections. The first section, Body Builders, illustrates and describes four sets of specific exercises to meet specific needs for different parts of your body. The exercises in this section help you build good posture, steady balance, and strong legs, feet, and hands. These are exercises that you can do at home using this book, and illustrations and instructions are included for each exercise. The second section, Community Programs, provides information and tips on various classes and programs in tai chi, yoga and water exercise that are available in many communities and online. The third section, The Moving Easy Program (MEP), provides complete instructions for 26 gentle exercises that make up a program that promotes flexibility and relaxation. The MEP exercises are illustrated, and there is an audio CD that will help you perform the exercises. The fourth section, Self-tests for Checking Your Progress, shows some ways you can check your exercise progress.

Deciding what you want to be able to do—feel less tense, be more flexible, have better balance, or be stronger—and making your own plan are the first steps to finding and doing the activities that work for you. There are many choices in each section of the chapter. You can choose one way to begin, add or subtract an activity as you go along, and mix and match to meet your needs.

For example, you could choose to do the balance exercises every morning and Moving Easy Program (MEP) in the afternoon. Or you could do posture exercises three days a week, MEP twice a week, and attend a weekend yoga class. By adding some exercises in this chapter to your endurance exercise habit, you are building a comprehensive fitness program. Experiment, see how you feel, and suit yourself. It is your choice and your plan.

Body Builders

This section is divided into four sets of exercises.

- **Very Important for Posture (VIP).** Seven exercises for your back and trunk and that remind your body of good posture.

- **Strong Legs (SL).** Five exercises to strengthen your legs.

- **Better Balance (BB).** Seven exercises to improve your standing and walking balance.

- **Hands and Feet (HF).** Six exercises that are helpful for stiff or weak wrists, hands, ankles and feet.

General Instruction for Body Builder Exercises

If you are limited by pain, muscle weakness, or joint tightness, do these exercises as completely as you can. *The benefit of doing an exercise comes from moving toward a certain position, not from being able to complete the movement perfectly.* In some cases, you may find that after a while you can complete the movement and increase your available range of motion. At other times you may need to keep doing it your own modified way.

As you begin to exercise, keep the following tips in mind:

- Move at a comfortable speed. Do not bounce or jerk.
- Maintain good posture. Imagine a string at the top of your head being gently tugged up toward the ceiling.
- Stop if your body starts to hurt. Stretching should feel good, not painful.
- Start with no more than five repetitions of a new exercise. Increase the number of repetitions gradually as you figure out what works for you.
- Always do the same number of exercises on both your left and right side.
- Breathe naturally. Do not hold your breath. Count out loud to make sure you are breathing.

Exercises That Are Very Important for Posture (VIP)

As we learned in Chapter 6, *Organizing and Pacing Your Life for Pain Self-Management and Safety*, good movement starts with good posture. Proper body mechanics and proper posture during daily activities help you manage pain. If you have neck or back pain or are not sure if these exercises are right for you, check with your doctor, physical therapist, or other health care provider before you begin.

1. Heads Up (VIP)

This exercise relieves jaw, neck, and upper back tension or pain and helps you learn and maintain good posture. You can do the Heads Up while driving, sitting at a desk, sewing, reading, or exercising. Just sit or stand straight and gently slide your chin back. Keep looking forward as you move your chin backward. You'll feel the back of your neck lengthen and straighten. To help do it correctly, put your finger on your nose and pull your head straight back away from your finger.

(Don't worry about a little double chin—you will look much better with your neck straight!)

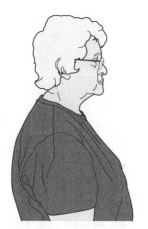 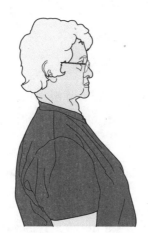

Clues for Finding the Correct Heads-Up Position:

- ears over shoulders, not out in front
- head balanced over neck and trunk, not out in front
- back of neck vertical and straight up and down, not leaning forward
- bit of double chin

2. Good Morning (VIP)

This exercise can be done sitting or standing. Start with your hands in front of you in gentle fists, palms facing your body and wrists crossed. Breathe in and stretch out your fingers while you uncross your arms and reach up for the sky. Stretch. Breathe out and move your arms back down and relax.

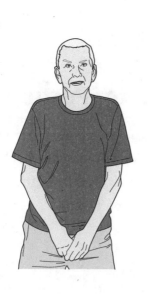 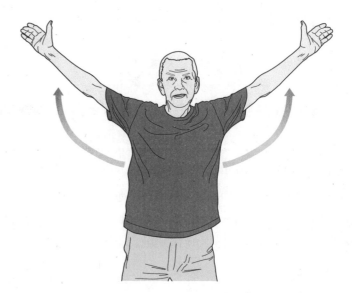

3. Shoulder-Blade Pinch (VIP)

This is a good exercise to strengthen the middle and upper back and to stretch the chest. Sit or stand with your head in Heads Up position (see page 159) and your shoulders relaxed. Raise your arms out to the sides with arms bent at the elbows and your fingers pointed to the ceiling. Pinch your shoulder blades together by moving your elbows as far back as you can. Hold briefly, and then slowly move your arms forward to touch elbows. If this position is uncomfortable, lower your arms or rest your hands on your shoulders as you move your elbows back and forth.

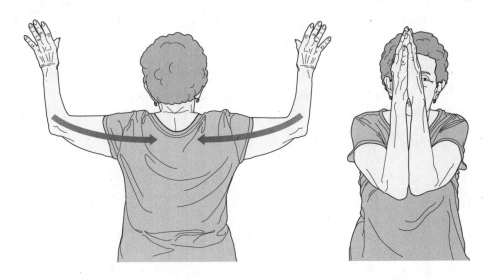

4. Curve and Arch (VIP)

This exercise improves back flexibility. When you first start doing this exercise, keep your movements small so that you do not strain your lower back. Start by sitting slightly forward in a straight-backed chair or bench. Sit up straight with your head over your shoulders and shoulders over your hips. Place your feet flat on the floor. Exhale slowly and reach forward. Bring your belly toward your spine and move your lower back toward the back of the chair. Allow your back and shoulders to round, your head to come forward, and your chin to come toward your chest so your back is in a curve. Pause. Inhale and bring your chest forward as you straighten up and arch your back. As you do this, raise your head and gently look up as far as is comfortable. Repeat several times at your own pace.

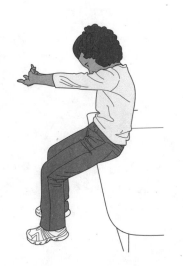
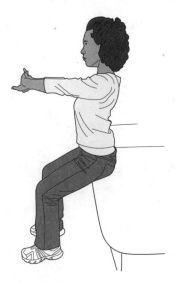

5. Pelvic Tilt (VIP)

The Pelvic Tilt is an excellent exercise for the lower back and can help relieve lower back pain. Lie on your back with knees bent, feet flat. Place your hands on your stomach. Flatten the small of your back against the floor by tightening your stomach muscles and your buttocks. Tilt your tailbone upward and pull your belly in. Think about trying to pull your stomach in enough to zip a tight pair of trousers. Hold the tilt for 5 to 10 seconds. Relax. Arch your back slightly. Relax and repeat. Don't forget to breathe! Count the seconds out loud. Once you've mastered the Pelvic Tilt lying down, practice it sitting, standing, and walking.

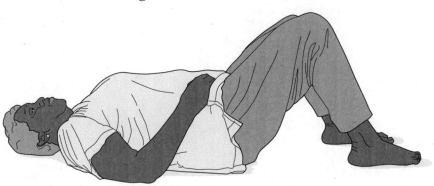

6. Back Lift (VIP)

This two-part exercise improves back and trunk flexibility. If you have moderate to severe lower back pain, do not do this exercise unless it has been specifically prescribed for you.

Part I: Lie on your stomach and rise up onto your forearms. Keep your back relaxed and your stomach and hips down. If this is comfortable, begin to straighten your elbows and raise your chest up away from the surface, arching your back as much as you comfortably can. Breathe naturally and relax for at least 10 seconds.

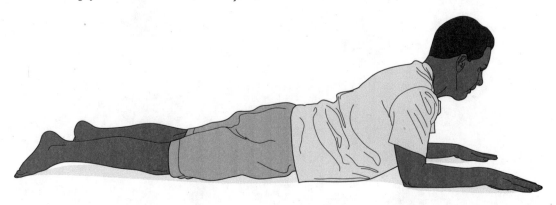

Part II: Lie on your stomach with your arms at your side or above your head. Lift your head, shoulders, and arms off the ground and hold them above the ground. Do not look up. Keep looking down with your chin tucked into a double-chin position. Count out loud to 10 as you hold this position. Relax. You can also lift your legs off the floor instead of your head and shoulders. Note that lifting both ends of your body at once is a fairly strenuous exercise and may not be helpful for a person with back pain.

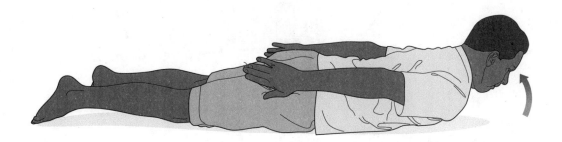

7. Back Kick (VIP)

The Back Kick increases the backward mobility and strength of your hip, making good posture easier. Hold on to a counter for support. Move your leg up and back, knee straight. Stand tall and do not lean forward. You probably will feel some stretching in front of your hip. Repeat with the other leg.

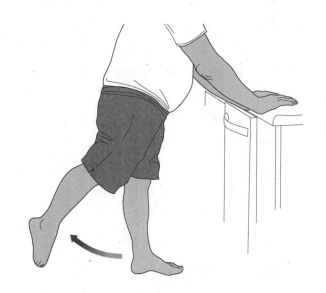

Exercises for Strong Legs (SL)

Strong hips, legs, and knees are important for walking and standing comfortably. These exercises improve your leg strength, which can help you be more safe when you are being physically active.

8. Straight-Leg Raise (SL)

Straight-Leg Raises strengthen the muscles that bend your hips and straighten your knees. Lie on your back, knees bent, feet flat. Straighten one leg. Tighten the muscle on the top of that thigh, and straighten that knee as much as possible. Keeping your knee straight, raise that leg off the ground. Do not arch your back. If your back starts to arch, lower your leg until you can hold your back flat. Hold your leg up, and count out loud for 10 seconds. Remember to breathe. Relax. Repeat with the other leg.

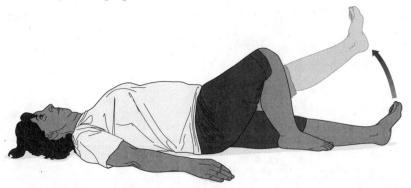

9. Knee Strengthener (SL)

Sitting in a chair, straighten your knee by tightening the muscle on the top surface of your thigh. Place your hand on your thigh and feel the muscle tighten. If you wish, draw circles with your toes while holding your foot up in the air. As your knee gets stronger, see if you can build up to holding your leg out for 30 seconds. Count out loud. Do not hold your breath. Repeat with the other leg.

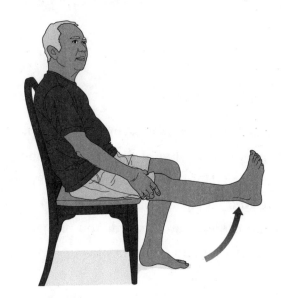

10. Power Knee (SL)

The Power Knee exercise strengthens the muscles that bend and straighten your knees. Sit in a chair and cross your legs at the ankles. Your legs can be almost straight, or you can bend your knees as much as you like. Try several positions. Push forward with your back leg, and press backward with your front leg. Exert pressure evenly so that your legs do not move. Hold and count out loud for 10 seconds. Relax. Switch leg positions. Be sure to keep breathing. Repeat.

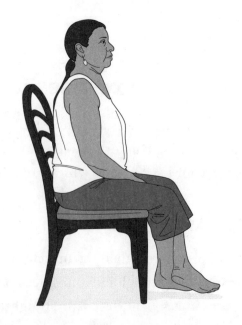

11. Sit-to-Stand (SL)

In this exercise you practice standing up without using your arms. Sit toward the front edge of a straight-backed chair that has arms and a firm seat. Bend your knees so that your feet are flat on the floor and behind your knees. Lean a bit forward and stand up. Practice moving from a sitting to a standing position using your arms as little as possible. At first you may need to push up with your arms. Stand up five times. Rest a bit and stand up five more times. As your hips and legs get stronger, you will be able to stand without using your arms.

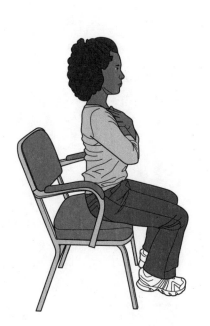
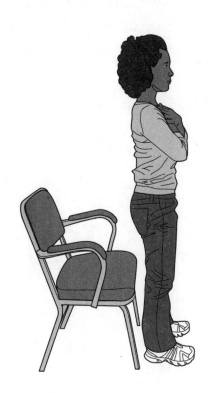

12. Ready-Go (SL)

Stand with one leg slightly in front of the other with your heel on the floor as if you are about to take a step down with the front foot. Now tighten the muscles on the front of your thigh, making your knee firm and straight. Hold to a count of 10. Relax. Repeat with the other leg. You can also do this exercise when you first stand up before you take your first step. It reminds your knees to be ready to bear weight and can make your first steps more comfortable.

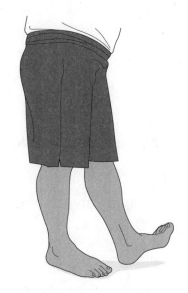

Exercises for Better Balance (BB)

The exercises in this section allow you to practice balance activities in a safe and progressive way. We list the exercises in order of difficulty. Start with the first exercises and work up to the more difficult ones as your strength and balance improve. If you feel that your balance is particularly poor, exercise with someone close by who can give you a supporting hand. Always exercise by a counter or stable chair that you can hold on to if necessary. Signs of improving balance include being able to hold a position longer or without extra support and being able to do the exercise or hold the position with your eyes closed.

13. Beginning Balance (BB)

Stand with your feet comfortably apart. Place your hands on your hips and turn your head and trunk as far to the left as possible and then to the right. Repeat five to ten times. To increase the difficulty, do the same thing with your eyes closed.

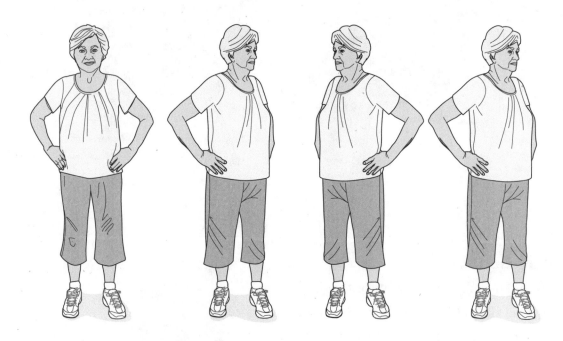

14. Swing, Sway, and March Away (BB)

With both hands on a counter or the back of a stable chair for support, repeat these two exercises five to ten times each:

1. Rock back on your heels and then rise up on your toes. Do this ten times. Don't hurry.

2. March in place for five to ten steps, first with eyes open and then with eyes closed.

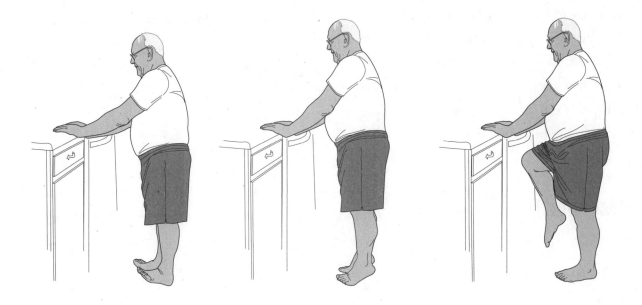

15. Walk the Line (BB)

Find a place to walk a few steps next to a kitchen counter or in a hallway with handrails (so you have support if you need it).

Walk a few steps in a line touching your heel to toe with each step (also called tandem walking). At first you will probably look down to watch your feet, but with practice you will be able to look straight ahead.

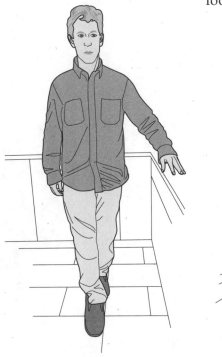

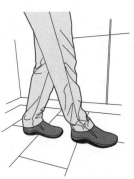

16. Base of Support (BB)

Do these exercises with someone nearby to help or standing close to a counter. The purpose of these exercises is to help you improve your balance by going from a larger to a smaller base of support. Repeat each of the three steps. Try to hold each position for 10 seconds. When you can do it with your eyes open, practice with your eyes closed.

1. Stand with feet together.
2. Stand with one foot out in front and the other back.
3. Stand heel to toe.

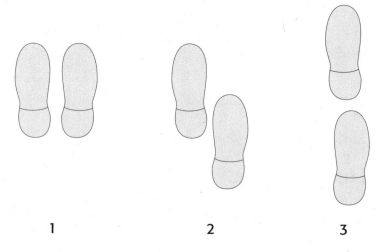

1   2   3

17. Toe Walk (BB)

The Toe Walk exercise increases ankle strength. It also helps you practice balancing on a small base of support while moving. Stay close to a counter for support. Rise up on your toes and walk along the counter. Once you are comfortable walking on your toes without support and with your eyes open, try the Toe Walk with your eyes closed. Always stay next to support.

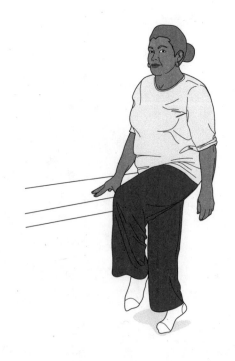

18. Heel Walk (BB)

The Heel Walk exercise increases your lower leg strength. It also helps you practice moving on a small base of support. Stay close to a counter for support. Raise your toes and forefoot and walk along the counter on your heels. Once you are comfortable walking on your heels without support and with your eyes open, try the Heel Walk with your eyes closed. Stay close to your support.

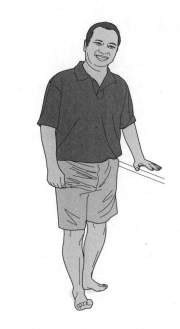

19. One-Legged Stand (BB)

Holding on to a counter or chair, lift one foot completely off the ground. Once you are balanced, take your hand off of the counter or chair. The goal is to maintain the position without holding on for 10 seconds. Once you can do this for 10 seconds without holding on, practice it with your eyes closed. Repeat for the other leg. Always stay close to support.

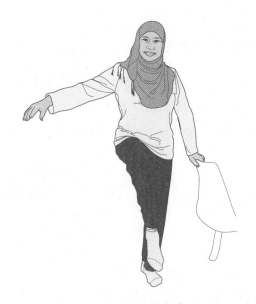

Exercises for Hands and Feet (HF)

Weak or stiff hands and feet can be a source of pain and frustration. Stronger wrists and hands make almost everything you do easier. Ankles and toes are important for moving and standing comfortably. These exercises can improve your flexibility and strength and may help you self-manage your pain.

20. Thumb Walk (HF)

Holding your wrist straight, form the letter O with one hand by lightly touching your thumb to each fingertip until your thumb has touched each one of your fingers. After you form each O, straighten and spread your fingers. Use the other hand to help if needed. Repeat with the other hand. It may be easier to start doing this with your forearms resting on a table.

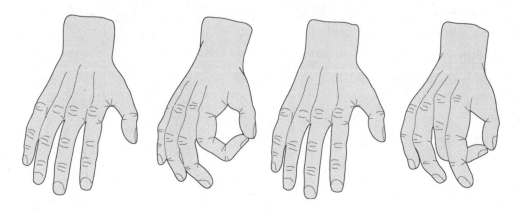

21. Wrist Stretch Down (HF)

Start with your arms at your sides, elbows straight and hands relaxed. Make a fist with each hand and bend at the wrists to lower your knuckles down toward the floor until you feel a stretch in your forearms. Hold for 5 seconds. Repeat several times.

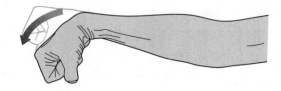

22. Wrist Stretch Up (HF)

Start with an arm out in front of you, elbow straight and palm facing away from you. Put your opposite hand over the away-facing palm. Gently stretch your hand back toward you until you feel a stretch. Hold for 5 seconds. Repeat several times. Repeat with the other hand and arm.

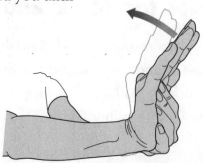

23. Towel Grabber (HF)

Sit on a sturdy chair with bare feet. Spread a towel in front of your chair. Place one foot on top of the towel, with your heel near the edge of the towel that is closest to you. Keep your heel on the ground. Now curl and then straighten your toes repeatedly to grab the towel and pull it back underneath your foot. When you have done this as much as you can, reverse the toe motion and scoot the towel forward again. Repeat with the other foot.

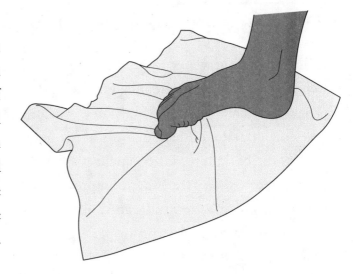

24. Marble Pickup (HF)

Place several marbles on the floor between your feet. Do this exercise one foot at a time. Using one foot, keep your heel down and pivot your toes and forefoot toward the marbles. Pick up a marble with your toes and pivot your foot to drop the marble as far as you can to the other side. Repeat until all the marbles have been moved. Reverse the process, returning all the marbles to the starting position. Repeat the entire exercise with the other foot. If marbles are difficult, try other objects, such as jacks, dice, or small wads of paper.

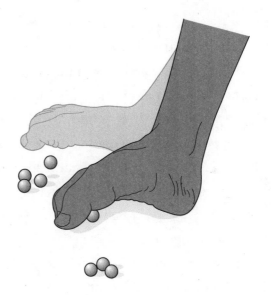

25. Foot Roll (HF)

Place a rolling pin (or a large dowel, closet rod, or bottle) under the arch of your foot and roll it back and forth. This feels great, like a massage, and stretches the ligaments in the arch of your foot. Repeat with the other foot.

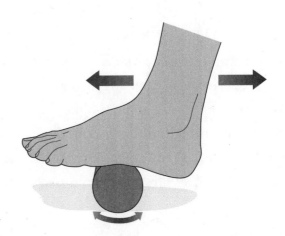

Community Programs: Water Exercise, Tai Chi, and Yoga

Exercising in the water is another gentle way to be more active and introduce variety to your program of activities. The buoyancy of water takes the pressure off painful areas of the body such as the back, hips, knees, and feet. Shallow water exercise is a great way to improve your flexibility, strength, and endurance. You do not have to know how to swim to participate in water fitness classes.

In general, people with chronic pain should avoid jogging and hopping, whether on dry land or in water. Be sure to tell your water exercise instructor that you have chronic pain. They can modify exercises for you if needed. If you are a swimmer, know that certain swimming strokes may aggravate your pain problem, while other strokes may be ideal. Always consult with your health care provider to be sure that the exercise you choose is right for you. You can read more about water exercise in Chapter 7, *Exercising and Physical Activity for Every Body*, pages 149–150.

Tai chi and yoga are excellent forms of exercise that involve the mind and the body. Both combine strength and flexibility training with relaxation and aim to reduce stress and tension. Tai chi is suited to many people with chronic pain because it involves gentle, slow, relaxed movements that safely increase flexibility, build strength, and improve balance. In fact, tai chi is often referred to as "moving meditation." Tai chi is good for young and old alike, for those without chronic conditions, and those who have chronic health problems and chronic pain. Recent scientific studies have found that tai chi

and a related practice from Eastern traditions called qigong are beneficial for those with fibromyalgia and osteoarthritis as well as for general health and well-being. For more information, visit the website of the National Center for Complementary and Integrative Health (www.nccih.nih.gov/health/tai-chi-and-qi-gong-in-depth).

Yoga combines physical postures, breathing techniques, and relaxation. Recent studies have found that people with lower back pain improved their ability to walk and move and had reduced pain after they practiced an adapted set of yoga poses. Other studies have found that yoga helps relieve anxiety and depression, may reduce blood pressure, and improves balance and reduces falls in older adults.

Be aware that there are many types of yoga practice, and some are more demanding and difficult than others. If yoga is of interest to you, investigate the classes available in your community. Contact instructors to find out if they have knowledge of chronic pain and how to adapt yoga poses for your needs. To learn more general information about yoga's health benefits, visit the website of the National Center for Complementary and Integrative Health (www.nccih.nih.gov/health/yoga-what-you-need-to-know).

Again, always talk with your health care providers or physical therapists before starting a new movement or exercise program. Tell them about any complementary or alternative practices you use to manage your chronic pain and your overall health. This will help ensure you have the safest experience possible.

The Moving Easy Program (MEP)

The Moving Easy Program (MEP) will help you improve and maintain flexibility. Flexibility refers to the ability of muscles and joints to move comfortably through a full range of motion. As an example, think of your wrist. You can make a circle with your wrist going clockwise and counterclockwise. You can extend your wrist back and flex it forward. Holding your forearm straight in front of you, you can move your hand to the right and to the left by using your wrist. These moves keep your wrists flexible by putting your wrist through its range of motion. Range-of-motion exercises gently stretch the muscles that act on the joint. This kind of range-of-motion exercise and gentle stretching helps keep you flexible.

When in pain, people tend to hold their muscles in tension, which leads to restricted movement, and joints become stiff. As a consequence, you become less flexible and have limited range of motion of your joints. This becomes a vicious cycle because the less flexible you are, the less you do and the more your muscles shorten and weaken, which leads to even less flexibility and more discomfort and pain and so on.

Flexibility exercises, like the ones in the MEP, help loosen tight muscles and joints and reduce stiffness so it's easier to get going in the mornings. These exercises are gentle so they can be done every day, even on days when you are not feeling your best. Flexibility exercises help with relaxation by promoting body awareness, which leads to improved posture and better breathing. And because they increase circulation to muscles and joints, flexibility exercises are a great way to warm up or cool down before and after aerobic exercise.

Once you have learned the sequence of moves in the program, you can include the Moving Easy Program (MEP) in your exercise routine as a warm-up or cool-down to aerobic exercise. You can also do the MEP by itself to promote relaxation and relieve stress and tension.

Moving Easy Program Precautions and Suggestions

The Moving Easy Program is an enjoyable way to safely improve your flexibility. It gently loosens muscles and joints and increases circulation. It incorporates the whole body and is not meant to be strenuous. The MEP consists of 26 movements that take less than 15 minutes to do. Flexibility exercises and gentle strength training combine with better breathing to reduce stress and tension. The program is safe for almost all people with chronic pain. An audio CD of the 26 moves is included with this book. Use the CD and the illustrations on pages 175–189 as your guide when doing the MEP at home. You can also stream the audio online at www.bullpub.com/mep. The box on page 174 lists important tips to keep in mind as you get started with the MEP.

Read and follow these eight precautions and suggestions as you begin the MEP:

1. The MEP program contains gentle neck and back exercises. If you have neck or back

Moving Easy Program (MEP) Tips

Getting Ready

- Clear your mind of any worries or unnecessary thoughts. Focus your mind on the present.
- Monitor your breathing. Take deep, relaxed breaths.
- Be aware of your posture. Maintain good posture by imagining a string at the top of your head being gently tugged up toward the ceiling.

Being Mindful

- Pay attention to your joints as you move. Move gently but with purpose.
- Move slowly. Don't jerk or bounce.
- Relax as you move, paying special attention to your shoulders. Your shoulders should be soft and relaxed.
- Keep breathing as you move. Don't hold your breath.
- Never force beyond what is comfortable.

pain or are not sure if these exercises are right for you, check with your doctor, physical therapist, or other health care provider before doing these exercises.

2. If there are some moves in the MEP you know are not right for you, don't do them. Instead, modify the moves (see suggestion 7 in this list) or just imagine you are doing them. Scientific evidence suggests that imagining moving an area of the body actually activates areas of the brain and stimulates nerves that connect to that part of the body.

3. Loosen your joints and relax your muscles with the MEP before doing your aerobic endurance exercise.

4. You can do the MEP even on days when you don't feel your best because it is not a strenuous program. Do be sure, however, to modify the movements to avoid any increased pain or stress on days when you don't feel 100 percent.

5. Although your long-term goal should be to be able to do MEP exercises with your full range

of motion, always avoid straining or forcing beyond your comfort level. Your goal is not to be perfect but to reach a level of flexibility and fitness where moving feels good!

6. When moving from sitting to standing positions, avoid tipping your midsection/waist area backward, which may strain your lower back.

7. Modify any of the MEP movements if you are not able to perform the specific moves. For example, if you are unable to stand, you can modify most of the exercises so you can do them while sitting.

8. To gently increase the active range of motion of a specific joint, move the joint to the point of comfort, pause and relax, and then move it again without straining.

Moving Easy Program Instructions

Begin by placing a stable chair in an area where you have enough space to move freely. Sit down and get comfortable. Take a few moments to clear your mind. Start by focusing on your breathing. Take a few deep, relaxing breaths in and out before beginning. Remember to breathe naturally throughout the program and to not hold your breath.

1. Raise It Up (MEP)

Inhale, then lift your arms, raising them as high as you can, very gently and slowly. If you can, raise your arms past your shoulders. Bring your hands together and guide them down toward the center of your body in prayer position. Repeat this, lifting your hands and arms up, placing hands together, and guiding them down. Finish by guiding your arms back down to the side of your body.

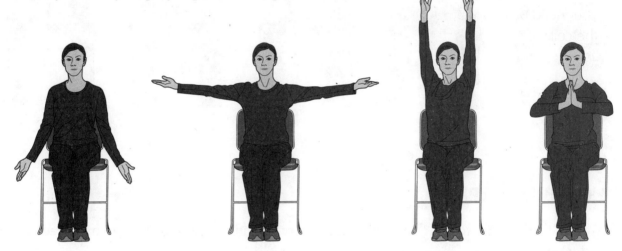

2. Ear to Shoulder (MEP)

Focusing on moving your head rather than your shoulders, bring your ear toward your shoulder. Hold this stretch for a few seconds and then return to center. Repeat on the other side, gently dropping your ear to your shoulder. Hold this stretch for a few seconds and then and return to center.

(Note: For every move in the MEP, "return to center" means "go back to the starting position.")

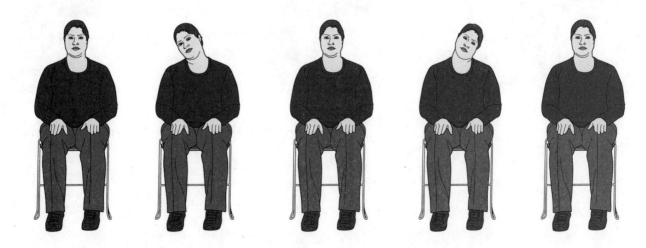

3. Side Look (MEP)

Gently turn just your head and look to the side. You may feel a stretch or tension release. Return to center. Repeat on the other side, gently looking to the other side, holding your stretch for a few seconds, and returning to center.

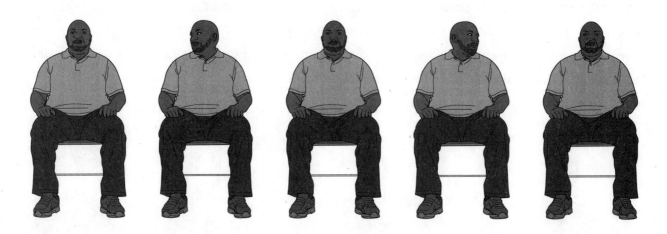

4. Head Bow (MEP)

Drop your head gently to your chest and hold your chin down for a few seconds to feel tension leave that area. Return to center. Repeat on the other side, gently dropping your head forward and returning to center.

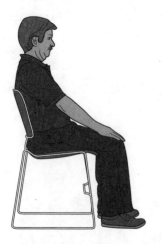 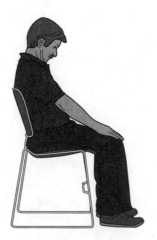 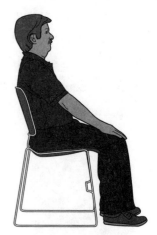

5. Shoulder Rolls (MEP)

Bring your attention to your shoulders and begin to make small, gentle circles forward. Start with small circles and increase them, remembering that even the smallest of movements can be beneficial. Reverse this circular movement, making small, gentle circles and increasing them and feel the tension start to ease. Repeat backward and forward a few times.

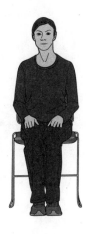 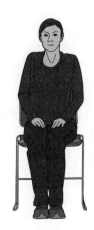 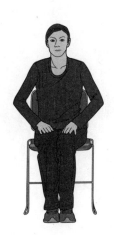 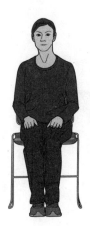

6. Side Turn (MEP)

Placing both hands on one thigh and using your body's midsection, gently look to the side by turning your head, shoulders, and chest. Hold for a few seconds. You should feel a lengthening of your spine. Come back to center. Now place your hands on the other thigh and gently turn your head, shoulders, and chest to the other side, feeling your body lengthen. Come back to center. Repeat these moves two more times, first to one side and then to the other.

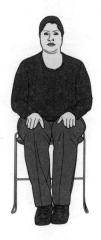 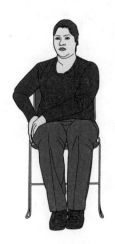 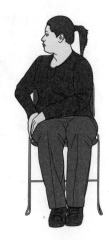 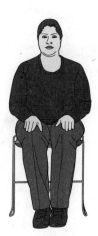

7. Scoop and Splash (MEP)

Reach your arms behind you with a large movement and move as if you are scooping water from beneath you. Slowly sit back up, splashing the water over your shoulders. Be sure to bend forward from the hips, keeping your back straight. Move to the best of your ability, with comfort and no pain. Do this two more times.

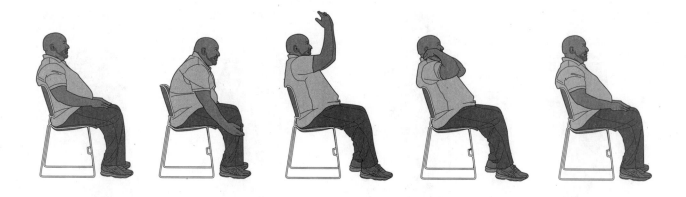

8. Squat Up (MEP)

If you are able to stand, using your hands, lean forward and lift yourself out of the chair. Focus on the large muscle groups in the tops of your legs and stand up. (Note: Avoid tipping your body backward since this may strain your lower back.)

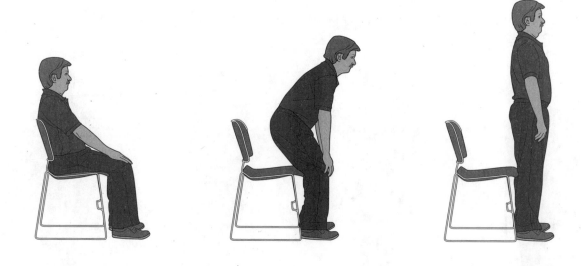

9. Leg Kicks (MEP)

Stand next to your chair. Holding gently on to the chair for balance, extend one leg forward as if moving your foot through a shallow pool of water . . . back and forth . . . back and forth . . . Repeat this a few more times.

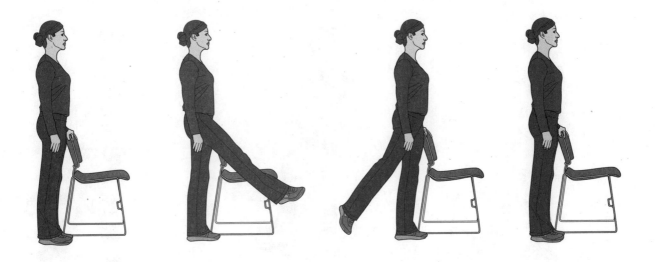

10. Leg Swing (MEP)

Continue standing next to your chair on the same side. Holding gently on to the chair for balance, gently glide the same leg from side to side in front of you as though moving it through a shallow pool of water. Repeat with gentle, slow, easy movements a few more times.

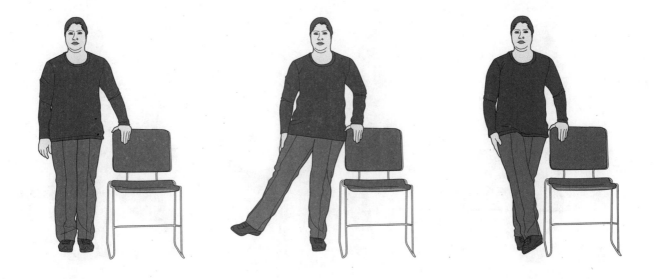

11. Flex and Point (MEP)

Continue standing next to your chair on the same side. Extend the same leg in front of you. Flex your toes up and then point your toes down. Feel the tension in your calf flexing up and releasing by pointing down. Repeat this again . . . up . . . and down . . . up . . . and down.

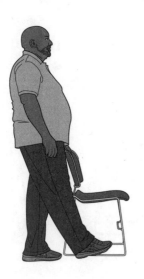 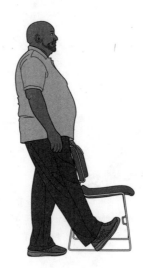 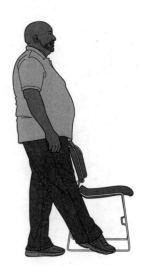

12. Leg Kicks (Other Side) (MEP)

Move to the other side of the chair. Holding gently on to the chair for balance, extend your other leg forward as if moving your foot through a shallow pool of water. Back and forth . . . back and forth. Repeat a few more times.

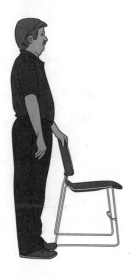 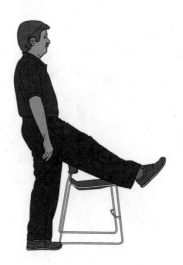 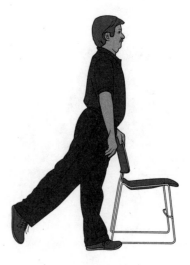

13. Leg Swing (Other Side) (MEP)

Standing on the same side of the chair and using the same leg, glide your leg through the imaginary water from side to side in front of you.

Repeat with gentle, slow, easy movements a few more times.

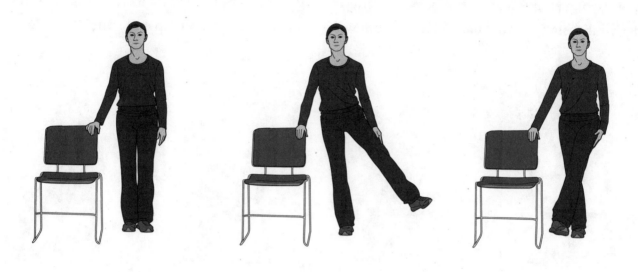

14. Flex and Point (Other Side) (MEP)

Standing on the same side of the chair and keeping the same leg extended in front of you, flex your toes up and point your toes down. Feeling the tension in your calf, flex up . . . and release by pointing down. Repeat a few more times.

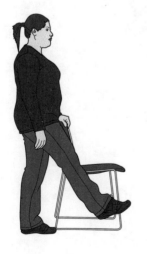
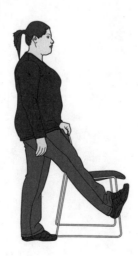
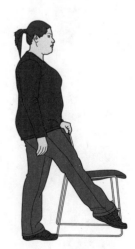

15. Squat Up and Down (MEP)

Return to the front of your chair so you can use the large muscles in the tops of your legs to squat up and down. Leaning slightly forward, slowly lower yourself into your chair, being mindful to let your weight sit on your heels as you lower yourself down. Now leaning forward slightly, lift yourself up out of your chair to a standing position, concentrating on your large muscle groups. Repeat this by slowly sitting back down and raising yourself up and sitting back down.

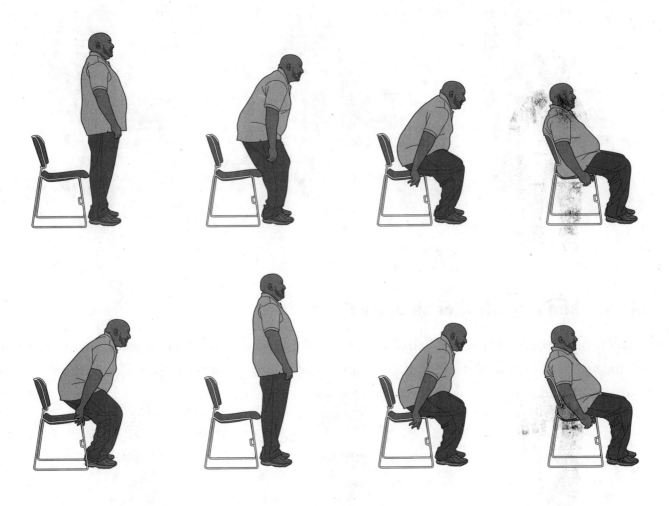

16. Knee to Chest (MEP)

While sitting, place both **hands under one** knee and gently bring your knee **up toward your** chest while sitting up straight **and keeping an** erect posture. (If you have a hip **or back problem**, you may want to lift your knee *without* **using** your hands.) **Feel a gentle stretch in your hip** and buttock area. Hold for two or three seconds and then place your leg back on the floor. Change legs and put your hands under your other knee and lift up and then place your leg back on the floor. Do this one more time on each side. Remember to keep your erect posture.

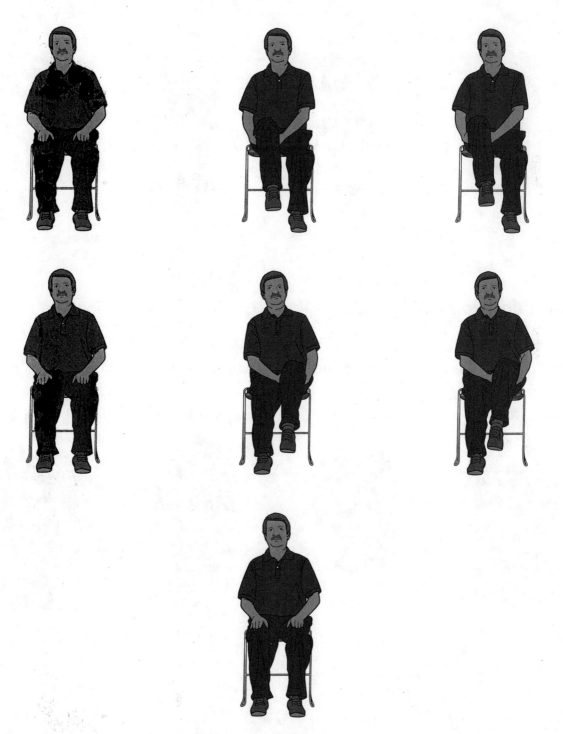

17. Abdominal Lean (MEP)

Sit down and slide slightly forward in your chair. Crossing your arms in front of your chest or holding on to the sides of your chair, lean back *very slowly*, to about 45 degrees, using your abdominal muscles. Hold for a few seconds and slowly return to center. Repeat a few more times. Lean back *very slowly*, to about 45 degrees. You should feel your abdominal muscles tighten, but only lean as far as is comfortable.

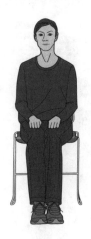 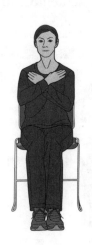 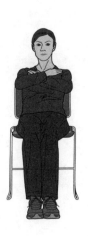 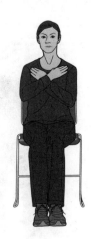

18. Ankle Rotation (MEP)

Sit on your chair and extend one foot in front of you, then rotate your ankle in one direction. Feel the tension release. Now rotate in the other direction. Do this a few times.

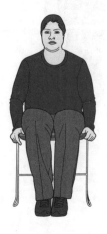 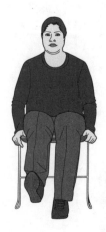 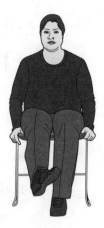 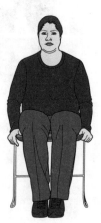

19. Hamstring Stretch (MEP)

Staying seated and placing your foot on the floor slightly in front of you, gently lean forward as if making a little bow to stretch the hamstring in the back of your knee. Move slowly, gently, and comfortably. Hold this stretch for a few seconds. Return to center. Do this one more time, going a little deeper if you can. Return to center.

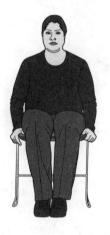 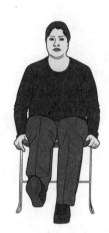 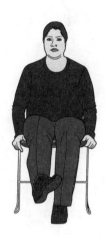 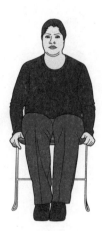

20. Ankle Rotation (Other Side) (MEP)

Still in a seated position, extend your other leg in front of you for ankle rotations. Rotate your ankle in one direction and then in the other direction. Repeat a few times.

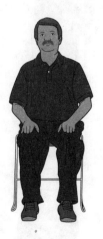 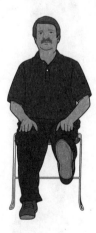 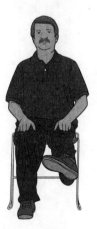

21. Hamstring Stretch (Other Side) (MEP)

In the same seated position, place the foot you did not extend last time slightly in front of you. Gently lean forward as if making a little bow. You should feel a stretch in the back of the knee.

Move slowly, gently, and comfortably. Hold this stretch for a few seconds. Return to center. Try this one more time, and if you can, bow a little deeper. Return to center.

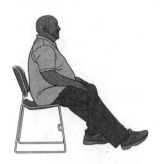 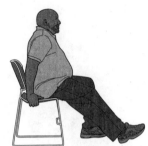 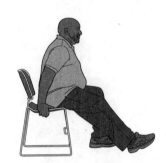 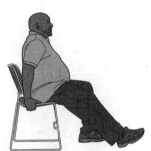

22. Side Stretch (MEP)

Take a deep breath in and a deep breath out. Lift both arms up over your head if you can and then gently lower one arm to your side. Move the lifted arm toward the center of your body, giving you an added stretch. Hold for a few seconds. Now gently lower the arm you have lifted and lift the other arm up. Move it toward the center and hold that stretch. Return to center. Repeat this again on both sides and return to center.

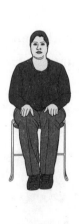 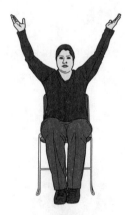 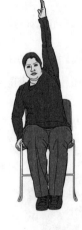

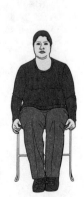 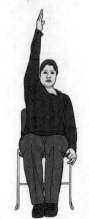 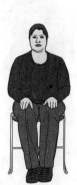

23. Bicep Curls/Wrist Flexion (MEP)

While seated, bring your arms in front of your body and bend your arms at the elbows, moving your hands up and in toward your shoulders. Make a gentle fist and extend your arms back out. Hold this position and feel the stretch in your forearms and the back of your hands. Repeat this a few more times, bringing your arms forward, curling your fists inward and up, and extending your fists out.

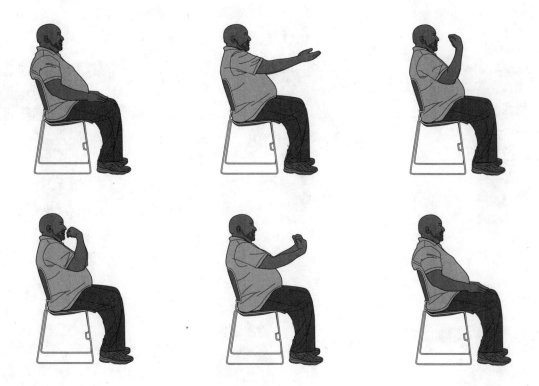

24. Wrist Rotations (MEP)

While seated, extend your arms (or lower them to rest on your legs if you wish). Rotate both wrists in a circular direction one way, then rotate them the other way.

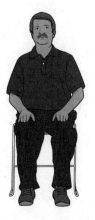 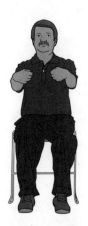 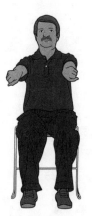 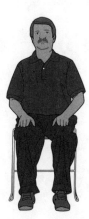

25. Wing Span Stretch (MEP)

While seated, lift your arms out to the side of your body as if they were wings. Move your hands back, opening your chest and holding this stretch for a few seconds. Keep your shoulders soft and relaxed. Bring your arms to the front of your body and hold your hands out in front. Lower your arms.

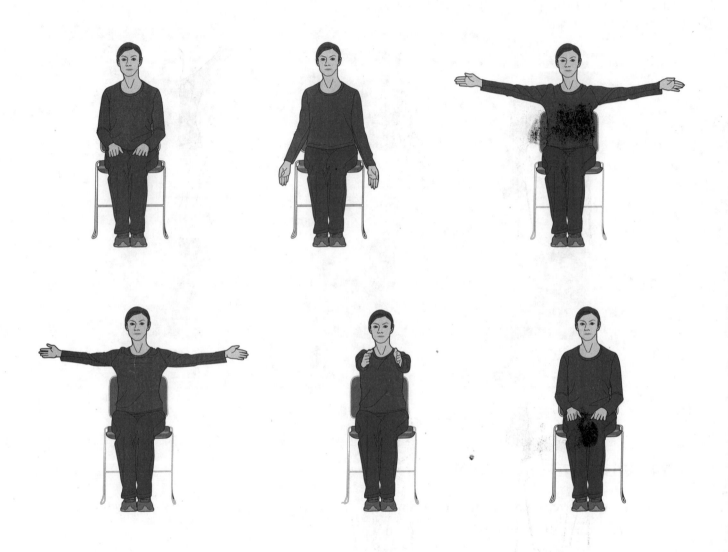

26. Raise It Up (MEP)

Take a deep, relaxed breath in and out. Lift your arms, raising them as high as is comfortable, very gently and slowly. Bring your hands together and guide them down toward the center of your body into prayer position. Finish by bringing your arms down through the center, exhaling as you do.

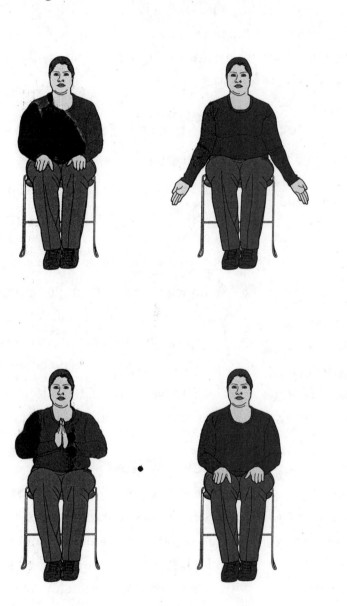

Self-Tests for Checking Your Progress

Most of the exercises in Body Builders, Community Programs, and the Moving Easy Program improve general strength, flexibility, and balance after a few weeks. Everybody wants to know that their efforts are making a difference, but change is gradual and it's often hard to see improvement. To monitor your progress, choose from these self-tests or design your own self-tests to measure progress toward your goal. Test yourself before you start your exercise program. Record the results. After two or three weeks, take the test again to check your improvement.

Arm and Shoulder Flexibility Self-Test

Stand facing a wall with your body almost touching the wall. One arm at a time, reach up the wall in front of you. Hold a pencil and mark the highest point you can reach, or have someone mark how far you can reach. Also do this reaching out sideways, standing about 3 inches (8 cm) away from the wall. *Goal:* To reach higher.

Hamstring Flexibility Self-Test

Do MEP Exercise 19 or 21, the Hamstring Stretch (page 185), one leg at a time. Keep your thigh (upper leg) perpendicular to your body. How much does your knee bend? How tight does the back of your leg feel? *Goal:* To have straighter knees and feel less tension in the back of the leg.

Ankle Flexibility Self-Test

Sit in a chair with bare feet flat on the floor and knees bent at a 90-degree angle. Keep your heels on the floor. Raise your toes and the front of your foot as high as you can while keeping your heels planted. Ask someone to measure the distance between the ball of your foot and the floor. *Goal:* For the distance between your foot and the floor to be 1 to 2 inches (2.5 to 5 cm).

Ankle Strength Self-Test

This test has two parts.

1. Stand at a table or counter for support. Stand on one foot and rise up on your toes as many times as you can without stopping. How many can you do before your tire?

2. Stand with your feet flat. Put most of your weight on one foot and quickly tap the floor with the front part of your other foot. How many taps can you do before you tire?

   Goal: To do a total of 10 to 15 repetitions of each movement without stopping.

Balance Self-Test

Do BB Exercise 19, One-Legged Stand (page 169). Time yourself and write down how long you can stand on each foot without needing to reach for support. Try with your eyes open and with your eyes closed. When you are ready to test your balance again, see if you can stand on one foot longer than you did last time. Also see if you can stand without support or balance with your eyes closed. *Goal:* To be able to balance on one foot with your eyes open for 30 seconds.

■ ■ ■

Whatever exercise you choose to do, how often you change what you do, or how long it takes you to do it, you know that successful self-management comes when you decide what you want to do, make a realistic plan, and do it. Success with even a small plan leads to confidence and more success. The quote at the beginning of this chapter—"the miracle is not that I finished, the miracle is that I had the courage to start"—rings true for most of us. It is courageous to begin when we are not sure what to do and not sure that we can be successful. But when we keep going and are successful, it is not a miracle. It is the well-earned benefit of making action plans and learning self-management skills.

**For a complete list of suggested further readings,
useful websites, and other helpful resources, please see**

www.bullpub.com/resources.

CHAPTER 9

Healthy Eating and Pain Self-Management

WHAT DOES NUTRITION HAVE TO DO WITH CHRONIC PAIN? Does what you eat really matter? Yes, nutrition and pain are related, and yes, what you eat is important. Although research on the relationship between nutrition and chronic pain is still at a relatively early stage, experts already agree that the best eating pattern or plan is a balanced and varied diet. We know that good nutrition is necessary for a healthy body and healing. More recent research also suggests that there are some foods that may help reduce inflammation. And, as we have discussed earlier, in some chronic pain conditions, inflammation is a factor. For example, there are some types of osteoarthritis where inflammation may occur. For some

Special thanks to Emily Clairmont, MS, RDN, CD, Ann Constance, MA, RDN, CDCES, FAADE, Robin Edelman, MS, RDN, CDCES, and Yvonne Mullan, MSc, RD, CDE, for their thoughtful and thorough contributions to this chapter.

193

About This Chapter

To write this chapter, we referenced the latest scientific research and used the USDA Dietary Guidelines, as well as information from the Centers for Disease Control and Prevention, the Academy of Nutrition and Dietetics, the American Heart Association, and the American Diabetes Association.

For Canadian information, we referenced Canada's Dietary Guidelines and information from the Public Health Agency of Canada, Dietitians of Canada, Heart and Stroke Foundation of Canada, and Diabetes Canada. (Please note that most Canadian-specific content is shaded.)

The overall focus is on scientific, evidence-based, nationally established nutrition guidelines.

people, a balanced and varied diet may be a diet that helps you maintain or reach a healthy weight (see Chapter 10, *Healthy Weight and Pain Self-Management*) and reduces inflammation (see *A Diet That Helps Fight Inflammation* on page 213).

In this book we present information about healthy eating, but we do not say there is one best way to apply these guidelines to your life. That is something you decide. There are different roads to healthy eating, and only you will know the best ways to do it for yourself. We offer suggestions that are working for other people and are based on research by nutrition experts.

There are many paths to healthy eating and many ways to learn about healthy eating. Some people prefer a less-detailed high-level view, and others want to know more details. We have tried to give you a little of both. And usually, we give high-level guidelines before providing details. You may want to read the chapter from beginning to end, or you may want to look at the topic headings and read only about the topics you find most interesting. If you just want quick tips for healthy eating, for example, read pages 217–219. This information is for you. Use it as you wish.

What Is Healthy Eating?

Healthy eating means making healthful food and drink choices most of the time. It does not mean being inflexible or perfect. Healthy eating can involve finding new or different ways to prepare your meals and snacks. If you have chronic pain, healthy eating may mean that you need to be choosier about what you eat and how much you eat. Healthy eating does not mean never enjoying your favorite foods. There is room in healthy eating to sometimes eat less healthy foods.

Why Is Healthy Eating So Important for Everyone?

Human bodies are complex and marvelous machines. Like an automobile, your body needs the proper mix of fuel. Without this, your body might "run rough" or even stop working. Healthy eating is important to every part of your life. It is linked to how you move, think, sleep, how much energy you have, and even your enjoyment of life. What you eat may also help prevent illnesses and promote healing from illnesses.

When you give your body the right fuel, you:

■ have more energy and feel less tired

■ increase your chances of preventing health conditions such as heart disease, diabetes, kidney disease, and cancer and lessen problems linked with health conditions you may already have

■ feed your brain, which can help you to better handle life's challenges

■ possibly sleep better

■ prevent weight gain that puts excess pressure on your hips, knees, ankles, and feet and can add to pain and loss of mobility

■ reduce inflammation, which in turn may affect chronic pain

■ possibly reduce some of the side effects of opioid pain relievers (see page 217)

Guidelines for Healthy Eating

There is no such thing as a perfect way to eat, but here we suggest some general guidelines to help you eat healthy:

■ Follow a healthy eating pattern no matter what your age, health conditions, or current weight. Healthy eating is for everyone.

■ Eat a variety of whole, unprocessed or less processed foods, especially fruits, vegetables, and whole grains, that are rich in vitamins, minerals, and other nutrients. (Nutrients are substances that provides nourishment essential for growth and the maintenance of life.)

■ Eat the right amount of food for your weight and health conditions. (See Chapter 10, *Healthy Weight and Pain Self-Management*.) Eat recommended portion sizes (what you actually put on your plate) and keep an eye on how many servings you eat. (A serving is a set amount determined by regulatory agencies such as the US Department of Agriculture.)

■ Use the USDA MyPlate (or Canada's Eat Well Plate) to help you choose the right amounts of healthy meals or snacks. Learn more about the plate method on pages 211–212.

- Limit added sugars, saturated fats, trans fats, and sodium (salt). Choose healthier fats (see page 212) and salt-free seasonings (herbs and spices).

- Eat a variety of lean protein foods, including seafood, lean meats and poultry, and legumes (dried beans, lentils, and split peas).

- Quench your thirst with beverages that you enjoy, but opt for choices without extra calories from sugar, such as unsweetened water, coffee, or tea.

- If you drink alcohol, limit the amount to one drink a day for women and two drinks a day for men. One alcoholic drink is 5 fluid ounces (148 mL) of wine, 12 fluid ounces (355 mL) of beer, or 1.5 fluid ounces (44 mL) of rum, vodka, whiskey, or other liquor.

- Allow yourself small occasional treats even if they are not the healthiest choices.

- If you are trying to improve your eating, shift gradually to healthier foods and drinks.

- Support others by being a model for healthy eating, and consider joining a support group (in person or online) to encourage your own healthy eating.

A real concern is the amount of less nutritious foods that people eat in place of healthy foods. This may be because less nutritious foods often cost less, are more available, are easy to fix, and taste good. About 75 percent of North Americans do not eat enough vegetables, fruits, and dairy. At the same time, many North Americans eat too many foods that are high in added sugars and sodium (salt); trans fats like stick margarine and hydrogenated oil; saturated fats from meats and coconut and palm oils; and high-fat dairy products such as butter, ice cream, and cheese. People in the United States and Canada also eat a lot of food that is made from white flour and other refined grains. These foods and added sugars, fats, and salt may be linked to health problems such as obesity, high blood pressure, diabetes, heart disease, and chronic pain.

The best evidence suggests that healthy eating focused on plant-based foods is best for both general health and pain. The Mediterranean diet is a good example of a dietary pattern for healthy eating. It is also an anti-inflammatory diet (see more about inflammation and food on page 213). Whatever you decide, do not make big changes in your daily food intake all at once. Make changes gradually.

The Mediterranean-Style Dietary Pattern

The Mediterranean diet is based on the traditional diet of Italy, Spain, and Greece. Consider the pyramid with four layers in Figure 9.1. The base of the pyramid shows the foods that should form the base of your eating. Most people benefit from eating more of these foods more of the time.

1. The base of the pyramid includes:
   - fruits
   - vegetables
   - dried beans and other legumes (such as lentils, navy beans, pinto beans, and split peas)
   - nuts and seeds
   - whole-grain bread, cereal, rice, and pasta

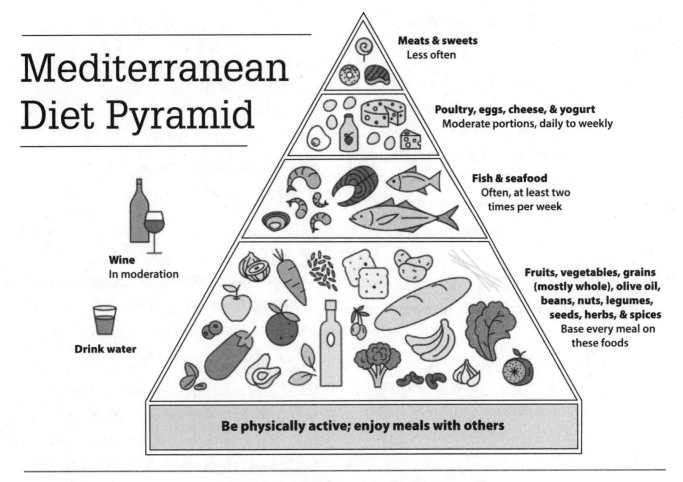

Figure 9.1 **Mediterranean Diet Pyramid**
©2017 America's Test Kitchen, www.americastestkitchen.com

- plant-based oils such as olive oil

- spices (without added salt)

2. The next layer in the pyramid is fish and seafood. These foods are OK to eat in moderate amounts often, at least twice a week.

3. The third layer is poultry, eggs, cheese, and yogurt. You can eat these foods daily to weekly. Eat these foods in moderate portion sizes.

4. At the very tip of the pyramid are red meats and sweets. Eat moderate portions of these foods no more than a few times per month.

Legumes

An essential food in the Mediterranean region, legumes contain anti-inflammatory nutrients and a good amount of protein. To boost plant-based foods in your diet, eat legumes in place of meat. Legumes include lentils, garbanzo beans, black beans, navy beans, pinto beans, and split peas.

5. Finally, the pyramid suggests you drink plenty of water and, if you drink wine (or any alcohol), do so in moderation.

Eating the Mediterranean Way

The Mediterranean diet advises you to:

- Work toward eating seven to ten servings of plant-based food a day. At least five of these servings should be from vegetables and fruit. (A serving of fruits or vegetables is 4 to 6 ounces, or 112 to 168 g—for more information on serving sizes, see page 200.)

- Eat fish and other seafood at least twice a week.

- Pass on the butter; instead, use olive oil or other plant-based oils for dipping bread and cooking.

- Eat nuts. Not only are they good for you, they also help fill you up. Do not go overboard, however. Eat small amounts, such as one serving (1/3 cup or 75 mL), a few times per week.

- Eat red meat less often (no more than a few times a month), and when you eat meat, choose small portions. Avoid fatty processed meats, such as bacon and sausage. Choose

Olive Oil

Extra-virgin olive oil (the least refined oil) has many benefits, including:

- Helping to prevent heart disease
- May help avoid blood clots
- Lowering blood pressure
- Reducing inflammation that my cause pain

poultry, eggs, and cheese more often than red meat on a daily to weekly basis.

- When you eat or drink dairy products and milk, choose low-fat options.

The Mediterranean diet may look quite different from how you eat now. Remember this motto: *"Go for the real, not the ideal."* You will be surprised at how small changes add up to big health gains. You can learn more about the Mediterranean-Style Dietary Pattern by visiting the Dietary Guidelines for Americans 2020–2025 website.*

---

*www.dietaryguidelines.gov/sites/default/files/2020-12/Dietary_Guidelines_for_Americans_2020-2025.pdf (table A3-5).

Healthy Vegetarian Eating

The Healthy Vegetarian Dietary Pattern is very similar to the Mediterranean-Style Dietary Pattern. In place of animal meat or fish, the vegetarian pattern suggests eggs, legumes (dried peas and beans), soy products, and nuts and seeds. You can learn more about the Healthy Vegetarian Dietary Pattern by visiting the Dietary Guidelines for Americans 2020–2025 website.†

---

†www.dietaryguidelines.gov/sites/default/files/2020-12/Dietary_Guidelines_for_Americans _2020-2025.pdf (table A3-4).

Knowing What and How Much to Eat

Eating well means knowing something about *what* you eat. It also means being mindful about *how much* you eat.

Portions and Servings

Many people make good food choices in terms of nutrients but eat more food than they need to maintain a healthy weight. Weight is a key factor in pain control, as excess weight puts extra pressure on bones, muscles, and joints. (To read more about weight and health, see Chapter 10, *Healthy Weight and Pain Self-Management*.) To understand healthy eating and to use the Nutrition Facts labels on packages and the charts in this book, you also need to know about portions and servings.

A portion is how much you actually eat. Another way you can remember this is that the word *portion* starts with the letter *p*, and a portion is what you put on your plate. If you eat a cup of ice cream, that is your portion. However, if you eat a half carton of ice cream, that is also your portion (and a likely cause of extra weight gain).

A serving is a standard amount used on a Nutrition Facts label or in the food charts of this book. A serving may be a different amount than the portion size you usually eat. For example, a serving may be half a cup or 4 ounces (118 mL). If you eat a full cup or 8 ounces (236 mL), you need to use math to figure how much calories and nutrients you are eating when you eat that portion. In this example, you are eating two servings (and therefore two times the calories and nutrients). Serving size also differs from one product to another. For some breakfast cereals, a serving is 1 cup (250 mL) and for others, a serving is 1/2 cup (125 mL). You can find out what a product's serving size is by reading the Nutrition Facts label on the food packaging.

The Nutrition Facts Label

Knowing what you are eating means knowing what nutrients are in foods. On pages 201–209, you can find a discussion of specific nutrients. There are several ways to find out what nutrients you are eating. You can read the Nutrition Facts labels on food packaging, which is the approach we discuss in this section of the chapter. (In Canada, these labels are referred to as Nutrition Facts tables.) You can also use the plate method for healthy eating explained on pages 211–212. And you can use the charts we have included at the end of this chapter in Appendix A: *Healthy Eating Patterns for 1,600 and 2,000 Calories* and Appendix B: *Food Groups for Meal Planning*. Or you can follow general guidelines provided by governmental agencies. We will discuss all of these. Feel free to use one or more of these ways, and mix and match as you choose. There are many different ways to help you make healthy food choices.

Labels such as the one shown in Figure 9.2 on the next page, along with the ingredients lists, can help you learn more about what is in the packaged foods you eat. The Nutrition Facts and the ingredients list are two key parts of food packaging. They tell you more about what you are eating and help you make informed choices.

Nutrition Facts/Datos de Nutrición

8 servings per container/8 raciónes por envase
Serving size/Tomaño por recíon   **2/3 cup/2/3 taza (55 g)**

Amount per serving/Contidad por recíon
Calories/Calorias   230

	% Daily value*/Valor Diario*
Total Fat/Grasa Total 8g	**10%**
Saturated Fat/Grasa Saturada 1g	**5%**
Trans Fat/Grasa *Trans* 0g	
Cholestero/Colestero 0mg	**0%**
Sodium/Sodio 160mg	**7%**
Total Carbohydrate/Carbohidrato Total 37g	**13%**
Dietary Fiber/Fibra Dietetica 4g	**14%**
Total Sugars/Azúcares Total 12g	
Includes10g Added Sugars/Incluye 10g azúcares añadidos	**20%**
Protein/Proeínas 3g	
Vitamin D/Vitamina D 2mcg	18%
Calcium/Calcio 260mg	20%
Iron/Hierro 8mg	45%
Potassium/Potasio 235mg	6%

*The % Daily Value (DV) tells you how much a nutrient in a serving of foods contributes to a daily diet. 2,000 calories a day is used for general nutrition advice

*El % Valor Diario (VD) le indic cuánto un nutriente en una porción de alimentos contribuye a una dieta diaria. 2,000 calorías al dia se utiliza para asesoramiento de nutrición general.

Figure 9.2 **US Nutrition Facts Label**

The Canadian Nutrition Facts table in Figure 9.3 differs slightly from the US Nutrition Facts label. In the next section we present the US label and discuss key differences in the Canadian table.

Some US labels are in both English and Spanish, such as the one in Figure 9.2. In this section of the chapter, we explain the information provided on the label in detail.

Servings per Container and Serving Size

You can find serving information at the very top of the label. All the other information on the label is based on serving size. Remember, a serving may be more or less than what you usually eat. You must compare the serving size to what you are actually eating. If you eat a cup (250 mL) of cooked rice and the serving size is half

Nutrition Facts
Valeur nutritive
Per 1 cup (250 mL)
pour 1 tasse (250 mL)

Calories 110	% Daily Value* % valeur quotidienne*
Fat / Lipides 0 g	0 %
Saturated / saturés 0 g + Trans / trans 0 g	0 %
Carbohydrate / Glucides 26 g	
Fibre / fibres 0 g	0 %
Sugers / sucres 22 g	22 %
Protein / Protéines 2 g	
Cholesterol / Cholestérol 0 mg	
Sodium 0 mg	0 %
Potassium 450 mg	10 %
Calcium 30 mg	2 %
Iron / Fer 0 mg	0 %

*5% or less is **a little**, 15% or more is **a lot**
*5% ou moins c'est **peu**, 15% ou plue c'est **beaucoup**

Figure 9.3 **Canadian Nutrition Facts Table**

a cup (125 mL), you have eaten two servings. This is neither good nor bad, but it does mean that when you look at calories, fats, sodium, and carbohydrates, you must consider that you have eaten twice as much of what is shown on the label. If the label says 25 grams of carbohydrates per serving and you eat two servings, you have eaten 50 grams of carbohydrates.

Calories

The label lists total calories for the stated serving size. Calories are a measure of energy. The numbers of calories you eat and the number of calories you burn largely determines your body weight. When a person eats too many calories, the extra energy is stored as fat and the result is being overweight. The number of calories you need per day depends on your body size as well as your activity level. An average diet of 1,400 to 2,000 calories a day results in a steady weight for many people. However, weight also depends on how active each person is. The calories you need for your body weight goals may be different from those a person who is more or less active than you needs to maintain a constant weight. If you are very active, you may need more calories. If you are very inactive, you may need fewer. Also, smaller, older women generally need fewer calories, while larger, younger men need more. See Appendix A: *Healthy Eating Patterns for 1,600 and 2,000 Calories* starting on page 221, which includes a guide for lower and higher calorie levels.

Percent (%) Daily Value

There are daily recommendations for some nutrients on the label. The percent daily value tells you what percentage of that nutrient is in each serving. This percentage is based on a 2,000-calorie-a-day diet. Even if you don't eat 2,000 calories each day, this information can still help you make decisions. The percentage indicates if there is a small or large amount of that nutrient in the food. In general, 5 percent or lower daily value means that the food is low in that nutrient. If the daily value is 20 percent or higher, the food is high in that nutrient. Please note that there are no percent daily values for trans fats and proteins. It is best to eat little or no trans fats.

> In Canada, the percent daily value is calculated in the same way as the US, although Health Canada uses the terms "a little" or "a lot." A food with a daily value of 15 percent or higher of any nutrient has "a lot" of that nutrient.

Total Fat

Fats, by weight, have twice as many calories as proteins and carbohydrates. An ounce is about 30 grams. An ounce of flour (which is mostly carbohydrate) has about 100 calories, while an ounce of butter (which is all fat) has about 200 calories. An ounce of chocolate chip cookie (about a 3-inch or 7.6 cm cookie) has about 140 calories. Part of that ounce of cookie is fat and part is carbohydrate with a little protein. Ounce for ounce (or gram for gram), foods with fat have more calories than those with little or no fat.

The number of grams listed under Total Fat includes the healthier fats (polyunsaturated and monounsaturated) and the less healthy fats (saturated and trans). Note that the label also lists saturated fat and trans fat amounts. Some people think that all fat is bad. This is not true. For your body to work well, you need

Healthy Fats

When Choosing Foods

- Eat cooked portions of meat, fish, and poultry that are 3 to 5 ounces (85 to 140 g). A portion is about the size of a deck of cards or the palm of your hand.

- Do not eat poultry skin. It contains bad saturated fat.

- Eat more cold-water fatty fish, such as salmon, tuna, and mackerel.

- Choose leaner cuts of meat (lean ground beef, round, sirloin, or flank cuts).

- Trim all the fat you can see from meat before cooking.

- Choose lower-fat milk and dairy foods (cheese, sour cream, cottage cheese, yogurt, and ice cream).

- Choose fats from plant-based whole foods, including nuts, nut butters, seeds, and avocados.

When Preparing Foods

- Cook in a nonstick pan or a pan with small amounts of sprayed cooking oil or broth.

- Broil, barbecue, or grill meats.

- Avoid frying or deep-frying foods.

- Skim the fat from stews and soups. (If you refrigerate them overnight, solid fat condenses at the top and lifts off easily.)

- Use less butter, gravies, meat-based and cream sauces, spreads, and creamy pasta sauces and salad dressings.

- Consider using extra-virgin olive oil or grapeseed oil in place of butter on vegetables and in spreads, sauces, and salad dressings.

- When cooking and baking, use oil (such as olive or canola oil) and plant-based margarines (olive oil, flax, soy) instead of shortening, lard, butter, or stick margarine.

- Use avocado, canola, peanut, and olive oils when cooking at medium or high heat. Extra-virgin olive oil is best for cooking at low heat or using uncooked (such as on a salad).

some fat—about a tablespoon (15 mL) per day. Although all fats have the same number of calories, some fats are more healthful and anti-inflammatory than others. In this book we sometimes refer to the healthy fats as "good" and the less healthy fats—which can be harmful—as "bad." We do this to encourage you to eat healthier fats. For people with chronic pain, there is an extra reason to eat healthy fats: They also help reduce inflammation.

Good healthy fats include oils that are usually liquid at room temperature. These fats help keep our cells healthy, and some of these fats can help reduce blood cholesterol. Oils rich in good fats include olive, canola, soybean, safflower, corn, peanut, and sunflower. Foods rich in good fats include nuts, seeds, and olives (and their oils), as well as avocados.

There is ongoing research about whether another group of good fats—the omega-3s—may be helpful for some people in reducing the risk of heart disease and may help with chronic pain symptoms. (Learn more about omega-3s on page 214.)

Bad fats are saturated fats and trans fats. Bad fats are usually solid at room temperature. Think about shortening, butter, lard, and bacon grease. Bad fats can increase blood cholesterol and the risk of heart disease. The source of much of these fats is animal foods such as butter, beef fat (tallow, suet), chicken fat, and pork fat (lard).

Other foods high in bad fats include stick margarines, red meat, regular ground meat, processed meats (sausage, bacon, pepperoni, and other cured, luncheon, and deli meats), poultry skin, and whole and low-fat milk and cheeses, including cream cheese and sour cream. Palm kernel oil, coconut oil, and cocoa butter are also bad fats because they are high in saturated fat.

The most unhealthy fats are trans fats. Trans fats raise blood cholesterol and the risk of heart disease more than other bad fats. Be warned! Food companies can legally claim "no" or "0 grams" trans fats on the label even when the food has up to half a gram (0.5 g) per serving. You can tell if a food contains trans fats if "hydrogenated or partially hydrogenated oils" is in a food's ingredients list. Eat as few trans fats as possible. Again, notice that the food label lists saturated fats and *trans* fats separately.

There are no specific daily recommendations for how much fat you should eat. Most people get more than enough through their normal diet. The best recommendation is to eat very little bad fats and replace them with good fats. When making this healthy switch, do not increase the overall amount of fat you eat.

In Canada, they list "Fat" and not "Total Fat" in the Nutrition Facts table. Also note that in Canada, if a food has less than 0.2 grams of trans fat it can be labeled as "trans-fat free." Cholesterol information is optional in Canada and may not appear on a food's label.

Cholesterol

Cholesterol is a part of the cells in the human body. Your body makes cholesterol, and you also get cholesterol from food. Too much cholesterol is a problem because it can clog the blood vessels and cause heart attacks and strokes. Some cholesterol in your body comes from the foods you eat. Cholesterol is only present in foods from animals, including shellfish, beef, eggs, milk, and cheese. Plant foods do not contain cholesterol. Foods highest in cholesterol are often those highest in saturated fat. However, most of the cholesterol that is in your body comes from the cholesterol your body makes rather than from the food you eat.

To tell if a specific food is high or low in cholesterol, look at the % Daily value column on the Nutrition Facts label. Any food with a value of 20 percent or more is high in cholesterol. If you want to eat less cholesterol or if you tend to eat more than one serving of foods, choose foods with cholesterol values of 5 percent daily value or lower.

Sodium

An average adult needs only about 500 milligrams (mg) a day of sodium. This is the amount of sodium in less than a fifth of a teaspoon of table salt. Most people eat more than six times that much. Most of the salt in people's diets comes from processed and refined foods rather than from the salt shaker at the table. Too much sodium can raise blood pressure, and high blood pressure can lead to heart disease, stroke, and kidney failure. Cutting back on sodium can help lower blood pressure. Adults should limit sodium to 2,300 mg a day (about 1 teaspoon of table salt). Some people may benefit from even lower levels of sodium (1,500 mg a day).

> In Canada, the recommendations for sodium are 1,500 to 2,300 mg per day. Foods labeled as "low in sodium or salt," "low sodium," and "low source of sodium or salt" contain less than 140 mg of sodium per serving.

You get sodium from the foods you eat—from tiny amounts in some plant foods to higher amounts in some animal foods (red meat, chicken, fish, eggs, and dairy products). You do not have to worry about sodium in foods that you eat in their natural unprocessed form. To control your sodium intake, limit processed foods in your diet. Processed foods, which often have different forms of sodium added to them in large amounts, contain high amounts of sodium.

A love of sodium comes from eating salty foods. When you eat food with less salt, your tastes adjust, and you can learn to like food with less salt. Cutting back on sodium can take some getting used to, but over time you learn to enjoy the natural flavors of food. Here are some tips to help you reduce your sodium intake:

- **Always taste your food before salting it.** It may taste good without adding more salt.

- **Cut down on the salt in recipes when cooking.** Add one half of the salt that the recipe calls for. Season food with spices, herbs, pepper, garlic, onion, or lemon.

- **Use minimally processed fresh or frozen poultry, fish, and lean meat instead of canned, breaded, or prepared packaged food.**

- **Choose foods labeled "low" or "reduced" sodium or those with 140 mg or less per serving.** Check the Nutrition Facts label (see Figure 9.2) for this information.

- **Save high-sodium food for special occasions.** Eat the following only once in a while rather than every day: canned soups, packaged mixes, bacon, luncheon or deli meats, salted snacks (like chips, nuts, and pretzels), and pepperoni or sausage pizza.

- **In restaurants, ask that your food not be salted.** Sauces, breading, rice, pasta or potato dishes, stuffing, and foods containing ham, sausage, or bacon are often high in sodium. Salad dressings can be high in sodium as well. Ask for sauces and dressings on the side. In addition, most soups at restaurants are high in sodium.

Total Carbohydrate

Carbohydrates are your body's main source of fuel. Your body breaks down carbohydrates (except for fiber) into glucose (sugar). Glucose is the energy source for your brain and the rest of your body. Carbohydrates—more than protein or fat—largely determine your blood glucose (blood sugar) level. They also do much more: Carbohydrates are the building blocks of nearly every part of your body.

There are two types of carbohydrates: sugars and starches. Carbohydrates are found in

Choosing Healthy Carbohydrates and Eating More Fiber

- Fill at least half of your plate with whole, fresh, or frozen vegetables and fruits.

- At least half of the grains you eat should be whole grains (brown rice, whole-grain breads and rolls, whole-grain pasta, and corn tortillas).

- Choose foods that list whole wheat or a whole grain (such as oats) first on the ingredients list.

- Choose dried beans, split peas, and lentils instead of meat or as a side dish at least a few times a week. Add cooked dried beans to your vegetable salads and pasta dishes.

- Choose whole fruit rather than fruit juice. Whole fruit contains fiber, takes longer to eat, fills you up better than juice, and may help keep you from overeating.

- Limit added sugars, especially sugar-sweetened beverages. (Learn more about added sugars on page 206.)

- Choose higher-fiber breakfast cereals (such as All-Bran®) or oatmeal.

- Eat higher-fiber crackers such as whole-rye or multigrain crackers and whole-grain flatbread.

- Snack on whole fruit, raw vegetables, and whole-grain crackers or breads rather than chips, sweets, or ice cream.

- When you add higher-fiber foods to your diet, do it gradually over a period of a few weeks.

- Drink plenty of water to prevent constipation.

plant food (grains, fruits, vegetables). Milk and yogurt also have carbohydrates.

Sugars occur naturally in foods, such as fruits (fructose) and milk/yogurt (lactose). Other packaged and processed foods, such as soda, candy, and crackers, often have added sugar. The added sugar adds extra calories. It is also common for healthful nutrients to be missing from these processed and packaged products.

Vegetables such as green peas, potatoes, winter squash, dried beans, and peas contain starchy carbohydrates. Lentils and other legumes and grains such as rice, corn, and wheat also have starchy carbohydrates. Because the grains they are made of are high in starchy carbohydrates, pasta, bread, tortillas, and baked goods are high in carbohydrates.

Some grain-based foods are more processed and refined than others. Processing does not change the amount of carbohydrates. However, processing does remove healthful nutrients (such as vitamins, minerals, and other nutrients and fiber). It is better to eat brown rice and whole grains than white rice and other processed grains, because they are more nutritious and include more fiber. Your body changes some carbohydrates to glucose more quickly than others. The carbohydrates in most high-fiber foods get converted into glucose more slowly than the carbohydrates in low-fiber foods. (Learn more about the health benefits of fiber on page 206.)

If you have diabetes, your body has trouble using all the carbohydrates you eat, and higher levels of glucose build up in the blood. If left untreated, diabetes causes many problems and can lead to painful nerve damage.

In some countries, including Canada, diabetes education materials refer to glycemic index (GI), which measures how quickly different carbohydrates are absorbed into the blood, and glycemic load (GL), which estimates approximately how much a food will raise blood glucose. To learn more about GI and GL, see the resources available at https://www.diabetes.ca/DiabetesCanada Website/media/Managing-My-Diabetes /Tools%20and%20Resources/glycemic -index-food-guide.pdf?ext=.pdf and www.bullpub.com/resources.

Dietary Fiber

Fiber is a carbohydrate that is not absorbed by the body. Fiber occurs naturally in whole and minimally processed plant foods with skins, seeds, and strings (like those found in celery and string beans). Whole grains, dried beans, peas, lentils, fruits, vegetables, nuts, and seeds all have fiber. Some foods have added fiber (for example, when pulp is added to juice). Animal foods (red meat, chicken, fish, eggs, and dairy products) and refined foods (white flour, bread, many baked and snack foods) have little or no fiber unless the manufacturer adds it to the product.

Even though it is not absorbed by your body, fiber helps your body. There are two types of fiber: soluble and insoluble fiber. Most plants contain both soluble and insoluble fiber, but in different amounts. Insoluble fiber, such as wheat bran, found in some fruits and vegetables, and whole grains act as "nature's broom." These foods keep your digestive system moving and help prevent constipation. This is especially important if you are taking opioid medications for chronic pain. The soluble fiber in oat bran, barley, nuts, seeds, beans, apples, citrus fruits, carrots, and psyllium seed can help regulate blood sugar. This form of fiber slows the amount of time it takes for sugar to get into the bloodstream. Foods that contain soluble fiber can help lower blood cholesterol. High-fiber diets may also help reduce the risk of rectal and colon cancers. The US daily recommendation for fiber for adults ranges from 22 to 34 grams, generally more for men than women and less for older adults than younger adults. If you are eating the recommended amounts of whole, plant-based foods you likely are getting enough of both types of fiber.

In Canada, the fiber recommendation is 25 grams for women and 38 grams for men.

Total Sugars and Added Sugars

The Total Sugars information on the Nutrition Facts label lists the amount of sugar in one serving of the food. Many foods, such as fruit, contain natural sugar. But in many other cases, such as carbonated drinks, sugar is also added.

Are natural sugars and added sugars different? No, your body uses natural sugars and added sugars the same way. They both have the same number of calories for the same weight (grams, ounces, etc.). However, processed foods tend to have more added sugars. A sugar—whether it is natural or added—is a sugar, but foods with natural sugar usually also contain healthy ingredients.

Added sugars contribute extra calories to your diet. If you are trying to lose weight or lower your blood glucose, eat as little added sugar as possible. A 12-ounce (355 mL) can of cola has nearly 40 grams (almost 10 teaspoons) of added sugar and no beneficial nutrients. Twelve ounces (355 mL) of orange juice with no added sugar has 33 grams of natural sugar but also lots of vitamins and other nutrients. It is clear that the juice is a better choice than the cola. An even better choice is a fresh medium orange. An orange has approximately 12 grams of carbohydrate, and it provides healthy nutrients and fiber. To quench your thirst, choose water, coffee, and tea. These drinks have no added sugar and no carbohydrates.

Both US and Canadian recommendations suggest you limit added sugar to no more than 10 percent of your total daily calories. For example, if you consume 2,000 calories in a day, your added sugar intake should not exceed 200 calories or 50 grams. In the United States, this is the equivalent of about 12½ teaspoons. The American Heart Association takes this public health message further and recommends not exceeding 6 teaspoons (24 grams, 96 calories) for women and 9 teaspoons (36 grams, 144 calories) for men per day. This may seem like a lot, but it can be surprising how much sugar is in foods and beverages, and this is why it's so important to read food labels. In addition to the information on the Nutrition Facts label, the ingredient list provides information on the sugar content of a food.

Protein

Protein is part of every cell in your body and helps control the way your body works. Protein helps your immune system fight infection. Your body also uses protein to build tissues, including muscles and bones, and repair damaged tissues. Protein provides a feeling of comfortable fullness after you eat. It satisfies your appetite and prevents you from getting hungry again too soon after you have eaten. Most people eat more than enough protein. However, many people get most of their protein from meat, which tends to be high in bad (saturated) fats. Getting your protein mainly from plant foods along with small amounts of lean meat, poultry, or fish, or eating a variety of plant-based foods, is better for your health.

There are two types of proteins: complete and incomplete.

Your body uses complete proteins just as they are. Complete proteins are found in fish and animal foods—meat, poultry, eggs, milk, and other dairy products—as well as in foods made from soybeans, such as tofu and tempeh.

Incomplete proteins do not contain one or more parts of a complete protein. Incomplete proteins are found in plant foods such as grains, dried beans and peas, lentils, nuts, and seeds. Nearly all plant proteins are incomplete proteins. (Most fruits and nonstarchy vegetables have little, if any, protein.)

Even though plant proteins are incomplete, they are at the heart of eating healthy. Scientists once thought that we had to eat two or more incomplete plant proteins at the same meal to get the complete protein we need every day. But now we know that our bodies store a supply of spare protein parts, and these parts are available to transform incomplete plant proteins after we eat them. In addition, we now know that by eating a small amount of an animal protein (such as chicken) with a plant protein (such as lentils or black beans), you get all the benefits of a complete protein. Casseroles and stir-fries are tasty ways to do this. Common incomplete proteins that pair up to form a complete protein when eaten together include rice with beans and peanut butter with bread.

In addition to containing protein, some plant foods, such as nuts and seeds, are sources of the good fats. Many plant foods are also sources of fiber and other nutrients. Plant foods have no cholesterol and little to no bad fats. For these reasons, plant foods are often the best choice for healthy eating.

Vitamin D, Calcium, Iron, and Potassium

Vitamins and minerals keep your body functioning properly and are needed for survival and health. Most people get all the vitamins and minerals they need from eating healthy foods.

Only vitamin D (see information on vitamin D on page 214) and four minerals are listed on Nutrition Facts labels: sodium (see information on sodium on page 203), calcium, iron, and potassium. You will find information about other vitamins and minerals on a food's packaging only if these are added or if a health claim about these is made on the package. The four minerals that are always listed on the label are linked to current health problems. Many of us eat either too much (sodium) or too little (calcium, iron, and potassium) of these minerals.

Vitamins and Minerals

Because vitamins and minerals are important to health, we discuss them in more detail in this section.

Potassium

The mineral potassium helps regulate our heartbeat and can lower blood pressure. Many kinds of vegetables and fruits are good potassium sources. These include broccoli, peas, dried beans (white, adzuki, and pinto), tomatoes, potatoes, sweet potatoes, avocados, winter squash (acorn, delicata, and butternut), citrus fruits, plantains, bananas, prunes, apricots, and nuts. Some fish (salmon, tuna, mackerel, and halibut), milk, and yogurt are also good sources of potassium.

Calcium

Calcium helps build bones, but did you know that it is also needed for blood clotting and helps with blood pressure? It may also protect against colon cancer, kidney stones, and breast cancer.

Unfortunately, some people, especially older women and young children, may not get enough calcium in their diets. Most women under 60 should get the amount of calcium found in 3 cups (750 mL) of milk every day. Another reason to eat less salt is because salt can cause your body to lose calcium.

Core Nutrients

In Canada, there are 13 core nutrients listed on the Nutrition Facts table. For vitamins and minerals, Canada lists vitamin A, vitamin C, calcium, and iron. A new Nutrition Facts table introduced in 2017 is being phased in over a five-year transition period. The new label removes vitamins A and C and adds potassium.

More Is Not Better

When it comes to vitamins and minerals, some people think that if a little is good, then more is better. This is not true. Too much of a good thing can cause harm. This is because everything in your body must be in balance, and too much of anything throws off the balance. (Think of baking. If you put too much of almost any ingredient into cookies, cakes, or pies, they do not come out right.) If you stick to eating mostly whole foods and limit processed foods, you will likely consume vitamins and minerals in the quantities your body needs.

Good sources of calcium are yogurt, cheese, and kefir (a fermented beverage that's similar to yogurt); calcium-fortified soy, rice, oat, and almond milks and orange juice; calcium-fortified cereal and breads; and canned salmon and sardines with bones. Brussels sprouts, kohlrabi, and leafy greens (bok choy, kale, collards, beet greens, turnip greens, and spinach) have calcium, but our bodies cannot use some of it because these plant foods contain natural chemicals that are not harmful but partially block calcium absorption. Most fruits are low in calcium. The exceptions are dried figs (there's not much in fig cookies, though) and tropical cherimoya (custard apple).

If you do not get enough calcium from what you eat and drink, talk to your health care provider about calcium supplements (pills).

Iron

Iron is a mineral that helps your body use oxygen. If you do not have enough iron in your diet, you can feel tired, weak, dizzy, and generally unwell. Iron is found in both plant and animal foods. In the United States and Canada, grain products (such as breads, pasta, and cereals) have iron added to them. Iron from animal foods is easier for our bodies to use than iron from plants. Eating foods with vitamin C at the same time that we eat plant foods with iron allows our bodies to better absorb the iron. Excellent sources of vitamin C include citrus fruits (grapefruit, orange, lemon, lime), sweet red peppers, and broccoli.

Water

Water, which makes up more than half of our bodies, is the most important nutrient. Water fills the spaces in and between body cells. All the natural chemical reactions in your body require water. Water keeps your kidneys working, helps prevent constipation, and helps you eat less by making you feel full. Water also helps prevent medication side effects.

Most adults lose about 10 cups of water a day through urine, sweat, and breathing. However, people usually have no problem getting enough water. The exact amount you need differs depending on the weather, your activity, and your weight. To determine if you are drinking enough water, check the color of your urine. If it is light colored, you are fine. If it is darker, you probably need more water. When you feel thirsty, your body needs more water. Milk and many fruits and vegetables are good sources of water. Coffee, tea, and other drinks with caffeine are also good sources of water, but speak with your health care provider about drinking decaffeinated drinks instead since caffeine may worsen pain. Alcohol is not a good source of water. Do not depend on alcohol to meet your need for water.

Pain and Water

Not getting enough fluids may make pain symptoms worse. Being hydrated may also improve how well you respond to pain management therapies.

If you have kidney disease or congestive heart failure or are taking special medications, you may need to drink less water. Talk to a registered dietitian or your health care provider.

The Ingredients List

An ingredients list is usually found on food labels under the Nutrition Facts, but it may be elsewhere on food packaging. This list of all the ingredients in the food package starts with the most abundant or heaviest ingredient. The last ingredients listed are those that make up the smallest part of the food. The ingredients list uses common or usual names of the ingredients. An ingredients list gives you additional information about what you are eating. Reading the ingredients list is especially important if you are trying to avoid certain items, such as added sugar or an allergen like soy or gluten.

Another Easier Way to Make Healthy Food Choices: The Plate Method

Nutrition Facts labels and ingredient lists inform you about what and how much you are eating and how what you eat compares to a healthy diet. (To learn more about daily recommended values, see page 201.) However, not all foods have labels, and sometimes you may need easier guidelines to help you eat healthier. The plate method is another way of deciding what and how much to eat.

Added Sugar in the Ingredients

Sugar and similar natural or processed sweet ingredients are listed in this table. All these ingredients contain calories from carbohydrates. They can all be found on ingredient lists. There are differences among these ingredients, and any of them can be added as sweeteners to foods. When any one of them is added, it increases the amount of added sugar in the food. Some foods may have several of these ingredients. Always read the Nutrition Facts label and ingredients list so you know what you're eating.

Agave	Coconut sugar	Fruit juice concentrate	Molasses
Agave nectar	Confectioners' sugar	Glucose	Muscovado
Anhydrous dextrose	Corn syrup	High-fructose corn syrup	Nectar
Beet sugar	Date sugar	Honey	Raw sugar
Brown sugar	Dextran	Lactose	Sorghum
Cane juice	Dextrose	Malt syrup	Sucanat
Cane sugar	Evaporated cane juice	Maltose	Sucrose
Carob syrup	Fructose	Maple syrup	Sugar
			Treacle

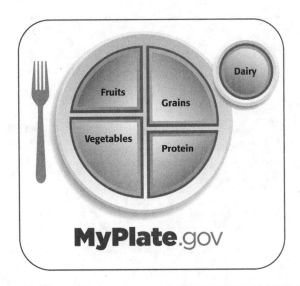

Figure 9.4 **MyPlate: A Map for Healthy Eating from the USDA**

MyPlate

MyPlate, a visual guide produced by the US Department of Agriculture (USDA) to help you make good food choices, is shown in Figure 9.4. This guide encourages you to cover one-half of your plate with vegetables and fruit, one-fourth with protein (lean meat, fish, or poultry, or better yet, plant foods such as tofu, cooked dry beans, or lentils), and the remaining one-fourth with grains (preferably at least half from whole grains) or other starches such as potatoes, sweet potatoes, yams, corn, peas, or winter squash. Finish off your meal with calcium-rich foods such as milk or foods made from milk (preferably low-fat), including cheese, yogurt, frozen yogurt, or calcium-fortified foods such as soy milk. Of course, your food choices and amounts should depend on what you like and need. A small amount of "good" fat (see page 202) is healthy at each meal. This fat may be oil you use to add flavor while cooking the food, dressing a salad, or seasoning food. It could also come from nuts mixed in with a grain, such as brown rice. Read more about suggestions for choosing healthy fats and seasonings on page 202.

Eat Well Plate

The Canadian government's recommendations from the Eat Well Plate are very similar to the US plate, with minor differences. As you can see in the Canadian Eat Well Plate in Figure 9.5 on the next page, Canada's Food Guide recommends water as your drink of choice with milk and other alternatives as a second choice. It also suggests that you choose protein foods that come from plants more often than animal proteins.

Portions and the Plate Method

Even with the plate method, the amounts (portion size) of food you eat are important. Plate sizes have grown over the years. As a result, people now tend to eat larger portions and more calories than we need. A plate that measures 9 inches (22.5 cm) across the center is a good size. Appendix A: *Healthy Eating Patterns for 1,600*

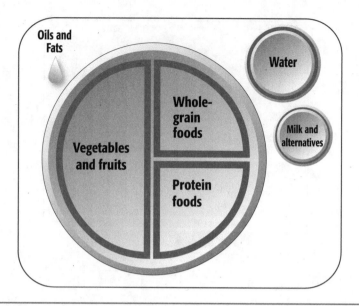

Figure 9.5 **Eat Well Plate from the Canadian Government**

and 2,000 Calories on page 221 and Appendix B: *Food Groups for Meal Planning* on page 222 list examples of recommended daily portions from different food groups. You can use these appendices to decide how much food to put on your plate. Note that these amounts may be different if you have special dietary needs. If you have questions, check with your health care provider or a registered dietitian.

Food Choices and Chronic Pain

Are some foods more helpful for chronic pain than other foods? The answer to this question is complex. There are some things that have been researched and there are some things that are generally accepted. If you have chronic pain, it makes sense to follow a good eating pattern as outlined above and maintain an appropriate weight to avoid putting excess pressure on your hips, knees, ankles, and other joints (see Chapter 10, *Healthy Weight and Pain Self-Management*). Drinking enough water and other fluids will help maintain your body chemistry and will also help medication work better.

Now we get to the complex part. Recently, scientists and others have looked at two more things (in addition to eating well, maintaining a healthy weight, and staying hydrated) that research may show us to be more important over time. These two additional factors have to do with the microbiome (all the bacteria in your gut) and the role certain foods play in inflammation. The information we discuss here is the best information we have as we write this book. This information will probably change in the years to come. Nothing that we suggest is harmful, and you may find it very helpful to follow these guidelines. It is important to remember that not all pain is accompanied by inflammation. It is also important to keep in mind that food alone will not stop chronic pain or inflammation. On the other hand, managing your diet may help you manage your pain. In this section, we also suggest how other nutrients may help with pain.

Your Intestines and Your Health

Your gut is your digestive system or digestive tract, including the mouth, stomach, and intestines. Trillions of microorganisms, including helpful bacteria and yeast, live in your gut. Your gut microbiome, which is all the microorganisms that live in your gut, plays an essential role in your health. Your microbiome helps you digest food and protects you from harmful bacteria.

Each person has their own unique microbiome. Each person's microbiome differs in both the kind of microorganisms and the number of organisms it includes. The foods you eat affect your microbiome. Some foods contain living healthy microorganisms known as probiotics. Fermented foods are the best sources of probiotics. Fermented foods are foods or beverages that have been transformed by age or by addition of a bacterial or yeast culture. Examples of fermented foods include yogurt, sauerkraut, and kombucha. Other foods contain prebiotics, a type of fiber that feeds the friendly bacteria in your gut. Prebiotics serve as healthy "food" for the microbiome. They allow healthy bacteria and yeast to thrive. Food sources of prebiotics include whole grains, onion, leek, asparagus, banana, garlic, honey, yogurt, and legumes (such as beans, peas, peanuts, etc.).

Scientists are not yet sure exactly how the microbiome works to help prevent and treat illness and pain. They believe that a good diet promotes a healthy microbiome, which in turn helps reduce pain. We will learn more about this in the coming years.

Your Gut: More Important Than You Think

Very recently, scientists have discovered that the millions of micro (very small) organisms in your gut are very important. It has been known for a long time that these organisms help with the digestion of food. What scientists are now learning is that they affect a large range of diseases and conditions, possibly including chronic pain. The content we include here is the most reliable information available as we publish this book.

A Diet That Helps Fight Inflammation (Anti-inflammatory Diet)

Some chronic pain conditions, such as rheumatoid arthritis, migraine headaches, and chronic colitis, are linked to inflammation. There are some chronic pain conditions, such as back pain or osteoarthritis, that may or may not produce inflammation. Researchers are still learning about inflammation and pain, and there is some evidence that what you eat may affect inflammation. If inflammation is part of your chronic pain condition, this information might help.

An anti-inflammatory diet features whole foods and some lightly processed foods while avoiding highly processed foods. This diet puts special emphasis on plant foods (vegetables, fruits, nuts and seeds, legumes, beans, whole grains, spices and herbs). It puts less emphasis on animal foods (red meat, chicken, fish, eggs, and dairy products). If you think this sounds a lot like the Mediterranean-Style Dietary Pattern (see page 196), you are right. Some anti-inflammatory diets limit foods that may increase pain and inflammation (see the list of foods that may cause inflammation on page 215). Anti-inflammatory diets may also include specific anti-inflammatory foods (see the list of foods that may help to reduce inflammation below). Foods that may help to reduce inflammation, which are also referred to as anti-inflammatory foods, are rich sources of dietary fiber, vitamins, minerals, and anti-inflammatory nutrients that are found in all plants.

Nutrients That May Help Chronic Pain

Sometimes in addition to eating healthy, it's helpful to focus on specific nutrients. A nutrient is a substance that provides nourishment essential for growth and the maintenance of life. There are many nutrients in foods that may be helpful for chronic pain. Your health care practitioner and a registered dietitian can help you decide which nutrients are best for you. Here we include information about some of these nutrients:

- Omega-3s are fats that should be consumed in moderation along with other fats in the diet (learn more about fats on page 201). They may help inflammation. Omega-3s are found in cold-water fatty fish (salmon, halibut, mackerel) and other seafood, nuts and seeds, and some plant oils.

- Vitamin D may help in pain regulation. It is estimated that as many as 50 percent of people with chronic pain have low levels of vitamin D. Scientists do not know for certain if vitamin D helps people with chronic pain, but they think it might. You get vitamin D from sunlight. For this reason, it is important

Foods That May Reduce Inflammation

- White meat (chicken, poultry, rabbit)
- Fish (bluefish, mackerel, anchovies, sardines, tuna, swordfish, salmon, hake)
- Legumes (dried or canned black beans, white beans, lentils)
- Soy (tofu, tempeh, miso, edamame)
- Nuts (walnuts, hazelnuts, almonds, pistachios, macadamias, Brazil nuts)
- Seeds (pumpkin, flax, sunflower, sesame, chia, hemp)
- Fruits and berries

- Plant oils (extra-virgin olive oil, grapeseed oil)
- Green vegetables and other colorful vegetables
- Yogurt and other fermented dairy such as kefir
- Spices, especially turmeric and ginger
- Water, seltzer water
- Herbal teas, decaffeinated green and black tea

A Note on Eggs: Eggs contain both inflammatory and anti-inflammatory nutrients. A rich source of vitamins, minerals, and high-quality protein, eggs are included in many anti-inflammatory diets. To eat eggs or to not eat eggs is a personal preference.

Foods That May Cause or Increase Inflammation

- Red meat (beef, pork, lamb, veal, goat)
- Processed meat (deli meat, fast food, frozen prepared meat, cured meat, bacon)
- Fried foods, trans fat (shortening, hydrogenated or partially hydrogenated oils)
- Refined grains (white bread, white pasta, white rice)
- Refined sweet foods and beverages (cookies, cake, candy, pastries, soda, sugar-sweetened drinks, added sugar)
- Caffeine
- Alcohol

to get outdoors every day when possible. Vitamin D is also found in some foods naturally, including fish (many of the same varieties of fish that are high in omega-3s), egg yolk, and cod liver oil. Most packaged foods containing vitamin D, including milk, yogurt, orange juice, soy milk and other non-dairy milk, and margarine, are fortified, meaning vitamin D is added to the food. Vitamin D can also be taken in supplement form. Everyone needs some vitamin D to keep bones healthy. The body cannot use calcium without vitamin D. If you do not get much sunlight or you are dark skinned or overweight, you may need a vitamin D supplement. This is especially true if you have a family history of osteoporosis. If you are not already taking a supplement recommended by your doctor, talk with your health care provider or a registered dietitian. The National Academy of Medicine suggests people under 70 get 600 IUs (international units) of vitamin D daily and people over 70 get 800 IUs. Health Canada recommends that men and women over 50 take a daily vitamin D supplement of 400 IUs. It is generally considered safe to take a supplement that provides 1,000 or 2,000 IUs. The recommendation is to stay below 4,000 IUs per day.

- Magnesium may reduce pain from migraine headaches and fibromyalgia, as well as some nerve pain. Magnesium-rich foods include flaxseed, sesame seeds, pumpkin seeds, Brazil nuts, almonds, pine nuts, cold-water fatty fish (salmon, halibut, mackerel), beans (black, lima, navy), black-eyed peas, green vegetables (cooked spinach and swiss chard), and wheat germ. Talk to your health care provider before you take a magnesium supplement, as too much magnesium in your diet may cause diarrhea.

- Zinc and selenium help to manage inflammation. Foods rich in zinc include oysters, chicken, tofu, hemp seeds, lentils, yogurt, oats, and mushrooms. Foods that are rich in selenium include Brazil nuts, tuna, shellfish, chicken, tofu, whole grains, and mushrooms.

- Vitamin B12 has many important functions for the health of the brain and nervous system, the heart, and overall energy. B12 may

Caffeine and Pain

Too much caffeine can increase anxiety, restlessness, irritability, chest palpitations, and stomach complaints and can interfere with sleep. These symptoms can further intensify your pain. Caffeine should be limited to about 400 mg—the equivalent of two to three 8-ounce (237 mL) cups of coffee a day. Caffeine isn't only in coffee; it is also in tea, colas and other sodas, chocolate, and some energy drinks. Cold remedies and some mild analgesics that you might take for pain may also contain caffeine. Always read the label.

If you want to use less caffeine, it's important to gradually reduce your intake over two to three weeks. If you withdraw too quickly, you might have symptoms such as headache, fatigue, irritability, and mood swings. If you reduce gradually, you should have no ill effects. Decrease your intake by substituting decaffeinated coffee and teas and caffeine-free drinks. Brewed decaf coffee, for example, has 5 to 10 mg of caffeine per 8-ounce cup compared to 100 to 150 mg of caffeine in the same amount of regular brewed coffee. An 8-ounce cup of green tea has about 33 mg of caffeine.

help manage nerve pain. B12 is found in animal proteins, such as red meat, eggs, fish, and chicken. It is also found in nutritional yeast.

■ Stay hydrated. Research indicates that there may be a link between chronic dehydration and muscle soreness.

Food Sensitivities and Chronic Pain Self-Management

Some foods trigger pain for some people. For example, the following foods have been reported as triggering migraines: sulfites (substances that naturally occur in some foods and the human body; they are also used as food additives and are found in dried fruits and some alcohol, especially red wine), tannins (substances found in wine and strong tea), various cheeses (especially cheeses that are aged or fermented), food additives such as nitrates and nitrites (found in processed meats), monosodium glutamate (MSG; a flavor enhancer in processed foods), aspartame and other artificial sweeteners, and fatty foods. Other reported migraine triggers include fasting or missing a meal and dehydration.

The exact cause of migraines is still not known. If you have migraines, it may be useful to experiment with avoiding foods you might suspect are triggers for you. Talk with your health care provider if you want to begin avoiding foods.

Many kinds of chronic pain (not just migraines) can be triggered by certain foods. To determine if you have an intolerance or sensitivity to any foods, keep a food and symptom list or fill in a behavioral worksheet (see Figures 4.1 and 4.2 on pages 56 and 57). Write down all the foods and beverages you consume in two weeks. Also, note if you miss a meal. And note each day whether your symptoms—your pain, mood, and emotions—are worse, better, or not affected. Look for patterns to see if certain foods make your symptoms better or worse. If you suspect any foods are problems, eliminate those foods one at a time to test your idea.

Opioids and Healthy Eating

Opioids are a family of powerful medications that help treat pain. For many people, opioids decrease appetite and cause constipation. Foods that contain high amounts of fiber, such as legumes, vegetables, and fruits, can decrease constipation. Other nutrients—including curcumin from turmeric root, prebiotics (a type of fiber that feeds the friendly bacteria in your gut; see page 213 to learn more about prebiotics) found in plant foods, and probiotics (living healthy microorganisms; see page 213 to learn more about intestines and your health) found in yogurt—may also have a beneficial role in maintaining health if you are taking opioids. People taking opioid medications often have reduced levels of zinc, an essential mineral required by the body for the immune system. Vitamin B12, an essential vitamin, may also be low in people taking opioid medications. Vitamin B12 is mainly found in animal protein. It can also be found in nutritional yeast (a vegan food product with a cheesy, nutty, or savory flavor), which can be bought in most health food stores. Improving your diet to include such healthier foods can decrease opioid side effects.

Eliminating foods is only part of the process. Always eat a balanced and varied diet. And don't forget to drink enough water! It is helpful to work with a registered dietitian or other health care provider to help you determine which food(s) to omit, for how long, and when to reintroduce.

Healthy Eating for Chronic Pain: Putting It All Together

You now know a lot about healthy eating and how the foods you eat might affect your pain. Now it is time to put all this information together. In this final section of the chapter, we include a number of tips to do just that. The two appendices at the end of this chapter will help as well. Appendix A: *Healthy Eating Patterns for 1,600 and 2,000 Calories* on page 221 lists the daily recommended number of servings, a sample menu, and lists of foods for meal planning. It includes the numbers of servings for a lower (1,600) and a higher (2,000) calorie level. Appendix B: *Food Groups for Meal Planning* on page 222 will help you choose healthy portion sizes of the foods you like. It is important to remember to start small. What you eat can have a great impact on your health and chronic pain, but do not make too many food and beverage changes too quickly.

Tips for Healthy Eating

You may decide that you want to eat more fruits and vegetables. You may want to move toward an anti-inflammatory diet. You might want to lose weight or make any number of other changes. No matter what you decide, the following tips will help.

- **Increase vegetables and fruit by one serving each day** until you are eating five (or more!) servings of vegetables and fruit each day.

Nutrition Experts

On the internet, there are many people who say they are nutrition experts who may not be. For reliable advice and information, seek out a registered dietitian (RD) or registered dietitian nutritionist (RDN). Note that "registered dietitian" is part of their professional credential. These health professionals are specially trained and are the best sources for diet and nutrition advice and information. In this book we refer to these experts as registered dietitians (RDs).

In Canada, look for a dietitian whose credentials include an RD, RDN, or PDt (in French DtP).

- **Include plant-based proteins in your meals**. The whole meal doesn't need to be from plants, but adding 1 tablespoon of nuts (pecans, cashews) and seeds (sunflower, sesame) to a meal will increase protein, fiber, and nutrients.

- **Choose the healthy foods you enjoy eating** from Appendix B: *Food Groups for Meal Planning* on page 222 and start adding more of these to your meals.

- **Eat dark-green leafy vegetables**, such as spinach, swiss chard, collard greens, and kale.

- **Include whole foods high in good fats** such as walnuts, pumpkin seeds, and olives.

- **Sprinkle ground flax on top of your meals** to add fiber, good fat, and other important nutrients.

- **Limit added sugar intake** to no more than 6 teaspoons/24 grams (women) and 9 teaspoons/36 grams (men) daily. Learn how much added sugars are in packaged foods by reading the Nutrition Fact label (see page 206) and ingredient list (see page 210).

- **Drink water**. If you are thirsty, or if your urine looks dark in color, drink more water and other calorie-free fluids that you enjoy. Increase your fluid intake in the heat and before, during, and after exercising.

- **Add herbs and spices to meals**. Remember, ginger and turmeric go well with many foods.

- **Eat one naturally fermented food each day** (yogurt, kefir, sauerkraut, kimchi, miso, tempeh, kombucha).

- **Choose foods that are close to the way nature made them**. In food stores, shop in the areas surrounding the middle aisles containing packaged foods. These surrounding areas are where you find fresh fruits, vegetables, meat, seafood, and dairy. Buy fewer items in the middle aisles that contain junk foods, snacks, and highly processed foods.

- **Eat a wide variety of colorful unprocessed foods**. The more variety in your food, the better. The more colors on your plate from vegetables and fruits, the better.

- **Eat foods that are minimally processed**. Choose grilled chicken breast instead of fried breaded chicken nuggets. Choose a baked potato (with skin) rather than french fries. And opt for whole grains, such as whole-grain bread, whole-wheat pasta, and brown rice.

■ **Get your nutrients from food, not supplements.** Dietary supplements cannot make up for unhealthy eating. Foods in nature have the right nutrient amounts and combinations for our bodies. Nutrients that are not naturally found in foods may be present in amounts in supplements that are not healthy, or they may not work the way they should. They may even have harmful side effects.

■ **There is a place for supplements in some diets.** Sometimes we cannot get all the nutrients we need from food. For example, older people may need a larger amount of calcium to help prevent or slow osteoporosis. If you are thinking of taking a supplement, talk to your health care professional or a registered dietitian first. It is important to know how supplements will interact with any medications you may take.

■ **Eat at regular, preferably evenly spaced times during the day.** This prevents you from getting overly hungry and maintains and balances your blood sugar level. Eating regularly means different things for different people. It can mean three regular-size meals or five small meals or whatever works for you and your health conditions. For overall health, meals eaten early in the day, including breakfast, are important.

Tips for Enjoying Cooking and Eating

■ **Cook something new.** Take a cooking class or watch videos on television or YouTube. If you have odds and ends or leftovers, search the internet for recipes that can help you figure out what to do with them.

■ **If you love to cook but are now cooking for one,** invite someone for dinner, plan a potluck, or prepare food for someplace like a Ronald McDonald House or a local bake sale or charity event.

■ **Illness, medicines, and surgery can change how food tastes.** Here are some things you might try if a lack of taste is keeping you from eating enough.

▶ Ask your health care team members about possible medication changes.

▶ Avoid smoking and limit alcohol.

▶ Practice good oral care. Ask your dentist or doctor about treatment for dry mouth, if that is a problem.

▶ Use herbs (basil, oregano, tarragon) and spices (cinnamon, cumin, curry, ginger, nutmeg).

▶ Squirt fresh lemon juice on foods.

▶ Use a small amount of vinegar in or on foods. There are many flavored vinegars. Try different ones.

▶ Add healthy ingredients (carrots or barley to soup, or dried fruits and nuts to salads) to make dishes tastier.

▶ Chew your food slowly and well to release more flavor.

▶ Make your food attractive. We really do eat with our eyes! Compare the appeal of a plate of white rice, white cauliflower, and white fish with one of baked sweet potato, bright green spinach, and grilled white fish with salsa. Which of these two meals is more appetizing?

■ **If pain gets in the way of shopping, cooking, or eating,** here are some hints.

▸ Cook enough for two or three and freeze for the future.

▸ Exchange meals with friends or family.

▸ Break your food preparation into steps, resting in between.

▸ Ask for help, especially for big holiday meals or family gatherings.

▸ Use a meal delivery service such as Meals on Wheels or many of the new food delivery services you can find on the internet.

▸ Use grocery delivery services. Ask if your grocery store offers this service.

■ **People who find it physically uncomfortable to eat meals tend to eat less.** For some, eating a large meal causes stomach problems such as indigestion, discomfort, or nausea. Chronic pain symptoms can also suppress appetite. If eating causes discomfort or shortness of breath, try these tips.

▸ Eat four to six small meals a day.

▸ Avoid foods that produce gas or bloating such as cabbage, broccoli, Brussels sprouts, onions, and beans.

▸ Eat slowly, take small bites, and chew your food well. Pause occasionally. Eating quickly to avoid shortness of breath might make breathing more difficult.

▸ Practice mindful eating. (See *Tips for Mindful Eating* in Chapter 10, *Healthy Weight and Pain Self-Management*, page 244.)

▸ Choose easy-to-eat foods such as yogurt, puddings, shakes, and fruit smoothies.

■ ■ ■

In the next chapter, Chapter 10, *Healthy Weight and Pain Self-Management*, we provide more of what you need to successfully address weight change and weight-related chronic pain concerns.

**For a complete list of suggested further readings,
useful websites, and other helpful resources, please see**

www.bullpub.com/resources.

Appendix A:
Healthy Eating Patterns for 1,600 and 2,000 Calories

These recommendations are based on the USDA Dietary Guidelines for Americans 2020–2025, table A3-2. See Appendix B: *Food Groups for Meal Planning* on page 222 for more information on the food groups referred to in the first column of the table.

Number of Servings per Day from Food Groups

Food Group	1,600 Calories	2,000 Calories	Sample Menu and Notes
Protein Foods	5 oz (140 g)	6 oz (168 g)	2 oz (56 g) of turkey for lunch sandwich, 3 oz (84 g) of broiled salmon for dinner (4 oz or 112 g for 2,000 calorie pattern)
Fats/Oils	6 choices	6 choices	6 almonds for a snack, 2 Tbsp (30 mL) of salad dressing for lunch, 3 tsp (15 mL) of olive oil for seasoning vegetables and fish
Lower Carbohydrate Vegetables	At least 2 cups (500 mL)	At least 3 cups (750 mL)	1 cup (250 mL) of salad greens at lunch (2 cups or 500 mL for 2,000 calorie pattern), 1/2 cup (125 mL) of cooked green beans at dinner
Higher Carbohydrate Vegetables	2 choices	3 choices	1/3 cup (75 mL) cooked lentils in soup at lunch (2/3 cup or 150 mL for 2,000 calorie pattern), 1/2 cup (125 mL) corn at dinner
Fruit	2 choices	3 choices	1/2 banana at breakfast (whole banana for 2,000 calorie pattern), 3/4 cup (175 mL) blueberries at dinner or evening snack
Bread, Cereals, and Grains (at least half should be whole grain)	5 choices	6 choices	1 cup (250 mL) cooked oatmeal at breakfast, 2 pieces of whole-wheat bread for lunch sandwich, 1/3 cup (75 mL) brown rice (2/3 cup or 150 mL for 2,000 calorie pattern)
Milk	3 cups (750 mL)	3 cups (750 mL)	1 cup (250 mL) plain yogurt at breakfast, 2 cups (500 mL) milk (1 at lunch and 1 at dinner)
Free Foods	As desired	As desired	Coffee at breakfast, tea at lunch, club soda at dinner, sugar-free gelatin for a snack
Extra Food with Calories	Approximately 100 calories	Approximately 200 calories	Choose additional foods from Appendix B: *Food Groups for Meal Planning*, page 222, or if you choose other foods use Nutrition Facts labels to determine the amount of extra food to eat.

Adapted from Healthy US-Style Dietary Pattern showing recommended amounts of food from each group at various calorie levels, available at: https://www.dietaryguidelines.gov/sites/default/files/2020-12/Dietary _Guidelines_for_Americans_2020-2025.pdf (table A3-2, accessed on 1/10/2021).

Household Measure Equivalencies

United States	Canada
1 teaspoon (tsp)	5 milliliters (mL)
1 tablespoon (Tbsp)	15 mL
1/4 cup	60 mL
1/3 cup	75 mL
1/2 cup	125 mL
2/3 cup	150 mL
3/4 cup	175 mL
1 cup	250 mL
1 ounce (oz)	28 grams (g)
1 fluid ounce (oz)	30 mL
1 inch	2.54 centimeters (cm)

Appendix B: Food Groups for Meal Planning

Protein

Protein from animal sources contains no carbohydrates. Protein from plant sources contains varied amounts of carbohydrate. Protein sources are listed according to how much fat they have.

Also note that this list shows protein sources in 1-ounce (28 gram) portions to make food comparisons and math easier when eating various portion sizes. Typical portion sizes for protein are closer to 3 ounces (84 grams), the size of a deck of cards.

Lean protein sources

1 ounce = 7 grams of protein, 0–3 grams of fat, and 21–45 calories

1 ounce equals:

Beef (fat trimmed, round, sirloin, flank), 1 oz (28 g)

Canned tuna (oil or water drained), herring (uncreamed), mackerel 1/8 cup (30 mL) or 1 oz (28 g)

Catfish, flounder, haddock, halibut, tilapia, perch, salmon (fresh or frozen), 1 oz (28 g)
Cheese (3 g fat or less per ounce), 1 oz (28 g)

Chicken, turkey, duck, goose (no skin, fat removed), 1 oz (28 g)

Game (buffalo, rabbit, venison, ostrich, dove), 1 oz (28 g)

Imitation crab meat (4 g carbohydrate), 1 oz (28 g)

Kidney, liver, heart (beef or chicken), 1 oz (28 g)

Oysters, 6 medium

Processed meats (3 g fat or less per ounce), 1 oz (28 g)

Sardines (oil or water drained), 6 small

Shrimp, lobster, scallops, crab, 1 oz (28 g)

Egg substitute (plain), 1/4 cup (60 mL)

Egg (large) whites, 2 or 1/4 cup (60 mL)

Low-fat or nonfat cottage cheese (2 g carbohydrate), 1/4 cup (60 mL)

Cooked dried beans, peas, lentils (20 g carbohydrate), 1/2 cup (125 mL)

Medium-fat protein sources

1 ounce = 7 grams of protein, 4–7 grams of fat, and 46–70 calories

1 ounce equals:

Corned beef, ground beef, meatloaf, 1 oz (28 g)

Cheese (reduced-fat cheese, mozzarella, feta, goat cheese; 4 to 7 g fat per ounce), 1 oz (28 g)

Edamame (without shells, 7 g carbohydrate), 2¾ oz (78 g) or 1/2 cup (125 mL)

Egg, 1

Fish (fried), 1 oz (28 g)

Pork cutlet (shoulder), 1 oz (28 g)

Pheasant, 1 oz (28 g)

Poultry with skin, 1 oz (28 g)

Reduced-fat sausage (4–7 g fat per ounce), 1 oz (28 g)

Ricotta cheese (made with part skim milk), 1/4 cup (60 mL) or 2 oz (56 g)

Tofu (3 g carbohydrate), 3 oz (84 g)

High-fat protein sources

1 ounce = 7 grams of protein, 8 or more grams of fat, and 80 or more calories

1 ounce equals:

Bacon, 2 slices

Cheese (regular), 1 oz (28 g)

Deli meats (bologna, salami, pastrami), 1 oz (28 g)

Mexican cheese (shredded queso blanco or crumbled fresco), 1/3 cup (75 mL)

Peanut (or other nut) butter (about 7 g carbohydrate), 2 Tbsp (30 g)

Pork ribs (small to medium), 1

Sausage, bratwurst, chorizo, 1 oz (28 g)

Tahini (8 g carbohydrate), 2½ Tbsp (37.5 g)

Turkey bacon, 3 slices

Fats/Oils

Per 1 teaspoon serving, fats and oils contain little or no carbohydrate, 5 grams of fat, and 45 calories. Some fat sources, such as nuts and peanut butter, also contain protein.

Choose unsaturated fats more often than saturated fats and trans fats.

Fat sources that are mainly unsaturated fats

Avocado, 1/4 cup slices

Mayonnaise, 1 tsp (5 mL)

Mayonnaise (reduced fat), 1 Tbsp (15 mL)

Nuts or seeds (6 almonds, 2 pecans, 5 peanuts in shell, 2 whole walnuts), 1 Tbsp (15 mL)

Olives, 10 small or 5 large

Peanut butter (or other nut butter), 1½ tsp (7 mL)

Salad dressings, 1 Tbsp (15 mL)

Salad dressings (reduced fat; may contain carbohydrates)*, 2 Tbsp (30 mL)

Soft margarine (with no trans fat), 1 tsp (5 mL)

Vegetable oil (olive, safflower, canola, corn, sunflower, peanut), 1 tsp (5 mL)

Fat sources that are mainly saturated fats or trans fats

Butter, 1 tsp (5 mL)

Bacon, 1 slice

Coconut (shredded), 2 Tbsp (30 mL)

Coconut oil, 1 tsp (5 mL)

Cream (half-and-half, whipped), 2 Tbsp (30 mL)

Cream (heavy, whipping), 1 Tbsp (15 mL)

Cream cheese, 1 Tbsp (15 mL)

Lard, 1 tsp (5 mL)

Margarine (stick; contains trans fats), 1 tsp (5 mL)

Nondairy coffee creamer (contains carbohydrates, may contain trans fats; check Nutrition Facts label), 2–5 Tbsp (30–75 mL)

Palm oil, 1 tsp (5 mL)

Salt pork, 1/4 oz (7 g)

Shortening (contains trans fats), lard, 1 tsp (5 mL)

Sour cream, 2 Tbsp (30 mL)

Lower-Carbohydrate Vegetables

For vegetables with a small amount of carbohydrate (5 grams or less), little or no fat, and less than 25 calories, serving size is 1/2 cup cooked or 1 cup raw; other serving sizes are noted.

Artichoke

Asparagus

Bamboo shoots

Bean sprouts

Beans (wax, green)

Beets

Broccoli

Brussels sprouts

Cabbage

Carrots

Cauliflower

Celery

Chayote (vegetable pear)

Chicory

Chilies, spicy

Eggplant

Fresh herbs (basil, cilantro, mint, parsley, sage, thyme)

Green onions

Greens (collard, kale, mustard, swiss chard, turnip)

Jicama

Kohlrabi

Mushrooms

Nopales (cactus)

Okra

Onion

Pea pods

Radishes

Rutabaga

Salad greens

Sauerkraut (high in sodium)

Snap peas

Spinach

Summer squash (yellow, zucchini)

Sweet peppers

Tomatoes (1 large)

Vegetable juice (usually high in sodium)

Watercress

---

*Avoid salad dressings that subtitute fat with added sugar and salt.

Higher-Carbohydrate Foods

Higher-Carbohydrate Vegetables and Legumes

Higher-carb vegetables contain about 15 grams of carbohydrate, little or no fat, and about 80 calories. Most have about 3 grams of protein and small amounts of fat.

Baked beans (higher in protein), 1/4 cup (60 mL)

Corn, peas, parsnips, plantain, potatoes (mashed), succotash (lima beans and corn), 1/2 cup (125 mL) cooked

Cassava root (yucca), 1/4 cup (60 mL)

Corn on the cob, 6-inch (15 cm) ear

Dried beans or peas (black-eyed or split peas; black, kidney, lima, or navy beans; lentils; cooked; higher in protein), 1/3 cup (75 mL)

Potato (baked or boiled), 1 small (3 oz or 84 g)

Sweet potato, yam, 1/3 cup (75 mL)

Taro root (cooked slices), 1/3 cup (75 mL) or 1½ oz (42 g)

Winter squash (acorn, butternut, pumpkin; cooked), 1/2 cup (125 mL)

Yautia slices, 1/2 cup (125 mL) or 2 oz (56 g)

Fruits

A serving of fruit contains about 15 grams of carbohydrate with little or no fat, no protein, and 60 calories. In general, 1/2 cup (125 mL) fruit or juice or 1/4 cup (60 mL) dried fruit is one serving.

Fresh fruit

Apple (small), 1

Apricots, 4

Banana (9 inch or 23 cm), 1/2

Berries (blueberries, raspberries), 3/4 cup (175 mL)

Cherries (about 12), 1/2 cup (125 mL)

Figs (small), 2

Grapefruit, 1/2

Grapes (small), 1/2 cup (125 mL)

Guava, 1½ or 1/2 cup (125 mL)

Kiwi (large), 1

Mango (cubed), 1/2 cup (125 mL)

Melon (honeydew, cantaloupe; cubed), 1 cup (250 mL)

Orange (small), 1

Papaya (small, cubed), 1 cup (250 mL)

Peach, nectarine (medium), 1

Pear (medium), 1/2

Persimmon (medium), 1½

Pineapple (cubed), 3/4 cup (175 mL)

Plum (small), 2

Pomegranate, 1/2

Strawberries (whole), 1¼ cups (310 mL)

Watermelon (cubed), 1½ cups (375 mL)

Dried fruit

Apples, 3 rings

Apricots, 7 halves

Dates (dried, pitted), 3

Figs, 2

Prunes (pitted medium), 3

Raisins, 2 Tbsp (30 mL)

Bread, Cereals, and Grains

Per serving, these bread, cereal, and grain items contain 15 grams carbohydrate, 3 grams protein, little or no fat, and about 80 calories. Products with added fat have more calories. Choose whole grains, which are good sources of fiber, as often as you can.

Breads, rolls, muffins, tortillas, and grains

Amaranth (cooked),* 1/3 cup (75 mL)

Bagel (medium), 1/4 (1 oz or 28 g)

Barley (cooked),* 1/3 cup (75 mL)

Biscuit (small),† 1/2

Bread (white, whole grain,* rye), 1 slice (1 oz)

Bulgur wheat (cooked),* 1/2 cup (125 mL)

Bun (hotdog or hamburger), 1/2

English muffin, 1/2

Horchata (drink), 1/2 cup (125 mL)

Pancake† (4 inches or 10 cm), 1

Pasta, white, whole wheat* (cooked), 1/3 cup (75 mL)

Pita bread (6 inches or 15 cm), 1/2

Quinoa (cooked),* 1/3 cup (75 mL)

Rice (white, brown,* or wild*; cooked), 1/3 cup (75 mL)

Roll (regular), 1/2

Tabbouleh* (cooked), 1 cup (250 mL)

Tortilla (corn* or flour; 6 inches or 15 cm), 1

Waffle (reduced fat; 4½ inches or 11 cm), 1

Wheat germ* (dry), 3 Tbsp (45 mL)

Cereals

Bran flakes,* corn flakes, spoon-size shredded wheat,* 1/2 cup (125 mL)

Granola,*† 1/4 cup (60 mL)

Oats* (cooked), 1/2 cup (125 mL)

Puffed, unfrosted wheat or rice cereal, 1½ cup (375 mL)

Crackers and snacks

Graham crackers (2½ inch or 6 cm square), 3 Matzo, 3 oz (84 g)

Melba toast (2 × 4 inches or 5 × 10 cm), 4

Popcorn (reduced fat),* 3 cups (750 mL)

Potato chips, 1 oz (28 g) or 15 chips

Pretzels, 3 oz (84 g)

Rice cakes (4 inches or 10 cm across), 2

Saltines, 6

Whole-wheat crackers* (reduced fat; 3 oz or 84 g), 2–5

---

*Good source of fiber
†Added fat

Sweets

Low-fat or nonfat sweets

Low-fat or nonfat sweets contain about 15 grams of carbohydrate, 0–3 grams of protein, and 60–80 calories. *Choose sweets less often.*

Gingersnaps, 3

Honey, 1 Tbsp (15 mL)

Jam or jelly, 1 Tbsp (15 mL)

Jelly beans (small), 15

Licorice sticks, 2

Pudding (skim milk), 1/4 cup (60 mL)

Sherbet, 1/3 cup (75 mL)

Soda, 1/2 cup (125 mL)

Syrup (regular), 1 Tbsp (15 mL)

Medium-fat sweets

Medium-fat sweets contain about 15 grams of carbohydrate, 0–3 grams of protein, 5 grams of fat, and 110–130 calories.

Cake with frosting (1 inch or 2½ cm square)

Cookies (small; 1¾ inches or 4 cm), 2

Granola bar (small), 1

High-fat sweets

High-fat sweets contains about 15 grams of carbohydrate, 0–3 grams of protein, more than 5 grams of fat, and more than 130 calories.

Chocolate candy bar (1½ oz or 42 g), 1/2

Danish pastry (4½ inches or 11 cm), 1/2

Fruit pie, 1/16 of 9 inch (23 cm) pie

Ice cream, 1/2 cup (125 mL)

Milk

Milk products contain both carbohydrate and protein. Fat content may be low or high depending on the item selected. Kefir's fat and calorie content varies based on the percent of milk fat used. Flavored milk and sweetened yogurt's fat, carbohydrate, and calories vary based on the percent of milk fat and added sugars. *Check Nutrition Facts labels for these products.*

Skim and very low-fat milk products

One serving contains 12 grams of carbohydrate, 8 grams of protein, 0–3 grams of fat, and about 80 calories.

Dry nonfat milk, 1/3 cup (75 mL)

Evaporated skim milk, 1/2 cup (125 mL)

Low-fat buttermilk, 1 cup (250 mL)

Plain nonfat yogurt, 8 oz (224 g)

Skim and 1% milk, 1 cup (250 mL)

Low-fat milk products

One serving contains about 12 grams of carbohydrate, 8 grams of protein, 5 grams of fat, and 120 calories.

2% milk, 1 cup (250 mL)

Plain low-fat yogurt, 8 oz (224 g)

High-fat milk products

One serving contains about 12 grams of carbohydrate, 8 grams of protein, 8 grams of fat, and 150 calories.

Evaporated whole milk, 1/2 cup (125 mL)

Whole milk, buttermilk, 1 cup (250 mL)

Whole, fresh, or evaporated goat milk, 1 cup (250 mL)

Whole-milk plain yogurt, 8 oz (224 g)

Milk substitutes

One serving contains about 6–9 grams of carbohydrate, 8 grams of protein, 5 grams of unsaturated fat, and 80–130 calories.

Calcium-fortified soy milk, 1 cup or 250 mL (15 g carbohydrate)

Calcium-fortified unsweetened soy milk, 1 cup or 250 mL (4 g carbohydrate)

Other milk substitutes generally have much less protein, calorie content varies, and they may or may not be fortified.

Cheese and cottage cheese are found in the protein section.

Sour cream and butter are in the fat section.

Alcoholic Beverages

Per serving most alcoholic beverages have no protein and fat. Calories and carbohydrate content vary.

Beer (lite), 12 oz (355 mL) (5 g carbohydrate, 100 calories)

Beer (nonalcoholic), 12 oz (355 mL) (about 20 g carbohydrate, 100 calories)

Beer (regular), 12 oz (355 mL) (about 13 g carbohydrate,160 calories)

Distilled spirits (80 proof), 1½ oz (44 mL) (0 g carbohydrate, 80–100 calories)

Liqueurs, 1½ oz (44 mL) (10–24 g carbohydrate, 140–240 calories)

Mixed drinks (margarita, mojito, gin and tonic, etc.), 1 drink (many are 20–30 g carbohydrate, 200–250 calories)

Wine (red, white, dry, sparkling), 5 oz (148 mL) (4 g carbohydrate, 125 calories)

Wine (sweet, dessert), 3½ oz (103 mL) (14 g carbohydrate, 165 calories)

Free Foods

Per serving, free foods contain up to 5 grams of carbohydrate and 20 calories. Enjoy moderate servings. Choose high-salt items less often.

Bouillon, broth, consommé*

Candy, hard (sugar-free)

Chewing gum (sugar-free)

Club soda, mineral water

Coffee or tea, black or with sugar substitute

Flavored ice pops (sugar-free)

Garlic

Gelatin (sugar-free or plain)

Herbs, spices

Hot pepper sauces

Seltzer water (unsweetened)

Soft drinks (sugar-free)

Soy sauce*

Water, plain

Worcestershire sauce*

_____

*high in sodium (salt)

Sugar Substitutes (approved by the US Food and Drug Administration)

Equal (aspartame)

Monk fruit in the raw (luo han guo)

Newtame (neotame)

NutraSweet (aspartame)

Splenda (sucralose)

Sugar Twin (aspartame)

Sunette (acesulfame potassium)

Sweet Leaf (stevia)

Sweet One (acesulfame potassium)

Sweet Twin (saccharin)

Sweet'N Low (saccharin)

Note: The sugar substitutes listed above, also called "nonnutritive sweeteners" or "low-calorie sweeteners," do not include all government-approved generic sugar substitutes. We also do not list all brand names. The list also omits sweeteners that are higher in carbohydrate (and calories) than sugar substitutes but lower than regular sugar. Examples of these sweeteners include fructose and sugar alcohols such as sorbitol, mannitol, and xylitol.

Health Canada has approved the following high-intensity nonnutritive sweeteners for use in foods and chewing gum and/or as tabletop sweeteners: acesulfame potassium, aspartame, cyclamate, neotame, saccharin, steviol glycosides, sucralose, thaumatin, and monk fruit extract.

Equal (aspartame)

Krisda (steviol glycosides)

Pure Via (steviol glycosides)

Stevia (steviol glycosides)

Sugar Twin (cyclamate)

Truvia (steviol glycosides)

Hermesetas (saccharin)

NutraSweet (aspartame)

Splenda (sucralose)

Sucaryl (cyclamate)

Sweet'N Low (saccharin)

CHAPTER 10

Healthy Weight and Pain Self-Management

Being overweight is a long-term chronic condition for many people. And being overweight makes chronic pain and most other chronic health conditions worse. The good news is that you can improve your health by losing even a small amount of weight. If a person with chronic pain is overweight, weight loss is often recommended for pain management along with other treatments and therapies.

Weight is important for many reasons. Excess weight is a risk factor for developing osteoarthritis of the hips, knees, ankles, and feet. Extra weight also puts extra stress on almost all joints. Imagine lifting a pound of rice—now think of lifting 20 pounds of rice.

Special thanks to thank Emily Clairmont MS, RDN, CD, Ann Constance, MA, RDN, CDCES, FAADE, Robin Edelman, MS, RDN, CDCES, and Yvonne Mullan, MSc, RD, CDE, for their thoughtful and thorough contributions to this chapter.

231

Which is more painful to lift? If you are overweight, extra weight could well be causing some of your pain.

When a person is overweight, the heart works harder and that can lead to high blood pressure, heart disease, and stroke. People with diabetes can have problems keeping blood sugar at healthy levels. If blood sugar rises, heart and nerve problems that come from diabetes may worsen. These nerve problems are often painful. For people with prediabetes who are overweight, losing 5 to 7 percent of current weight may delay or reverse the progression toward diabetes. Research shows that losing this small amount of weight (5 percent loss for a person who weighs 150 pounds or 68 kg is 7.5 pounds or 3.4 kg) prevents or delays many health problems.

But losing weight and maintaining a weight loss is often difficult. Studies show that people who lose weight and maintain their new weight usually have ongoing support from family, friends, health providers, or a group of people working together to lose weight and maintain the loss.

Although having excess body weight is a more common problem than being underweight, for people living with chronic pain, some may need help gaining a few pounds. In this chapter we provide information and tools to help you successfully manage your weight and weight-related chronic pain concerns. Although we mostly talk about losing weight, you will find some information about gaining weight on page 243.

What Is a Healthy Weight for You?

There is no such thing as an "ideal" weight. Instead, healthy weights span a range for each person. Finding your healthy weight range and deciding whether you want or need to change your weight depends on many things. These include your age, activity level, overall health, where your body fat is located, and your personal and family history of weight-related health problems, such as chronic pain, high blood pressure, and diabetes.

One way to understand a healthy weight is to figure out your BMI (body mass index). Your BMI summarizes your height and weight in a single number. Although not a perfect measure, BMI is a useful guide. In Table 10.1 from the National Institutes of Health (pages 234–235), find your height and follow that line to

the number nearest to your current weight. The heading on that column above your weight lists your BMI and indicates what range or group you are in: Normal, Overweight, Obese, or Extreme Obesity. (Note that these are standard medical terms, not our terms of choice.) One study found that people in the BMI overweight category compared to normal-weight people had 20 percent more pain, while those in the obese category had nearly 70 percent more pain. People whose BMI was over 40 had more than twice as much pain as normal-weight people. There is still much to learn, but when it comes to chronic pain, weight seems to matter.

Once you know your BMI, refer to Table 10.2 on page 235. It tells you more about what your BMI score means in terms of your health. If you are older than 65, your health care providers may recommend a healthy weight range that is a little higher than the numbers for "normal weight" and "overweight." Your BMI and weight goals depend on your health conditions and other items you can discuss with your health team.

Another way to consider if your weight is healthy is to measure the distance around your waist (your "waist circumference"). Measure your waist by standing up straight and placing a tape measure (one that is not old and stretched out) around your bare middle, just above your hip bone. Bring the tape measure all the way around your body, keeping it level with your belly button. Make sure it's not too tight and that it is straight and flat across your back. Do not hold your breath. Check the number on the tape measure just after you breathe out. A goal is a waist circumference measurement less than 40 inches (101 cm) for men and less than 35 inches (89 cm) for nonpregnant women. If your number is higher, this means that you have more health risks. If you are overweight and most of your body fat is around your waist (rather than on hips and thighs), you are at higher risk for heart disease, high blood pressure, and type 2 diabetes. Body fat around your waist also increases inflammation, which may add to your pain.

Making the Decision to Change Your Weight

Reaching and maintaining a healthy weight usually means making some changes. Deciding to make changes is your choice, not the choice of your friends, family, or health care provider. If you want to make changes, do it slowly, and only make changes that are realistic for you. The motto "go for the real, not the ideal" is a good one for weight management.

To get started, review the information about action planning in Chapter 2, *Becoming an Active Self-Manager*. If you think you want to change your weight, consider asking your primary care provider to refer you to a registered dietitian. You might also join a weight loss support group such as Weight Watchers. Managing your weight is not something you need to do alone. In fact, people who have ongoing support usually are better able to meet and maintain their goals.

When you are ready to consider weight change, ask yourself these two questions:

1. **Why do I want to change my weight?**
   Everyone has personal reasons for how and why they manage weight. Here are some examples:
   - to manage my symptoms (pain, fatigue, shortness of breath, etc.)
   - to manage my diabetes or other chronic disease
   - to prevent conditions such as diabetes, stroke, and heart disease
   - to have more energy to do the things I want to do
   - to feel better about myself
   - to change the way others think of me
   - to take more control of my health or my life

Table 10.1 **Body Mass Index Table**

	Normal						Overweight				
	19	**20**	**21**	**22**	**23**	**24**	**25**	**26**	**27**	**28**	**29**
4'10"	91	96	100	105	110	115	119	124	129	134	138
4'11"	94	99	104	109	114	119	124	128	133	138	143
5'0"	97	102	107	112	118	123	128	133	138	143	148
5'1"	100	106	111	116	122	127	132	137	143	148	153
5'2"	104	109	115	120	126	131	136	142	147	153	158
5'3"	107	112	118	124	130	135	141	146	152	158	163
5'4"	110	116	122	128	134	140	145	151	157	163	169
5'5"	114	120	126	132	138	144	150	156	162	168	174
5'6"	118	124	130	136	142	148	155	161	167	173	179
5'7"	121	127	134	140	146	153	159	166	172	178	185
5'8"	125	131	138	144	151	158	164	171	177	184	190
5'9"	128	135	142	149	155	162	169	176	182	189	196
5'10"	132	139	146	153	160	167	174	181	188	195	202
5'11"	136	143	150	157	165	172	179	186	193	200	208
6'0"	140	147	154	162	169	177	184	191	199	206	213
6'1"	144	151	159	167	174	182	189	196	204	212	219
6'2"	148	155	163	171	179	186	194	202	210	218	225
6'3"	152	160	168	176	184	192	200	208	216	224	232
6'4"	156	164	172	180	189	197	205	213	221	230	238

List your reasons for losing weight here (yes, you can write in the book):

_____

_____

_____

_____

2. **Am I ready to make lifelong changes?**
   The next step is to find out if this is a good time to start making changes. If you are not ready, you may be setting yourself up for failure. The truth is that there is never a "perfect" time. The following additional questions may help you figure out if you are ready:

   ■ Are there other things in my life that I can do now that might make losing weight easier? (To get more exercise, for example, is there a dog that needs walking, or can you get off the bus one stop earlier in your daily commute? Maybe you live somewhere close to stores and you can start walking for errands instead of driving. Maybe you can sign up for a meal service.)

   ■ What things may get in the way of not making eating or activity changes?

   ■ Will concerns about family, friends, work, or other things make it difficult to make changes?

   ■ Do I have support? Is there someone who will make it easier to begin and continue making changes?

   ■ Am I able to find and afford healthful food?

Table 10.1 **Body Mass Index Table (*continued*)**

	Obese										Extreme Obesity		
	30	**31**	**32**	**33**	**34**	**35**	**36**	**37**	**38**	**39**	**40**	**41**	**42**
4'10"	143	148	153	158	162	167	172	177	181	186	191	196	201
4'11"	148	153	158	163	168	173	178	183	188	193	198	203	208
5'0"	153	158	163	168	174	179	184	189	194	199	204	209	215
5'1"	158	164	169	174	180	185	190	195	201	206	211	217	222
5'2"	164	169	175	180	186	191	196	202	207	213	218	224	229
5'3"	169	174	180	186	191	197	203	208	214	220	225	231	237
5'4"	175	180	186	191	197	204	209	215	221	227	232	238	244
5'5"	180	186	192	198	204	210	216	222	228	234	240	246	252
5'6"	186	192	198	204	210	216	223	229	235	241	247	253	260
5'7"	191	198	204	211	217	223	230	236	242	249	255	261	268
5'8"	197	204	210	216	223	230	236	243	249	256	262	269	276
5'9"	203	210	216	223	230	236	243	250	257	263	270	277	284
5'10"	209	216	222	229	236	243	250	257	264	271	278	285	292
5'11"	215	222	229	236	243	250	257	265	272	279	286	293	301
6'0"	221	228	235	242	250	258	265	272	279	287	294	302	309
6'1"	227	235	242	250	257	265	275	280	288	295	302	310	318
6'2"	233	241	249	256	264	272	280	287	295	303	311	319	326
6'3"	240	248	256	264	272	279	287	295	303	311	319	327	335
6'4"	246	254	263	271	279	287	295	304	312	320	328	336	344

Table 10.2 **Weight Classifications Based on Body Mass Index**

Body Mass Index	Weight Classification	What It Means
Less than 18.5	Underweight	Unless you have other health problems, being in this weight class may not be an issue if you are small or petite.
18.5 to 24.9	Normal weight	This is the healthy range.
25 to 29.9	Overweight	This range suggests that you are carrying extra pounds. It may not be of much concern if you are healthy and have few or no other health problems or risk factors or you are very physically active and have a lot of muscle.
30 to 39.9	Obese	This range signals that it is likely you have a large amount of body fat. It puts you at increased risk for weight-related health problems.
40 and over	Extremely obese	This weight class pinpoints that a high proportion of your body weight is fat. It puts you at very high risk for developing serious health problems.

Refer to Table 10.3 on page 237 and think about what will help and what will get in the way of making changes. When you ask and answer these questions, you may find that now is not the best time to start. If this is true for you, you can revisit weight self-management in the future. No matter what you find, accept that this is the right decision for you now.

If you decide to start making changes, start with the changes that are easiest and the most comfortable. Take "baby steps." Work on changing only one or two things at a time. Do not try to do too much. Action planning tools are great tools for making change at a healthy pace. (See pages 33–39 in Chapter 2, *Becoming an Active Self-Manager*.) Slow and steady wins the race.

Getting Started with Weight Change

The good news is that eating for weight loss is very similar to eating for pain management. You can read more about food and pain in Chapter 9, *Healthy Eating and Pain Self-Management*. Start by keeping a diary of what you eat and your physical activity. Do this for at least one weekday and one weekend day (or one workday and one non-workday). If you can keep it for more days, all the better. Write down what you eat in the Food and Activity Tracking Diary in Figure 10.1 on page 238, or use an app or fitness tracker. You will find some health-related apps and trackers listed on our resource site, which is provided at the end of this chapter.

Here are the specific things you should list:

- what you eat and where you are eating

- why you are eating (Are you hungry or eating because you are bored or are with other people who are eating?)
- how you feel when eating (your mood or emotions)
- your exercise (the physical activities you do)

You might also have a section in your diary for ideas about what you would like to do differently. See an example on page 241.

When you have kept a diary for a few days or weeks, look at what you have written. You may be surprised to realize how much or little you exercise, that you drink a lot of soda, or that you eat ice cream every night. You can use what you learn about yourself and your habits to decide where to start making changes.

Making Eating and Activity Changes

The two basics of weight management are:

1. Take "baby steps."
2. Start by making changes you know you can accomplish.

There is no getting around it: to change your weight, you need to change the amount of food you eat as well as some of the things you eat and drink. Physical activity can help, but it is very

Table 10.3 **Factors Affecting the Decision to Change Your Weight Now**

Things That Will Help Me to Make Changes	Things That Will Make It Difficult for Me to Change
Example: I have the support of family and friends.	*Example:* The holidays are coming up, and I will be busy preparing for gatherings.

Figure 10.1 **Food and Activity Tracking Diary**

Date	Time	What I Ate/Drank	Where I Ate	Why I Ate	My Mood, Emotions, or Pain	My Exercise

difficult to exercise enough to lose weight without also changing what you eat. This may seem scary or even impossible, but by sticking to the basics you can do it!

What are "baby steps" and how do you know what you can accomplish? For instance, when you first get started trying to lose weight, a good first step is to cut your portions a small amount. Instead of eating a cup of rice or ice cream, eat a few tablespoons less. (Review the discussion of portions—what you put on the plate—on page 211 in Chapter 9, *Healthy Eating and Pain Self-Management*.) Another good first small step is a few days a week, instead of sitting on the couch after lunch, walk around the block. There are many more tips for losing weight on pages 241–242.

When you find things you want to change, choose only one or two things to change at a time. You have heard this before, but we repeat it here because it is important. Allow yourself time to get used to changes and then slowly change more things. If you tell yourself you are going to walk 5 miles (8 km) a day every day of the week and never eat potatoes or bread again, you probably won't be able to stick to that eating pattern very long. You won't lose weight, and you will feel frustrated and discouraged. Instead, plan to have only one piece of toast at breakfast instead of two, and take two 10-minute walks four times a week. This way you are more likely to stick to it, make long-term changes, and lose weight. By the way, if you are like many people, if you put on your shoes and make it out of your house to walk 5 minutes, you may find yourself walking 10 or 15 minutes. The hard part is getting out of the house.

When you change your weight slowly, you have a better chance of maintaining the change.

This is partly because your brain begins to recognize the changes as part of your regular routine and not just a passing fad. Remember, the best eating pattern combines healthy eating and exercise and is a slow, steady plan that feels right to you.

The 200 Plan for Weight Loss

One way to get started losing weight is the 200 Plan, which involves making small daily changes in your eating and physical activity. You change what you do by 200 calories a day. To lose weight, eat 100 fewer calories a day than you do now and burn off 100 calories a day more with a little bit of extra activity. This may add up to losing about 20 pounds (9 kg) a year. The 200 Plan is a good way to balance eating and exercise and helps you achieve long-term weight change.

Eat 100 Fewer Calories a Day

Look at your food log and see if there is anywhere you can easily cut back. Then check Appendix A: *Eating Patterns for 1,600 and 2,000 Calories* on page 221 and Appendix B: *Food Groups for Meal Planning* on page 222 for serving sizes and numbers of calories per serving. For example, a 1-ounce slice of bread has close to 100 calories. By eating one less piece of toast in the morning or by not eating one of the slices of bread on your sandwich, you cut out close to 100 calories.

Burn 100 More Calories a Day

Add 20 to 30 minutes to your regular activity routine, whether it is walking, bicycling, dancing, or gardening. Take the stairs and park farther away from the store or work. If time is an issue, burn your extra 100 calories in three 5- to 10-minute chunks of time over the day. This method works just as well as doing it all at once. Some people find that a fitness tracker can help them move a little bit more each day.

Physical Activity and Weight Loss

As we noted before, physical activity can help you lose weight and keep it off. However, it is very difficult to exercise enough to lose weight without also changing what you eat. It is important to understand that success comes from making both activity and eating changes that become part of your daily life. To help with weight loss, endurance (aerobic) exercise is the best. You can learn more about endurance exercises on pages 145–153 in Chapter 7, *Exercising and Physical Activity for Every Body*. Endurance exercises help you lose weight because they use your large muscles that burn the most calories. The exercise guidelines recommend moderate endurance (aerobic) exercise for at least 150 minutes (2½ hours) each week or vigorous intensity activity for at least 75 minutes each week. These guidelines are the same for general health, weight loss, and keeping weight off.

But remember, you do not need to exercise at these levels if you are just starting an exercise program. This is something you can work up to over time. If you can never achieve this, that is OK too. The idea is to add more activity to your day and do more than you used to do. Do your physical activities of choice four or five times a week. Do not go more than two days without exercising. And add to your activities a little each week.

Exercising in short bouts of 10 minutes or more works as well as longer workouts. If you can add more minutes, that is even better. Consider also including some strength training. Muscle-strengthening activities help you maintain your muscles during weight loss, plus muscle burns calories around the clock, even while you are asleep!

As you add exercise to your routine, follow the same advice we give you for making eating changes. Take "baby steps" to make small changes, and start with changes you know you can accomplish. If you exercise too hard or too long, you are more likely to have to stop because of an injury, fatigue, frustration, or loss of interest. You don't have to do it all at once.

At some point you might become discouraged. The pounds may stop coming off. There are many reasons why this might happen. Exercise may be building muscle as well as reducing fat. Muscle weighs more than fat, so you could be losing fat, but the scale is not showing it. If you keep track of body measurements such as waist and hips* or notice that your clothes fit better or are looser, this can be a signal that exercise is working. And remember, when you exercise regularly, even if you don't lose weight, you are doing good things for your body. Regular exercise can help give you more energy. As we noted at the beginning of the chapter, exercise can also help a person who has prediabetes avoid getting diabetes. Exercise can reduce blood glucose, blood pressure, and blood fat levels as well as increase good cholesterol, reduce the risk of heart disease, and help with depression and anxiety.

---

*For specific information on hip and waist measurement and healthy hip/waist ratios, please visit
https://apps.who.int/iris/bitstream/handle/10665/44583/9789241501491_eng.pdf?sequence=1

Tips for Losing Weight

The following are some additional tips for losing weight:

- **Set small, gradual weight loss goals.** Break the total amount of weight you want to lose into small, reachable goals. For most people, aiming to lose 1 to 2 pounds (0.5–1 kg) a week is realistic and doable, especially in the first several weeks. After a while, a smaller goal (such as 1/2 pound or 1/4 kilogram per week) may be more doable. Consider yourself successful if you continue to hold your lower weight steady without gaining any pounds back.

- **Identify your specific actions to lose weight.** For example, walking 20 minutes a day five days a week, not eating between meals, and eating more slowly. Review the information about action planning in Chapter 2, *Becoming an Active Self-Manager.*

- **Pay attention to what you eat.** Overeating is common when people are with friends, using the computer, or watching television. Set out the portion you want to eat and keep the other food out of sight. By focusing on what you are eating and not what you are doing (such as watching television), you will be more satisfied and you will eat less. For more on this, see *Tips for Mindful Eating* on page 244.

- **Know a serving size when you see one and choose appropriate portions.** A 3/4-cup (175 mL) serving is the size of a tennis ball or a small closed fist. A 3-ounce (84 g) serving of cooked meat, fish, or poultry is the size of a deck of playing cards or a checkbook. The end of your thumb to the first joint is about 1 tablespoon (15 mL). Using a measuring cup or a food scale is a great way to learn about appropriate serving size. Especially when starting to make changes, measure your portions—and do this frequently over time. It is amazing just how easily 1/2-cup (125 mL) of rice can "grow" to a 1-cup (250 mL) portion. Foods that come prepackaged as single servings can help you learn what you eat. Restaurants often serve oversized portions. When eating away from home, select appetizers or first courses over main entrées, or order a child's meal. This will help you eat fewer calories. Another trick is to order a carryout box with your food and put half of your meal in the box before you start to eat. Don't eat "family style" by putting serving dishes on the table. Put your meal on a plate and leave everything else in the kitchen. Put leftovers away as soon as you have finished eating or after you have dished out your meal.

- **Watch out for supersizing and portion inflation.** Portion sizes have grown over the years. The typical cheeseburger used to have about 330 calories; now it has 590 calories. Twenty years ago, an average cookie was about 1½ inches (3.8 cm) wide and had 55 calories; now it is 3½ inches (8.9 cm) wide and has 275 calories—*five times* the calories! In the past, soda came in 6½-ounce (192 mL) bottles. That amount contains just 85 calories. Today a typical soda bottle is 20 ounces (591 mL) and has 250 calories. Pay attention to the Nutrition

Facts printed on food packages to see if you are eating one or more servings when eating at home. Ask for calorie information about menu choices when eating out.

- **Do not skip meals.** Eat three meals per day, including breakfast. If you skip a meal, you may feel hungrier later and end up eating more than you need to satisfy your larger appetite.

- **Eat slowly.** If you take less than 15 or 20 minutes to eat a meal, you are probably eating too fast. Give your brain time to catch up with your stomach. If you find it hard to slow down, try putting your fork down on the table between bites. Pick it up again only after you have swallowed. Try not to be the first person at the table to be finished.

- **Clock yourself.** After you eat your single portion, make it a habit to wait about 15 minutes before either taking another portion or starting to eat dessert or a snack. You'll often find that the urge to continue eating will go away if you wait a little while.

- **Keep on top of what is happening.** Check your weight on a schedule that works for you. You may not need to check it every day. If you check your weight at the same time of day (usually first thing in the morning), it is easier to note changes.

- **Make sure you are drinking enough water.** Sometimes people think they are hungry when they are actually thirsty.

- **Join a support group (either in person or online) and stay with it for at least four to**

six months. Look for a group that does the following:

- ▶ emphasizes healthy eating
- ▶ emphasizes lifelong changes in eating habits and lifestyle patterns
- ▶ gives support in the form of ongoing meetings or long-term follow-up
- ▶ does not make miraculous claims or guarantees (Remember, if something sounds too good to be true, it probably is not true.)
- ▶ does not rely on special meals or supplements

Also check out the tips in the section *Healthy Eating for Chronic Pain: Putting It All Together* in Chapter 9, *Healthy Eating and Pain Self-Management* (see page 217).

Tips for Keeping Weight Off

Maintaining weight loss requires effort. If you begin to lose weight, make sure to keep your weight within healthy guidelines. If you are feeling well, have good blood sugar and cholesterol levels, and are managing other health issues well, you may not need to lose more weight. The following are some tips to help you move from weight loss to keeping the weight off:

- **Instead of focusing on weight loss,** focus on staying at the same weight and not gaining any weight for a few weeks; then check your progress and make midcourse corrections if needed and adjust your plans.

- **Increase your physical activity.** Your body may have adjusted to your lower weight and therefore needs fewer calories, so you may need to exercise more to burn more calories to keep the weight off.

- **Plan your meals ahead.** Take time once per week to plan meals (or at least dinners) for the week and make a grocery list. This can reduce food waste and save money. Dinner is the largest meal most people eat. Dinner planning helps you have the ingredients you need when you want them.

- **Log your foods in your food diary periodically to get back on track.** (See Figure 10.1, Food and Activity Tracking Diary. on page 238.)

- **Try different fruits to end your meals with something sweet but light and refreshing.** Use the food lists in the appendices of Chapter 9, *Healthy Eating and Pain Self-Management*, on pages 221–229 to check the serving sizes and control calories.

- **Allow yourself an occasional treat so you don't feel deprived.** Treat yourself to a higher-calorie food you don't usually eat. Be sure the treat is a small portion, and don't make this a daily habit.

- **Keep thinking positively.** Remind yourself of what you have already done. Write about your successes on sticky notes and post them where you will see them.

- **Set a personal weight gain "upper limit."** This could be perhaps 3 pounds (1.4 kg) higher than your current weight. Knowing when you are starting to put on weight can help you take action, if needed. Some people decide that when they regain, say, 3 pounds (1.4 kg), it is a signal to get back into eating less or moving more. If you hit

your upper limit, go back on your weight loss program. The sooner you start, the faster the newly added pounds will come off.

- **Plan to be active on most days.** Once you have lost some weight, exercising most days of the week improves your chances of keeping the weight off.

- **If something big is happening in your life,** weight management may need to take a back seat for a while. Set a date when you will restart your weight management program.

- **If you have not already done so, join a support group.**

Tips for Gaining Weight

Some people are told they need to gain weight by their health care providers. If this is an issue for you, consider the following strategies:

- **Eat dried fruit in place of some fresh fruit,** or drink nectars instead of regular fruit juice.

- **Choose whole milk, cheese, and yogurt** instead of lower-fat dairy products.

- **Add extra whole milk** or milk powder to sauces, gravies, cereals, soups, and casseroles.

- **Drink liquid supplements or smoothies** with or between meals.

- **Drink high-calorie beverages** such as shakes, malts, fruit whips, smoothies, and eggnogs.

- **Top salads, soups, and casseroles** with shredded cheese, nuts, dried fruits, or seeds.

- **Try waiting to drink beverages** 30 minutes after a meal so you have more room to eat food with higher calories. Or **sip high-calorie drinks with your meal** if you are thirsty. Try both options to find what works best for you.

- **Leave some nuts or dried fruit out** and eat a few pieces each time you pass the bowl.

- **Eat the highest-calorie foods on your plate first**, saving lower-calorie foods for later (for example, eat buttered bread before cooked spinach).

- **Add melted cheese** to vegetables and other dishes.

- **Use butter, margarine, or sour cream** as toppings. Add a flavored plant-based oil as a heart-healthy topping.

- **Keep a snack at your bedside** so that you can eat something if you wake in the middle of the night. Dried fruit and nuts are healthy snacks. Always sit up or get out of bed before you eat. To prevent dental issues, it is important to drink water and rinse your mouth out after a midnight snack.

- **Eat six small meals every 2 to 3 hours** instead of two to three big meals every 5 hours.

- **Do not skip meals.** Even if you need to eat something small, it is better than nothing at all.

Tips for Mindful Eating

Go for the real, not the ideal. Healthy eating is not all or nothing. Healthy eating is making small changes. Many people find that applying the concepts of mindfulness to eating can help them be more aware of what and how they eat.

To learn more about mindfulness, review Chapter 5, *Using Your Mind to Manage Pain and Other Symptoms* (page 112). Consider these mindful eating tips:

- **Be mindful while you eat.** Notice what you eat, how much you eat, and how you are enjoying it. Practice this without things that take your attention away, such as friends, the newspaper, a phone app, or television. When you eat, concentrate on eating. When something tastes good, savor the flavor.

- **Replace thoughts about foods that include** *never, always,* **and** *avoid.* Instead, tell yourself that you can enjoy things occasionally, "but a healthier choice is better for me most of the time."

- **Think about retraining your taste buds,** and know that making healthier choices can help you on the road to healthier eating. This is especially true when cutting back on salt. Your taste buds eventually adjust to less salty flavors and learn to enjoy them.

- **Do a relaxation exercise before eating.** Or pause for five deep breaths during your meal time. (See *Tools for Breathing Self-Management* in Chapter 4, *Understanding and Managing Common Symptoms and Problems.*)

- **Notice your food-mood connection in your food diary.** Review your food diary, especially your notes about your mood or emotions when eating (see Figure 10.1 on page 238). Look for patterns. Do you eat when you are bored? When you are stressed out?

Mindful Eating Exercise

For this exercise, you will need something to eat, such as a raisin, dried cranberry, grape, walnut, or carrot. Really, any food will work, but it works best if you choose something healthy that comes from a plant! For this example, we have chosen a grape.

1. Sit comfortably in a chair.
2. Place the grape in your hand.
3. Examine the grape as if you had never seen it before.
4. Imagine the grape growing, surrounded by nature.
5. As you look at the grape, think about what you see: the shape, texture, color, size, and ingredients. Is it hard or soft? Shiny or dull? Lumpy or smooth?
6. How does the grape feel?
7. Bring the grape to your nose and smell it.
8. Are you anticipating eating it? Is it difficult not to pop it in your mouth?
9. Place the grape in your mouth. Become aware of what your tongue is doing.
10. Bite ever so lightly into the grape. Feel the texture.
11. Chew three times and then stop. What is the response from your body?
12. Describe the flavor of the grape. Salty? Sweet? Spicy? Sour?
13. As you complete chewing, swallow the grape.
14. Sit quietly, breathing, aware of what you are sensing.

Use what you learn to make small changes. Try walking around the block or doing a few stretching exercises from Chapter 8, *Exercising to Feel Better*, when you get bored or frustrated instead of heading to the fridge.

- **When you are bored and are thinking about eating,** ask yourself, "Am I really hungry?" If the answer is no, make yourself do something else for a few minutes. Keep your mind and hands busy.

- **Stop eating when you first feel full.** This helps you control the amount you eat so you don't overeat. Pay attention to your body so you can learn what fullness feels like. Like all new skills, identifying fullness takes some practice. If it is hard to stop eating when you begin to feel full, remove your plate or get up from the table if you can.

- **Eat slowly.** Eating slowly gives you more enjoyment and helps prevent overeating. Make your meals last more than 15 or 20 minutes. It takes that long for the brain to catch up and tell your stomach that it is getting full. Put down utensils between bites. If you finish the food on your plate quickly, wait at least 15 minutes before getting more food.

Tips for Eating Out

- Select restaurants that have a variety of menu choices.

- Select foods that are grilled, baked, or steamed rather than fried.

- Before you go out, decide what you will eat. Look up menus on the internet.

- Order small plates of appetizers instead of main courses.

- When you are with a group, order first so that you aren't tempted to change your mind.

- Consider splitting an entrée or taking half home.

- Choose menu items that are low in fat, sodium, and sugar, or ask if food can be prepared with less salt, gravy, or sauce.

- Eat bread without butter or have the bread removed.

- Request salad with dressing on the side.

- Dip your fork into the dressing before each bite instead of pouring the dressing on your salad.

- For dessert, select fruit, nonfat yogurt, sorbet, or sherbet.

Tips for Healthy Snacking

- Rather than crackers, chips, and cookies, munch on fresh fruit, raw vegetables, or fat-free or plain popcorn.

- Measure out your snack in a single-portion size so you won't be tempted to eat more.

- Make specific places at home and work your "eating areas," and don't eat anywhere else. For example, eat in the kitchen or dining room but not in your home office or in front of the television.

- If you crave something sweet, try hard candy or gum drops (or frozen grapes) in small amounts instead of ice cream or cookies.

Eating and Moods and Emotions

Do you eat when you're bored, sad, or feeling lonely? Many people find comfort in food. They eat when they need to take their minds off something or have nothing else to do. Some people eat when they are feeling angry, anxious, or depressed. At these times, it is easy to lose track of how much you eat. It is also easy to make unhealthy choices. It can seem like when you're emotional, celery sticks, apples, or popcorn just won't do! Here are some ways to help control unhealthy urges and make healthier choices:

- Use your Food and Activity Tracking Diary (See Figure 10.1 on page 238) as a "food mood" tracking journal. Every day, make sure you are listing what, how much, and when you eat. Note how you feel every time you have the urge to eat. Look for patterns so you can anticipate when you tend to eat without really being hungry.

- If you catch yourself feeling bored and thinking about eating, ask yourself, "Am I really hungry?" If the answer is no, make yourself do something else for 2 to 3 minutes. Go for a short walk in the house or around the block, work on a jigsaw puzzle, brush your teeth, or play an educational game on your phone.

- Keep your mind and hands busy. Getting your hands dirty (as with gardening) is a great trick because you are less likely to eat with dirty hands.

- Write down an action plan (see Chapter 2, *Becoming an Active Self-Manager*) to have on hand for when emotional eating situations arise. Sometimes it is easier to refer to the written word than to remember what you said you would do.

For a complete list of suggested further readings, useful websites, and other helpful resources, please see

www.bullpub.com/resources.

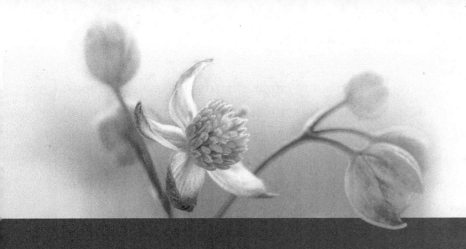

Communicating with Family, Friends, and Health Care Providers

"You just don't understand!"

T HIS STATEMENT OFTEN SUMS UP HURT FEELINGS and a frustrating discussion. Whenever you talk, your goal is for the other person to understand what you are saying. Like all people, you are frustrated when you feel misunderstood. Poor communication often leads to anger, isolation, and depression. This can be worse when you have chronic pain. Pain is often not visible to others. This can lead others to dismiss your pain or simply not realize it is an issue for you. So how can you communicate about your pain without being embarrassed or feeling that the other person is judging you as "complaining" or "wanting attention"?

Pain can get in the way of interactions with others. For example, pain can distract you so that you don't listen very well when others are talking to you. Pain can make you angry and irritable, and sometimes you may vent these feelings inappropriately—at family, friends, or coworkers. Pain can leave you so overwhelmed that your world

249

begins to shrink in size and revolve solely around you and your pain. In the long run, these styles of communication turn off the people you care about most. The result is poor relationships with family members, friends, coworkers, or members of your health care team. Building your communication skills can keep this from happening to you.

When communication breaks down, symptoms often get worse. Pain can increase, blood sugar and blood pressure levels may rise, and there is increased strain on the heart. When you are misunderstood, you may become irritable and unable to concentrate. This can lead to accidents. Clearly, poor communication is bad for your physical, mental, and emotional health.

Healthy communication is one of the most useful tools in your pain self-management tool box. It helps you use the rest of your tools better. It is the foundation to good relationships. Good relationships help people deal with stress. Poor communication is the biggest reason for poor relationships between spouses or partners, family, friends, coworkers, or health care providers.

In this chapter we discuss tools to improve communication. It is particularly important that you can communicate with your health care team about your pain, and we offer many tools and suggestions on how to do this. The tools in this chapter help you express your feelings to get positive results and to avoid conflict. We also discuss how to listen, how to recognize body language, and how to get the information you need.

Expressing Your Feelings

Communication is a two-way street. If you are uncomfortable expressing your feelings or asking for help, others probably feel the same. It may be up to you to make sure the lines of communication are open. Here are two keys to better communication:

- **Do not make assumptions.** We often think, *"They should know."* But people are not mind readers. If you want to be sure others know something about you, tell them.

- **You cannot change how others communicate.** What you can do is change your communication to be sure you are understood. Good communication starts with you.

When communication is difficult, it can help to review the situation. Ask yourself to identify what you are feeling. Identifying feelings and expressing them can make communication better. Consider the following example.

Manny and Carlos agreed to go to a football game. When Manny came to pick him up, Carlos was not ready. In fact, he was not sure he wanted to go because he was having back pain.

Carlos: "You just don't understand. If you had pain like I do, you wouldn't be so quick to criticize. You don't think of anyone but yourself."

Manny: "You are always complaining about your pain. I can see that I should just go by myself."

Communication Hurdles

When you have a long-term condition such as chronic pain, you may face communication problems. You may need support from your family and friends. And getting that support requires communication. At times other people may be trying to hide their feelings of anger, grief, and guilt. They may not know how to act toward you. These hurdles can come up during the following communication challenges:

- telling people about your chronic pain and how it affects your life
- deciding whom to tell about your condition
- talking about fear of the future
- becoming dependent on others

- talking to family about your condition
- asking for help
- being dropped by friends
- dealing with workplace issues
- talking about sexual difficulties
- talking about making decisions

The tools in this chapter can help in these situations. Remember that the first time you use them it might feel awkward. It will get easier over time.

In this conversation, neither Manny nor Carlos stopped to think about what was really bothering him or how he felt about it. Each blamed the other for an unfortunate situation.

The following is a conversation about the same situation, but in this example Manny and Carlos use more thoughtful communications.

Manny: "When we have made plans and then at the last minute you are not sure you can go, I feel frustrated and angry. I don't know what to do—go on without you, stay here and change our plans, or just not make plans."

Carlos: "When my back pain acts up at the last minute, I'm confused too. I keep hoping I can go and so I don't call you. I don't want to disappoint you and I really want to go. I keep hoping that my back will get better. I don't want my pain to cause problems for us."

Manny: "I understand."

Carlos: "Let's go to the game. You can drop me off at the gate so I won't have to walk far. I can take the steps slowly and be in our seats when you arrive. I really want to go to the game with you. In the future, I will let you know sooner if my back is acting up."

Manny: "Sounds good to me. I really do like your company and knowing how I can help. It is just that being caught by surprise sometimes makes me angry."

In this example, Manny and Carlos talked about the situation and how they felt. Neither blamed the other.

Unfortunately, situations where one person blames the other are common. Consider the following example from a workplace.

Elena: "Why are you always late when you say you are going to do something? I get stuck doing everything myself."

Sandra: "I understand. Having a deadline is difficult for me. I want to get things done on time, but sometimes I offer to do too much. I just never know when I am going to get a migraine. When I get one, I am not sure what to do. I keep hoping I can get everything done, and I don't tell you I'm behind because I don't want to disappoint you. I keep hoping that my headache will get better as the day wears on and I will catch up."

Elena: "Well, I hope that in the future you will call and tell me when you have a migraine that is slowing down your work. I don't like being caught by surprise."

Sandra: "I understand. I will start on my report and if the time is short and I'm not sure if I can get it done on time, I will let you know."

In this example, only Sandra is being thoughtful and expressing her feelings. Elena continues to blame. The outcome, however, is still positive. Both people got what they wanted.

The following are some suggestions for using good communications to express your feelings and create supportive relationships:

- **Show respect.** Always show respect. Try not to preach. Avoid demeaning or blaming statements such as, "Doctor, you don't seem to believe me when I tell you how bad my pain is." The use of the word *you* is a clue that blaming is happening. Rather, try using "I" statements, such as, "Doctor, I'm really frustrated that I may not be taken seriously about how bad my pain is. I know we both want to make things better. Is there a way I can explain it better?" (Learn more about using "I" messages in this chapter on page 253.) Courtesy can go a long way toward softening a situation. (Review the material on anger in Chapter 4, *Understanding and Managing Common Symptoms and Problems*, on pages 81–83.)

- **Be clear.** Describe the situation using facts. Avoid general words like *everything*, *always*, and *never*. For example, Sandra said, "I understand. I will start on the report and if the time is short and I'm in pain and not sure if I can get it done on time, I will let you know." She responded by clearly explaining her last-minute pain, as well as her hopes for completing her report.

- **Don't make assumptions.** Ask for more detail. Elena did not do this. She assumed that Sandra was being rude or inconsiderate and that was why Sandra did not get the report done. It would have been better if she asked Sandra why she was late and why she hadn't let her know earlier about the delay. Assumptions are the enemy of good communication. Many arguments arise from one person expecting the other person to be a mind reader. Ask questions if you don't understand why someone else is acting a certain way.

- **Open up.** Express your feelings openly and honestly. Don't make others guess what you are feeling—their guess might be wrong. Sandra did the right thing. She shared her plan to get started on the report and let Elena know early if she had pain problems.

- **Listen first.** Good listeners seldom interrupt. Wait a few seconds when someone is finished talking before you respond. They may have more to say.

- **Accept the feelings of others.** It is not always easy to understand or accept what someone else is feeling. Sometimes this takes time and effort. You can stall a bit by saying, "I'm trying to understand" or "I'm not sure I understand; could you explain some more?"

- **Use humor carefully.** Sometimes it helps to gently introduce a bit of humor. But don't use sarcasm or hurtful humor. Know when to be serious.

- **Don't play the victim.** You become a victim when you do not express your needs and feelings and those needs and feelings go unmet. Sometimes you may expect that the other person should act in a certain way, but unless you communicate about what you want, the person may not act that way. Unless you have done something to hurt another person, do not apologize. Apologizing all the time is a sign that you see yourself as a victim. You deserve respect, and you have a right to express your wants and needs.

Using "I" Messages

Many people have problems expressing feelings. This is especially true when people are being critical of someone else. When frustration mixes with high emotions, the result is often many "you" messages. "You" messages usually start with the word *you.* "You" messages often suggest blame. The person being addressed feels attacked and becomes defensive. Communication problems spring up everywhere when people use "you" messages. The result is more anger, frustration, and bad feelings. Everyone loses. No one wins.

One way to avoid this is to try using "I" statements instead of "you" statements. "I" statements are strong and direct ways to express your views and feelings. "I" messages start with the word "I."

Here are some examples of "I" statements to use instead of "you" statements:

- Say "I try very hard to do the best work I can" rather than "You always find fault with me."

- Say "I appreciate that you offered to cook tonight" rather than "It's about time you did some cooking around here."

Sometimes people think they are using "I" messages when they are really using "you" messages. For example, "I feel that you are not treating me fairly" is a disguised "you" statement. A true "I" statement is "I feel angry and hurt."

Here are some more examples of "I" statements and "you" statements:

- "You" message: *"Why are you always late? We never get anywhere on time."*

Exercise: "I" Messages

Change the following statements into "I" messages. (Watch out for hidden "you" messages.)

1. "You expect me to wait on you hand and foot!"
2. "You hardly ever touch me anymore. You haven't paid any attention to me since my accident."
3. "Doctor, you didn't tell me the side effects of all these drugs or why I have to take them."
4. "Doctor, you never have enough time for me. You're always in a hurry."

"I" message: *"I get really upset when I'm late. It's important to me to be on time."*

■ "You" message: *"There's no way you can understand how lousy I feel."*

"I" message: *"I'm not feeling well. I could use a little help today."*

Watch out for hidden "you" messages. These are "you" messages with "I feel . . ." stuck in front of them:

■ "You" message: *"You always walk too fast."*

■ Hidden "you" message: *"I feel angry when you walk so fast."*

■ "I" message: *"I have a hard time walking fast."*

The trick to "I" messages is to report your personal feelings using the word *I*. Do your best to not use the word *you*. Of course, like any new skill, using "I" messages takes practice. Start by listening to yourself and to others. In your head, take some of the "you" messages and turn them into "I" messages. You'll be surprised at how fast "I" messages become a habit.

If using "I" statements seems difficult, try starting out your sentences with these phrases:

■ "I notice . . ." (state just the facts)
■ "I think . . ." (state your opinion)
■ "I feel . . ." (state your feelings)
■ "I want . . ." (state exactly what you'd like the other person to do)

For example, imagine you baked a special bread to bring to a friend as a gift. A family member comes into the kitchen as it is cooling and cuts out a large slice. You're upset because, with a piece missing, the gift is ruined. You might say to the bread eater: "You cut into my special

Ensuring Clear Communication

Words That Help Understanding	Words That Harm Understanding
I, me, mine	You, yours
Right now, at this time, at this point	Never, always, every time, constantly
Who, which, where, when	Obviously, of course
What do you mean, please explain, tell me more, I don't understand	Why?

bread (observation). You should have asked me about it first (opinion). I'm really upset and disappointed because I can't give the bread as a gift now (feeling). I'd like an apology, and next time I would like you to ask me first (want)." Yes, this contains some "you" messages, but they state specific observations and opinions. This approach is better than the obvious "you" messages we talked about earlier. It gives the other person some specific details to help them understand your feelings and how to deal with them.

"I" messages are not a cure-all. Sometimes the listener may need time to hear them. This is especially true if the person is used to hearing blaming "you" messages. If "I" messages do not work at first, keep using them. As you gain new communication skills, old patterns of communication will change.

Beware! Some people use "I" messages to manipulate others. They express that they are sad, angry, or frustrated to gain sympathy from others. If you use "I" messages in this way, your problems can get worse. Good "I" messages report honest feelings.

Good communication skills help make life easier for everyone, especially those with long-term health problems such as chronic pain. The Ensuring Clear Communication table (page 254) lists some words that can help or harm communication. Finally, note that "I" messages are also an excellent way to express positive feelings and compliments. For example, "I really appreciate the extra time you gave me today, Doctor."

Reducing Conflict

In addition to using "I" messages, there are other communication strategies you can use to reduce conflict, including the ones listed here:

- **Refocus the discussion.** If you get off topic in a conversation and emotions are running high, shift the focus back to the original topic. For example, you might say, "We're both getting upset and drifting away from what we agreed to discuss." Or "I feel like we are bringing up things other than what we agreed to talk about. I'm getting upset. Can we talk about these other things later and just talk about what we originally agreed to discuss?"

- **Ask for more time.** For example, you might say, "I think I understand your concerns, but I need more time to think before I respond." Or "I hear what you are saying, but I am too frustrated to respond now. Let me find out more and then we can talk."

- **Make sure you understand the other person's viewpoint.** Do this by summarizing what you heard and asking for more information. You can also switch roles. Try arguing the other person's position the best you can. This will help you understand all sides of an issue. It also shows that you respect and value the other person's point of view.

- **Look for compromise.** You may not always find the perfect solution or reach total agreement. But you may find something on which you can agree (compromise). Agree to part of what you want and part of what the other person wants. Or decide what you'll do and what the other person will do. Another compromise is to do it your way this time and the other person's way the next time. These are all forms of compromise and can help you solve some disagreements.

■ **Say you're sorry.** We have all said or done things that have hurt others. Many relationships are hurt—sometimes for years—because people have not learned the powerful social skill of apologizing. Often all it takes to restore a relationship is a simple sincere apology. Rather than a sign of weakness, an apology shows great strength. For an apology to be effective, follow these four steps:

1. **Admit the specific mistake and accept responsibility.** Name what you did wrong. Don't gloss over it by saying something general like, "I'm sorry for what I did." Be specific. You might say, for example, "I'm very sorry that I spoke behind your back." Explain what led you to do what you did. Don't offer excuses or sidestep responsibility.

2. **Express your feelings.** A genuine, heartfelt apology involves some suffering. Sadness shows that the relationship matters to you.

3. **Admit to the impact of wrongdoing.** You might say, "I know that I hurt you and that my behavior cost you a lot. For that I am very sorry."

4. **Offer to make amends.** Ask what you can do to make the situation better or volunteer specific suggestions. Making an apology is not fun, but it is an act of courage, generosity, and healing. It brings the possibility of a renewed and stronger relationship, and it can also bring peace.

■ **Forgive others.** There are two sides to making up. When someone offers you an apology, accept it as graciously as possible and be ready to tell them how they can make amends. Sometimes you are wronged, and the other person does not apologize. Whatever happened can grow larger and larger in your mind. Maybe the relationship is over but the wrong still upsets you. In this case you need to work on forgiveness. That does not mean that you have to restart the friendship. What it means is that you can let go of the past wrong so it no longer weighs you down.

Receiving and Giving Help

Giving and receiving help are parts of life. Most people like to be helpful. It makes us feel useful. Providing help is a way to show friendship and to show that you care. But sometimes people ask for too much or for things you cannot give. Saying no can be a challenge. Many people also feel it is challenging to ask for help. When you need assistance, how can you make that need known? In this section of the chapter, we offer tools to help you ask for help, accept help gracefully, and refuse requests that you cannot meet.

Asking for Help

Even though most of us need help, few of us like to ask for it. You may not want to admit that you are unable to do things for yourself.

Telling People about Your Pain

Do you tell people about your long-term pain? Who needs to know, and whom will you tell? Pain can get in the way of relationships. Some people are fine with telling others about their health problems; others may not be comfortable doing so. Telling your family and friends is probably something you expect to do, but do you tell your employer?

It's up to you as a self-manager to think about and make decisions about whom to tell and when to tell them. It may take some self-reflection to decide how you feel about pain's effect on your life. Where do you draw the line? Do you draw a line at all? It can be liberating to get it out in the open. You don't have to worry about hiding your symptoms or keeping a secret.

When you want to make this decision, review pages 31–33 in Chapter 2, *Becoming an Active Self-Manager*, for some decision-making help. Then consider these issues:

- Take your time to decide whom to tell. Weigh the pros and cons.

- Think about who really needs to know.

- Decide how much you want to share with each person.

- Figure out why you want to tell each person.

- Prepare and think ahead about what you are going to say.

- Accept that not everyone will react positively, but remember that people's feelings often change over time.

- Trust your instincts. If a thought is nagging you, listen to it.

You may not want to burden others. You may not be direct or make a very vague request like, "I'm sorry to have to ask this . . . ," "I know this is asking a lot . . . ," and "I hate to ask this, but . . ." Being indirect tends to put the other person on the defensive (e.g., "Gosh, what's she going to ask anyway?"). To avoid this, be specific. A general request can lead to misunderstanding. The person being asked to help may react negatively if the request is not clear. This leads to a further breakdown in communication and no help. A specific request is more likely to have a positive result.

Here are some examples of specific requests you can use instead of general requests:

General request: "I know this is the last thing you want to do, but I need help moving. Will you help me?"

Reaction: "Uh . . . well . . . I don't know. Um . . . can I get back to you after I check my schedule?"

Specific request: "I'm moving next week, and I'd like to move my books and kitchen stuff ahead of time. Would you mind helping me load and unload the boxes in my car Saturday morning? I think it can be done in one trip."

Reaction: "I'm busy Saturday morning, but I could give you a hand Friday night."

If you are the kind of person who hesitates to ask for help, imagine yourself as the person being asked by a friend for help. How do you feel? Probably pretty good. Have you ever considered that maybe you are giving your friend or family member a gift? They probably want to help, they want to feel good, but they may not know what to do and may not want to offend you.

Sometimes you might get offers for help that you don't want or need. In most cases, these offers come from valued people in your life. These people care for you and genuinely want to help. Use a well-worded "I" message to decline the help without embarrassing the other person. For example: "Thank you for being so thoughtful, but today I think I can handle it myself. I hope I can take you up on your offer another time."

Saying No

What about when *you* are asked for help? It is probably best not to answer right away. You may need more information. If a request leaves you feeling negative, trust your feelings.

The example of helping a person move is a good one. "Help me move" can mean anything from moving furniture upstairs to picking up a pizza for the crew. Using communication skills to find out more specific information will help you avoid problems. It is important to understand any request fully before responding. Asking for more information or restating the request will help you understand. Start by saying, "Before I answer . . ." and then ask key questions. This will not only clarify the request but also prevent the person from assuming you are going to say yes.

If you decide to say no, acknowledge the importance of the request. In this way, people can see that you are rejecting their requests, not rejecting them. Your turndown should not be a putdown. For example, here is a polite way to say no: "That sounds like a worthwhile project you're doing, but it's beyond what I can do this week." Again, specifics are the key. Try to be clear about the conditions of your turndown. Give them information. Let them know if you will always turn down this request or that today or this week or right now is the problem. If you are feeling overwhelmed and imposed upon, saying no can be a useful tool. You may wish to make a counteroffer such as, "I won't be able to drive today, but I will next week." But remember, you always have the right to decline a request, even if it is a reasonable one.

Accepting Help

You may often hear, "How can I help?" And your answer may be, "I don't know" or "Thank you, but I don't need any help." All the time you may be thinking, "They should know . . ." One way to get out of this loop it to accept help by being specific. For example, "It would be great if we could go for a walk once a week" or "Could you please wheel the garbage can to the curb?" Remember that people cannot read your mind, so you'll need to tell them what help you want and thank them for it. Think about how each person who offers help in your life can help. If possible, give people tasks that they can easily accomplish. You are giving them a chance to help out and feel useful. People like being helpful and feel rejected when they cannot help you if they care about you. When people help you, do not forget to say thank-you. It is positive and healthy to express your gratitude. (Read more about expressing gratitude in Chapter 5, *Using* *Your Mind to Manage Pain and Other Symptoms*, on page 114.)

Listening

Good listening is probably the most helpful communication skill. Most of us are much better at talking than listening. For example, do you ever find that when others talk to you, you are only half listening as you prepare a response? Try following these steps to good listening.

1. **Listen to tone of voice and observe body language** (see pages 261–262). There may be times when words don't tell the whole story. Is the person's voice wavering? Are they struggling to find the right words? Do you notice body tension? Are they distracted? Do you hear sarcasm? What is their facial expression? If you start to notice some of these signs, you can pick up what speakers are communicating beyond just the words.

2. **Let the person know you are listening.** This may be a simple "uh-huh." Many times, the only thing the other person wants is to know you are listening. They may not even want your opinion or response. They may just need to talk to a sympathetic listener.

3. **Let the person know you hear both their content and the emotion.** You can do this by restating what you hear. For example, "Sounds like you are planning a nice trip." Or you can respond by acknowledging the emotions: "That must be difficult" or "How sad you must feel." When you respond on an emotional level, the results are often startling. These responses can lead to more expression of feelings and thoughts. Responding to either the content or the emotion can help communication. It discourages the other person from simply repeating what has been said. Don't try to talk people out of their feelings ("You shouldn't feel that way" . . . "That's not true"). Their feelings are real to them. Just listen and reflect.

4. **Respond by seeking more information.** This is especially useful if you are not completely clear about what was said or what is wanted. This is the subject of the next section of the chapter.

Getting More Information

The most straightforward way to get more information is to ask for it. Saying "tell me more" generally works to get you more information. Other phrases that work are "I don't understand; please explain," "I would like to know more about . . . ," "Would you say that another way?" "How do you mean?" "I'm not sure I got that," and "Could you expand on that?"

Paraphrasing

Another way to get more information is to paraphrase. Paraphrasing is repeating what a person says in your own words. When you paraphrase what someone says, it helps you understand the true meaning of what was said. This can be especially important with instructions from your health care provider.

But there is a trick to using this communication tool. Paraphrased *questions* help communications; paraphrased *statements* can harm communications. For example, imagine someone says:

"I don't know. I'm really not feeling well. This party will be crowded, there'll probably be smokers, and I really don't know the hosts very well."

Here is a poorly paraphrased statement you can make in response:

"Obviously, you're telling me you don't want to go to the party."

People don't like to be told what they meant. This response might get an angry response in return, such as, "No, I didn't say that! If you're going to be that way, I'll stay home for sure." Or their response might be no response—a total shutdown because of either anger or despair ("he just doesn't understand").

Here is a better paraphrased question:

"Are you saying that you'd rather stay home than go to the party?"

The response to this paraphrased question might be:

"That's not what I meant. Now that I'm moving so stiffly, I'm feeling a little nervous about meeting new people. I'd appreciate it if you'd stay near me during the party. I'd feel better about it, and I might have a good time."

As you can see, the paraphrased question helps communication. The question gets at the real reason for your friend's hesitation about the party. You get more information when you paraphrase with questions.

Asking Specific Questions

Be specific when you ask questions. If you want specific information, you must ask specific questions. People often speak in generalities. For example:

Doctor: "How have you been feeling?"

Patient: "Not so good."

The doctor has not gotten much information. "Not so good" isn't very useful. Here's how the doctor gets more information:

Doctor: "Are you still having those sharp pains in your lower back?"

Patient: "Yes. A lot."

Doctor: "How often?"

Patient: "A couple of times a day."

Doctor: "How long do they last?"

Patient: "A long time."

Doctor: "About how many minutes would you say?"

And so on . . .

Health care providers are trained to get specific information from patients, although they sometimes ask general questions. Most of us are not trained, but we can learn to ask specific questions. Simply asking for specifics often works, such as, "Can you be more specific about . . . ?" or "Are you thinking of something special?"

Avoid asking "Why?" "Why?" is too general. "Why?" makes a person think in terms of cause and effect and can put people on the defensive. Most of us have had the experience of being with a 3-year-old child who just keeps asking "Why?" over and over again. You don't have the faintest idea what the child has in mind and answer "Because . . ." in an increasingly specific order until the child's question is answered. Sometimes, however, your answers are very different from what the child really wants to know, and the child never gets the information they want. Rather than using *why*, begin your responses with *who*, *which*, *when*, or *where*. These words usually get a more specific response.

Sometimes you may not get the correct information because you do not know what question to ask. This is especially true when you are responding quickly. In important situations, consider thinking about and writing down your questions before you ask them. For example, imagine you are seeking legal services from a senior center. You call and ask if there is a lawyer on staff. When the receptionist says no, you hang up. If instead you had asked where you might get low-cost legal advice, you might have gotten some referrals.

Being Aware of Body Language and Conversational Styles

Part of listening to what others are saying includes watching how they say it. We discussed this in the steps to good listening on page 259. Even when people say nothing, their bodies are talking; sometimes they are even shouting! Research shows that people communicate more than half of what they are saying through body language. If you want to communicate well, be aware of your body language, facial expressions, and tone of voice. These should match the words you say. If you do not do this, you are sending mixed messages and creating misunderstandings.

For example, if you want to make a firm statement, look at the other person, and keep your expression friendly. Stand tall and confident, relax your legs and arms, and breathe. You may even lean forward to show your interest. Try not to sneer or bite your lip; this might indicate discomfort or doubt. Don't look away, move away, or slouch. Movements like these communicate disinterest and uncertainty.

When you notice that the body language and words of others do not match, gently point this out. Ask for clarification. For example, you might say, "Dear, I hear you saying that you would like to go with me to the family picnic, but you look like you are in pain. Would you rather stay home and rest while I go alone?"

In addition to reading people's body language, it is helpful to recognize and appreciate that everyone expresses themselves differently. Our conversational styles vary according to where we were born, how we were raised, our occupations, and our cultural backgrounds. Accept that people have different communication styles, and do not expect everyone to communicate in the exact same way. By doing so, you can reduce the misunderstanding, frustration, and resentment that sometimes occur when talking with others.

Communicating across cultures can also be confusing. This is true even if everyone is fluent in the same language. In England a "corner" is a "turning." In some places on the East Coast of the United States, a "soda" is a "tonic," and in the Midwest, the same drink might be "pop." Body language can also be different. For example, it may be accepted for people from some cultures to stand closer to strangers than you are used to. This might be uncomfortable for you. If you move away, they might see you as standoffish. These are a few examples of how communication can differ across cultures. The topic is too complex for this book to address in detail. But the one piece of advice we can share is this: when in doubt about what someone is trying to communicate to you, ask for more information or an explanation.

Communicating with Members of Your Health Care Team

Communicating about your pain to your health care provider can be challenging. Good communication is a necessity when you have a long-term condition like chronic pain. Your health care team must understand you. And you must understand them. When you don't understand advice or recommendations from your health care providers, serious problems can result.

The self-management skill of communication can be a challenge to master. You may be afraid to talk freely, or you may feel that there is not enough time whenever you are in a health care setting. Health care providers may use words you do not understand. You may not want to share personal and possibly embarrassing information. These fears and feelings can block communication with providers and harm your health.

Providers share the responsibility for poor communication. They sometimes feel too busy to take the time to talk with and know their patients. They may ignore or tune out questions. Sometimes they are reluctant to prescribe pain medication. It may seem that some don't believe you. Their actions or inaction might offend you. Although your providers may not become your best friends, they should be attentive and caring. You also want them to be able to explain things clearly.

Explanations aren't always easy with chronic pain conditions. Providers are often perplexed about this complex health problem. Establishing

Your Health Care Provider

Note that in this book and this chapter we use both the terms "doctor" and "health care provider" to refer to primary health care professionals you may encounter. Although you may be seeing a nurse practitioner or a physician's assistant for many of your health care needs, to simplify the discussion and save words we sometimes simply refer to the person who is diagnosing and treating you as "doctor."

and maintaining a long-term relationship with a primary provider may take some effort, but it can make a large difference to your health. You may think that you can only get the best care by going to specialists. This may be true in some cases, but it can also greatly complicate the care you receive. If you see several specialists, they may not really get to know you, and each may not be aware of what your other care providers are doing, thinking, or prescribing. These are good reasons to have a primary provider, or a medical "home."

Your provider probably knows more personal details about you than anyone else, except perhaps your spouse, partner, or parents. You, in turn, should feel comfortable expressing your fears, asking questions that you may think are "stupid," and negotiating a treatment plan that satisfies you both.

To successfully communicate with your health care providers, you must be clear about what you want. Many people would like their providers to be warmhearted computers—gigantic brains, stuffed with knowledge about the human body and mind. You may want your providers to analyze the situation, read your mind, come up with a treatment plan, and tell you exactly what to expect. At the same time, you may want them to be warm and caring and to make you feel as though you are their most important patient.

Most providers wish they were just that sort of person. Unfortunately, no one provider can be all things to all patients. Providers are human. They have bad days, they get headaches, they get tired, and they get sore feet. Many have families who demand their time and attention. Paperwork, insurance companies, electronic record keeping, and large bureaucracies may frustrate them just like they frustrate you.

Most health care providers enter the health care system because they want to help people, and they undergo extensive training in order to be able to do so. Despite their years of training, many times they must be satisfied with improvements rather than cures for their patients. Undoubtedly, you have been frustrated, angry, or depressed from time to time about your pain, but bear in mind that your health care providers have probably felt similar emotions because they cannot make your pain go away. In this, you and your health care providers are truly partners.

Taking PART

One source of unclear communication between health care providers and patients can be the lack of time. This is an obstacle to a good patient-provider relationship. Health care providers are typically on very tight schedules. This becomes painfully clear when you have to wait in the office because of an emergency or a late patient that has delayed your appointment. An overcrowded appointment schedule sometimes causes both patients and providers to feel rushed. Both you and your provider would probably greatly welcome more face-to-face time. When time is short, the resulting anxiety can bring about rushed communication. "You" messages and misunderstandings are common in these situations. (See pages 253–255.)

One way to get the most from your visits to health care providers is to take PART. PART is an acronym that stands for Prepare, Ask, Repeat, Take action. In this section, we explain more about taking PART.

Take PART

Prepare

Ask

Repeat

Take action

Prepare

Before visiting or calling your health care provider, prepare. People with chronic pain are often referred to multiple health care providers. That's because no single provider has all the answers. This means that you may have appointments with people who do not know your pain history. It is very helpful to communicate clearly and directly with all these providers. Doing so is a key part of self-managing your chronic pain.

Describing Your Pain

Pain is a personal experience. The pain you have is only felt by you. Your pain can't be compared to another person's. Only you can know how much pain you feel, when you feel it, and how it affects you physically, emotionally, and socially. Although this may sound very basic, think about the frustration you feel when you try to describe your pain to your provider. Not easy, is it? At the same time, your providers can be frustrated because they are desperately trying to understand your pain problem better. Very often, there are no blood screens, X-rays, or other tests to help them sort out your problem. Providers can use these tools to rule out other diseases, but they cannot use them to assess your pain. They are relying on your communication to help them. No matter what kind of pain you have, describe it and any related symptoms precisely. Accurate and clear descriptions reduce everybody's frustration level. The following guidelines can help you gather detailed information about your pain that will make your visits with a health care provider more productive:

- **Pain Profile:** When you go to a provider's office, have a written "pain profile" with you so you are ready to answer questions about your pain. Whether you have had pain for six months or six years, it can be hard to remember details if you are not prepared. Before going to a new appointment, answer the questions in Figure 11.1. Preparing a pain profile will help you help your provider better understand the nature of your pain. This is part of being a good self-manager, because you are helping to develop the best plan of care for you. Once your health care provider knows your pain history, you usually will not need to review your entire pain profile except to report changes.

- **Pain Language:** Although the word *pain* means many things to many people, specific kinds of words are commonly used for specific types of pain conditions. For example, *throbbing*, *pounding*, and *splitting* are words frequently used by people who have headaches. *Burning*, *tingling*, and *jumping* can describe pain that is associated with nerves. People with arthritis sometimes use the words *achy*, *sore*, or *tiring*. The words

Figure 11.1 **Your Pain Profile**

1. When did the pain start? _____
_____

   Was there a specific cause (e.g., a fall) or did it just seem to develop over time?
_____
_____

2. Has it gotten worse with time or has it remained the same?

3. Is it intermittent or constant? _____
   Does it come in waves and then subside?
   Yes ☐ No ☐

4. What does the pain feel like? (Refer to Figure 11.2 on the next page.)
_____
_____

5. Is there a time of day when the pain is worse? _____
_____

   Does it wake you from sleep? Yes ☐ No ☐
   Does it cause insomnia? Yes ☐ No ☐

6. Have you ever had this type of pain before? Yes ☐ No ☐
   When _____
_____

   Why?_____
_____

7. What increases the pain? Sitting? _____
   Lying down? ____ Mild massage? _____
   Other? _____
_____

8. Does the pain radiate to another part of your body such as your back, shoulder, or legs? _____
_____

9. How severe is the pain? On a 0 to 10 scale, with 10 being the most severe, how does this pain rate? _____
_____

10. Can you distract yourself from the pain either partially or completely? Or is the pain so intense that distraction is impossible? _____
_____

11. How does it affect the quality of your life? Have you stopped visiting friends? Are you irritable, angry, depressed?
_____
_____

12. Is the pain accompanied by symptoms such as nausea, sweating, shortness of breath? _____
_____

13. Which, if any, medications have you taken? _____
_____
_____

   Have they relieved the pain?
   Completely?   Yes ☐ No ☐
   Partially?   Yes ☐ No ☐
   Not at all?   Yes ☐ No ☐

14. Are you sensitive or allergic to any pain medication?_____
_____

15. Miscellaneous comments:
_____
_____
_____
_____

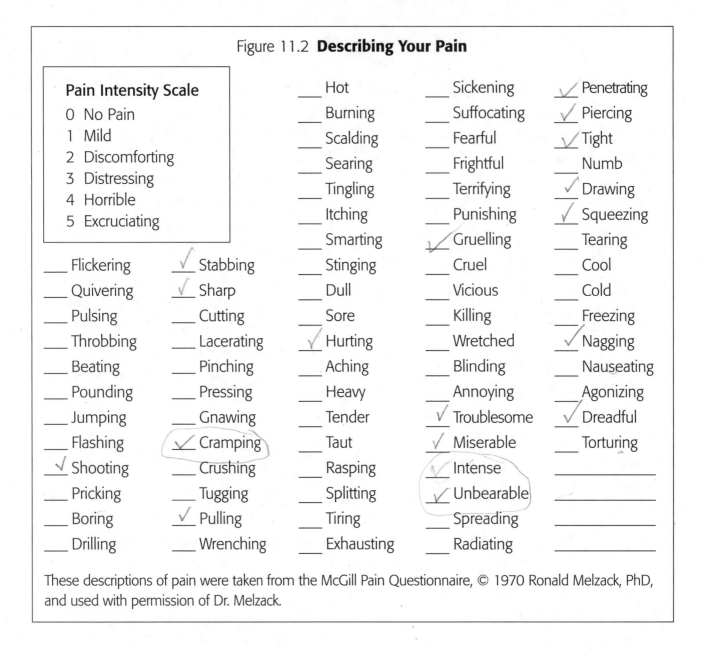

Figure 11.2 **Describing Your Pain**

Pain Intensity Scale

0 No Pain
1 Mild
2 Discomforting
3 Distressing
4 Horrible
5 Excruciating

___ Flickering	✓ Stabbing	___ Hot	___ Sickening	✓ Penetrating
___ Quivering	✓ Sharp	___ Burning	___ Suffocating	✓ Piercing
___ Pulsing	___ Cutting	___ Scalding	___ Fearful	✓ Tight
___ Throbbing	___ Lacerating	___ Searing	___ Frightful	___ Numb
___ Beating	___ Pinching	___ Tingling	___ Terrifying	✓ Drawing
___ Pounding	___ Pressing	___ Itching	___ Punishing	✓ Squeezing
___ Jumping	___ Gnawing	___ Smarting	✓ Gruelling	___ Tearing
___ Flashing	✓ Cramping	___ Stinging	___ Cruel	___ Cool
✓ Shooting	___ Crushing	___ Dull	___ Vicious	___ Cold
___ Pricking	___ Tugging	___ Sore	___ Killing	___ Freezing
___ Boring	✓ Pulling	✓ Hurting	___ Wretched	✓ Nagging
___ Drilling	___ Wrenching	___ Aching	___ Blinding	___ Nauseating
		___ Heavy	___ Annoying	___ Agonizing
		___ Tender	✓ Troublesome	✓ Dreadful
		___ Taut	✓ Miserable	___ Torturing
		___ Rasping	✓ Intense	_____
		___ Splitting	✓ Unbearable	_____
		___ Tiring	___ Spreading	_____
		___ Exhausting	___ Radiating	_____

These descriptions of pain were taken from the McGill Pain Questionnaire, © 1970 Ronald Melzack, PhD, and used with permission of Dr. Melzack.

you use to describe your pain can sometimes point to a type of pain problem, so a rich vocabulary can be very helpful. Figure 11.2 lists typical words to describe pain sensations and the emotions that pain can cause. Place a mark next to each word that describes your pain. If there are other words that you use to describe your pain, add them to the list. Bring the list with you when you see your providers.

- **Pain Intensity:** Just as words describe the quality of your pain, numbers can help describe the intensity or strength of your pain. There are several ways to measure or monitor pain intensity with numbers. One is a 0 to 5 scale (see Figure 11.2, top left). Another is to use a 0 to 10 scale, with 0 indicating no pain at all and 10 as the worst pain you have ever experienced (see Figure 11.3). When your provider asks, "How bad

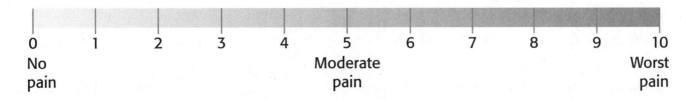

Figure 11.3 **Pain Intensity Scale**

is your pain now?" you can answer, "Well, on a scale from 0 to 10, I'd say it's a 5 or 6 right now." That is much more precise than saying, "Well, it's bad but not as bad as it gets." A numbered scale provides a point of comparison. It is also a good way for you to monitor your pain levels when you are trying to pace your activities (see Chapter 6, *Organizing and Pacing Your Life for Pain Self-Management and Safety*, page 133). Your rating only applies to your pain, not anyone else's. Your rating of 6 might be very different from another person's rating of 6.

■ **Pain Effects:** Think about how pain affects your everyday physical, mental, and social functioning. This is addressed somewhat in your pain profile. Does it affect your ability to walk, sit, do personal care, or get in and out of bed or a chair? Can you complete job responsibilities, prepare and enjoy meals, participate in leisure and family activities, and enjoy sexual intimacy? This is all useful information for your health care provider. Come to your appointments prepared to talk about the specifics of how pain affects your activities and your life.

Making an Appointment Agenda

If you have a chronic pain condition, you likely have regular appointments with your primary care doctor or other members of your pain team. To get the most out of these appointments, prepare an agenda before each appointment. The agenda explains what the reasons are for the visit and what you expect from your health care provider.

Before every appointment, write a list of your concerns or questions. After you walked out of the provider's office, have you ever thought to yourself, "Why didn't I ask about . . . ?" or "I forgot to mention . . ." Making a list beforehand helps ensure that your main concerns get addressed. Be realistic. If you have 13 different problems, your provider probably cannot deal with all of them in one visit. Star or highlight the two or three most important items.

Give the list to your health care provider at the beginning of the visit and explain that you have starred your most important concerns. By calling attention to the starred items, you let the provider know which items are the most important to you. But by providing the complete list, you let the provider see everything in case there is something medically important that is not starred. If you wait until the end of your appointment to bring up concerns, there will not be time to discuss them.

Here is an example. Your doctor asks, "What brings you in today?" You might say something like, "I have a lot of things I want to discuss this visit" (glancing at his or her watch and thinking of the appointment schedule, the doctor immediately begins to feel anxious), "but I know that we have a limited amount of time. The things that most concern me are my shoulder pain, my dizziness, and the side effects from one of the medications I'm taking" (the doctor feels relieved because the concerns are focused and potentially manageable within the appointment time available).

Listing Your Medications

In addition to your starred list of concerns, take a list of all your medications and the dosages to all your appointments. If writing down a list is difficult, put all your medications in a bag and take them with you. Do not forget to list vitamins and over-the-counter medications, supplements, ointments, suppositories, and eye drops.

You may be able to download your medications list from your electronic medical record (EMR) on your providers' website. (For more on EMRs, see page 273.) If all your providers use the same electronic medical record system, this can be easier.

Preparing Your Story

The final thing to prepare for your appointments is your story. Visit time is short. When the provider asks how you are feeling, some people go on for several minutes about this and that symptom. It is better to be specific and succinct. Sum up your story, and make it short and clear. Say, for example, "I think that overall my pain is about the same, but now I have more trouble sleeping and I'm feeling a bit depressed about things."

As part of your story, be prepared to describe your symptoms in detail, including:

- When symptoms started
- How long symptoms last
- Where symptoms are located
- What makes symptoms better or worse
- Whether you have had similar problems before
- Whether you have changed your diet, exercise, or medications in a way that might contribute to symptoms
- What worries you most about symptoms
- What you think might be causing symptoms

If you were given a new medication or treatment during a previous visit, be ready to report how it went. If you are going to several providers, bring the results of all tests you have had in the past six months.

In telling your story, talk about trends: Are you getting better or worse, or are you the same? Also talk about frequency and degree: Are your symptoms more or less frequent or intense? For example, "In general, I am slowly getting better. I mostly feel the pain first thing in the morning and after I go grocery shopping. Last week, though, my pain did not get better over the course of the day, which is why I'm here."

Be as open as you can in sharing your thoughts, feelings, and fears. Remember, your provider is not a mind reader. If you are worried, explain why: "I'm worried that I may not be able to work," or "I'm worried I have cancer because no one can find the cause of my pain," or "My father had similar symptoms before he died." The more open you are, the more likely your provider can help. If you have a problem, don't wait for the provider to "discover" it. State your concern immediately. For example, "I'm worried about this mole on my chest."

Share your hunches or guesses about what might be causing your symptoms, as they often provide vital clues to an accurate diagnosis. Even if it turns out that your guesses are not correct, it gives your provider the opportunity to reassure you or address your hidden concerns.

The more specific your story is (without overdoing it with irrelevant details), the better the picture your health care provider will have of your problem. And a clear story means less time is wasted for both of you.

Ask

Your most powerful tool as a self-manager is the question. By asking questions, you can fill in critical missing pieces and close gaps in communication. And asking questions shows that you are an active participant in your care. Being a participant is critical to getting the most out of your health care. Getting answers and information is a cornerstone of self-management.

Be prepared to ask questions about your diagnosis, tests, treatments, and follow-up. The following are some guidelines for asking questions.

Diagnoses. Ask what's wrong and what caused your problems and issues. At the same time, remember that sometimes it is very difficult or impossible to pinpoint the exact cause of chronic pain. This does not mean it cannot be treated, but it does mean your health care provider may

not be able to answer all your questions about why you are in pain. (See Chapter 1, *Chronic Pain Self-Management: What It Is and How to Do It*, pages 3–6, to learn more about what causes pain.)

Tests. If the doctor wants to do tests, ask how the results are likely to affect treatment and what will happen if you are not tested. If it will not affect your treatment, there may not be a need for the test. If you decide to have a test, find out how to prepare for the test and what the test will be like. Ask how and when you will see test results.

Treatments. Ask if there are any choices in treatments and the advantages and disadvantages of any options. Ask what will happen if you have no treatment. Ask what you can do to manage at home. (See Chapter 14, *Managing Your Treatment Decisions and Medications*.)

Follow-ups. Find out if and when you should call or return for a follow-up visit. Ask what symptoms to watch for in between visits and what to do if they occur.

Repeat

One way to check that you have understood everything that comes up in your appointment is to briefly report back key points to your provider. For example, "You want me to take these three times a day." Repeating gives the provider a chance to quickly correct any misunderstandings.

If you don't understand or remember something the provider said, say that you need to go over it again. For example, you might say, "I'm pretty sure you told me some of this before, but I'm still confused about it." Don't be afraid to ask what you think might be a stupid question. Such questions may prevent misunderstanding.

Sometimes it is hard to remember everything. Take notes or bring another person to important visits. You can even record the visit with a smartphone if the health care professional grants permission. Many providers give you a printed summary of your visit. Your provider may share this at the end of your appointment, or you may be able to access it online in your electronic medical record.

Take Action

At the end of a visit, you need to understand what to do next. What action do you need to take? This may include picking up or ordering medications, scheduling treatments and tests, and booking follow-up appointments. You should also know any danger signs and what you should do if they occur. If necessary, ask your provider to write down or print out instructions. You can also ask for providers to recommend reading material or online resources.

If for some reason you can't or won't follow the provider's advice, say so. For example, you might say, "I can't take aspirin; it gives me stomach problems," or "My insurance doesn't cover that much therapy, so I can't afford it," or "I've tried to exercise, but I can't seem to keep it up." If your providers know why you can't or won't follow advice, they may be able to make alternative suggestions. If you don't share that you are unable or unwilling to take action and the reasons why, it's difficult for providers to help.

Asking for a Second Opinion

Sometimes you may want to see another provider or get a second opinion. Asking about getting a second opinion can be hard. This is especially true if you and your provider have had a long relationship. You may worry that asking for another opinion will anger your provider or that maybe your provider will take your request the wrong way. Requests for second opinions seldom bother providers. If your condition is complicated or difficult, the provider may have already consulted with another health care expert (or more than one). This is often done informally. Asking for a second opinion is perfectly acceptable, and providers are taught to expect such requests. However, asking for third, fourth, and fifth opinions may be unproductive.

Ask for a second opinion by using a nonthreatening "I" message such as the following:

> "I'm still feeling confused and uncomfortable about this treatment. I feel that another opinion might reassure me. Can you suggest someone I could see?"

Express your own feelings without suggesting that the provider is at fault. Also confirm your confidence in your provider by asking for a recommendation. You are not bound by your doctor's suggestion, though. If there is a pain clinic near you, this may be a good place for a second opinion about a chronic pain or related issue.

Giving Providers Positive Feedback

When you are pleased with your care, let your providers know. Everyone appreciates compliments and positive feedback, especially members of your health care team. They are human, and your praise can help nourish and console these busy, hardworking professionals. Letting them know that you appreciate their efforts is one of the best ways to improve your relationship with them—plus it makes them feel good! Likewise, if you do not like the way you have been treated by any members of your health care team, let them know.

Your Role in Medical Decisions

Many medical decisions are not clear-cut. Often there is more than one option. The best decisions, except in life-threatening emergencies, depend on your values and preferences. The decision should not be left solely to your health care team members. For example, you might say, "I'm concerned about taking medications and their side effects. Is there a complementary treatment option, like relaxation or biofeedback, to try before I start taking the medication?"

No one can tell you which choice is right for you. But to make an informed choice, you need information about the treatment options. Informed choice, not merely informed consent, is essential to quality medical care. The best medical care for you combines your health care team's medical expertise with your own knowledge, skills, and values.

To make an informed choice about any treatment, you need to know the cost and risks of the treatment. This includes the likelihood of possible complications such as drug side effects and reactions, including constipation, dizziness, fuzzy thinking, bleeding, infection, injury, or death. It also includes personal costs, such as absences from work, and financial considerations, such as how much of the treatments your insurance will cover. You also need to understand how likely it is that the proposed treatments will benefit you in terms of relieving your pain and improving your ability to function. Sometimes the best choice may be to delay a decision about treatment in favor of "watchful waiting."

Making decisions about treatments can be difficult. Read more about making decisions on pages 31–33 in Chapter 2, *Becoming an Active Self-Manager.* See Chapter 14, *Managing Your Treatment Decisions and Medications*, for advice on evaluating new treatments.

Working with the Health Care System

Today most providers work in larger systems such as clinics. Someone other than your provider usually decides on appointment times, billing, and telephone and email use. If you are unhappy with your health care system, don't suffer in silence. Do something about it.

Find out who is running the organization and who makes decisions. Then share your feelings in a constructive way by letter, phone, or message through your provider's online portal. The problem is that the people who make the decisions tend to isolate themselves. It is easier to express our feelings to the receptionist, nurse, or doctor. Unfortunately, these people have little or no power to change the system. But they can tell you whom to contact. If something is a problem for you, it might also be a problem for your provider and other consumers. If you work together, you and your provider may be able to improve the system.

> In Canada, the province or territory sets health care policies. Provincial and Territorial Departments of Health can direct people to the most appropriate office or agency to address a complaint.

If you do decide to write or message, here are some suggestions. Keep your letter short and factual. Share what actions you would find helpful. For example:

> Dear Ms. Brown:
>
> Yesterday I had a 10:00 a.m. appointment with Dr. Zim. The doctor did not see me until 12:15 p.m., and my total time with her was 8 minutes. I was told to make another appointment so I could get my questions answered at another time.
>
> I know that sometimes there are emergencies. I would appreciate being called if my doctor is running late so I don't make the trip to the clinic. If I am already at the clinic, I would like to

> be told I can leave and when to return. I would also like 15 or more minutes with my doctor.
>
> I would appreciate a reply within two weeks.
>
> Thanks for your consideration.

In this section of the chapter, we address some common issues that people regularly have with health care systems. We offer a few hints for addressing these issues and working with the health care system to get more positive results. Not all problems and suggestions will apply to all systems, but most do.

- **"I hate the phone system."** Often when you call for an appointment or information, you reach an automated system. This is frustrating. Unfortunately, you cannot change this. However, phone systems do not change often. If you memorize the numbers or keys to press, you can move more quickly through the menu of options. Sometimes pressing the pound key (#) or 0 will get you to a real person. Once you do get through, ask if there is a way to do this faster next time. Many organizations now let you make appointments online. This often saves time and prevents frustration.
- **"It takes too long to get an appointment."** Ask for the first available appointment. Take it. Then ask about how you can be added to a list to be called when other people cancel their appointments. Some organizations are happy to call or text you when they have an empty spot. There may even be an automated system in place to do this and the system texts you with a short time limit to respond "yes" if you want a

last-minute appointment. In others, you may have to call them once or twice a week or look online to check for cancellations. Ask the scheduler what you can do to get an earlier appointment. Ask for a telephone number so you can reach the person making appointments directly. Some organizations set time aside each day for same-day appointments. If these appointments do become available, know when to call to get one. It is usually early in the morning. If you are in pain or believe that you must see a doctor right away, tell the scheduler. No matter how frustrated you are, be nice. The scheduler has the power to either give you an appointment or not.

■ **"I have so many providers; I do not know which one to ask."** One provider is in charge. Your job is to find out which one. Ask each provider you see who is coordinating your care. It is most likely your primary care doctor or general practitioner (GP). Check with that provider's office to confirm that they are coordinating your care. Ask how you can help coordinate your care. It may be a good idea to let this provider know when someone orders a test or new medication. This is especially important if you see two providers who do not use the same electronic medical record system.

■ **"What is an electronic medical record (EMR) anyway?"** Your EMR is your electronically stored health information in a digital format. Your medical information is stored on a secure system. Any provider who is in the same system can see your information. Very few doctors today keep paper charts. You should know what information is in your EMR. In some systems, the EMR includes just test results. In other systems, the EMR has test results and medication information. In most systems it has everything your provider knows about you. An EMR is just like a paper record: It does no good if your providers don't read it. For example, when you have a test, the doctor ordering the test knows when the test results are ready. However, your other doctors don't know anything about the test unless you tell them to read the results. Learn about the medical records system your provider uses so you can help all your providers use it more effectively.

In the United States, Canada, and many other countries, you have the right to a copy of almost everything in your record. Many times, you can get this information online through such apps as MyHealth or MyChart. Before you visit a provider outside your regular health care system, download your tests and medications to give to the new provider. If you cannot do this yourself, ask your regular provider for copies of all your tests.

Currently, a small percentage of Canadians have access to their medical records online. These records are incomplete because they are not shared among the medical institutions where people get care. Provinces are developing systems to improve the sharing of information, such as LifeLabs in BC and Ontario, which allows patients to access their lab tests online.

- **"I can never reach my doctor."** It is hard to get a provider on the phone, but you might be able to email. Many systems now have ways for health care providers and patients to communicate by secure text or email. The next time you see your provider, ask about this. Or visit your care provider's internet portal to review your options. One good thing about electronic systems is that routine things such as prescription refills can be done quickly. It may mean requesting it on your patient portal, calling a special number, or talking to the nurse. Learn how to do this.

In a medical emergency, do not waste time getting online or trying to contact your health care provider directly. Call 911 (in the United States and Canada) or go to a hospital emergency department.

- **"I have to wait too long in the waiting room or the examination room."** Delays caused by emergencies happen. Or when each patient before you takes an extra 5 minutes, it can also cause a wait. If your schedule is tight and it may cause a problem if your appointment is delayed, call your health care provider's office or clinic before you leave home and ask how long you will have to wait. If you learn that your provider is running late, you can decide whether to take a book or ask to reschedule. You can also show up with your book and ask about the wait. Rather than getting upset, let the receptionist know that you are going to step out for a little while to run a short errand, make a phone call, or get a cup of coffee. Tell the receptionist that you will return at a specific time.

- **"I don't have enough time with my provider."** This may be a system problem since someone other than your provider often decides how many patients to schedule and for how long. The decision is sometimes based on what you tell the scheduler. If it's a regular follow-up visit, you will be given a short visit. If you say you are having severe pain and are very depressed and cannot function, you may be given a longer appointment. When making the appointment, ask for the amount of time you want, especially if you want more than 10 or 15 minutes. Be prepared with reasons why you need more time. You can also ask for the last appointment in the day. You may have to wait awhile, but at least your provider will not rush your visit to get to other waiting patients.

There are also ways you can act to prevent this problem. First, use your time with the provider wisely. Be prepared for your visit. Try hard not to take extra time. If every patient takes 5 extra minutes, it means extra hours of work for the provider and extra waiting time for the patients whose appointments are later in the day. If you do not need all your time, do not chitchat. When you have what you need, thank the doctor. Say you have gotten what you needed and that you are going to give your extra 5 minutes to the next patient. This is a very big gift and will be appreciated and long remembered.

The following are a few parting words of advice for dealing with the health care system:

- **If something in the health care system is not working for you, ask how you can help make it work better.** Very often, if you learn how to navigate the system, you can solve or at least partially solve your problems.

- **Be nice—or at least as nice as possible.** If the system or your provider sees you as a difficult patient, life will become more difficult for you.

Many people think that things should not be this way. It is not fair to place this burden on the patient. Health care systems should be responsive and patient-friendly. Many health care systems are striving to be better. In the meantime, use the suggestions in this chapter to help you deal with difficult situations.

For a complete list of suggested further readings, useful websites, and other helpful resources, please see

www.bullpub.com/resources.

CHAPTER 12

Managing Pain during Employment and Unemployment

MANAGING CHRONIC PAIN CAN FEEL LIKE A JOB all by itself. Yet many people with chronic pain also have a full- or part-time job. If you are one of those people, you have the added challenge of balancing your work and home lives while also taking care of your health. On the other hand, many people with chronic pain do not work outside the home. This may be because of the pain or for other reasons. When you have pain, you may not be able to work or at least not work at your chosen occupation. Not being able to work may require a major readjustment and self-management skills just as working does. In this chapter, we talk about the challenges of employment and unemployment and self-management tools to help you with your personal employment situation.

Special thanks to Heather Zuercher, MPH, for contributions to this chapter.

Being Employed and Managing Chronic Pain

Work is a large part of many people's lives. If you are working full-time, you may spend more time at work than you do at home. In fact, for many people who are employed, the only thing that they do more than work is sleep! People work for a variety of reasons, primarily financial. But many people also work because their jobs benefit them mentally and physically as well as financially. Work can provide social interactions, a sense of accomplishment, and distraction from other challenges in your life. At the same time, a job can also be a source of stress, challenges, and conflict. Because work has both positive and negative effects and makes up a significant part of our life, it is important to think about how work impacts pain and pain impacts work.

Being employed and managing chronic pain presents special challenges, including:

- **Physical challenges.** At work, physical challenges include dealing with symptoms such as pain or fatigue. Your pain may limit what you can do at work. Or what you do at work may add to your pain.

- **Missed work.** You may miss work because of your symptoms or because of health care appointments.

- **Dealing with what others think.** What your coworkers or supervisors think about you can affect how you deal with your condition. Pain cannot be seen, and your coworkers may think you are taking it easy or not doing a good job. They may not see your symptoms or know why you miss work. Coworkers may have to take on responsibility for things you cannot do. All of these can lead to misunderstanding, confusion, and resentment.

- **Time management.** Everyone who works must balance home and work responsibilities.

A chronic pain condition can make finding a balance with your work life much more difficult. Managing chronic pain at work is a challenge because many things at work are out of your hands. In most jobs, there are schedules, responsibilities, and expectations that employees must meet. There are many things about your job or things at work that you cannot control or change.

Imagine someone with joint pain with a job in an office. For them, sitting and typing at a computer is part of their responsibilities and can't be avoided, even though it can make their pain worse. Or consider people who experience pain-related fatigue. Fatigue can make it difficult to focus and accomplish tasks, making those tasks take longer. For most people it is not possible to take a rest or nap breaks during work. An employee who is fatigued or in pain may find it difficult to deal with coworkers, customers, and clients.

Unfortunately, you can't leave your symptoms at home when you go to work. Many people with jobs and chronic pain just put up with their pain and work through it. This leaves them exhausted and in the long run can add to their pain. More pain can lead to poor job performance and poor work attendance. Everything can start to add up and make everything worse, including your home and family life.

Despite these challenges, there are things that you can do and choices that you can make to be a better self-manager at work. This chapter includes information about managing stress at work, communicating about your symptoms, staying physically active, and making healthy eating choices at work. Instead of toughing out the symptoms, focus on taking care of yourself. This can improve your quality of life and make you a better employee.

Finding Work/Life Balance

Balancing your work life and your home life is complex for everyone. It is even more so when you are dealing with chronic pain. The term *work/life balance* can be misleading because getting that perfect balance is very difficult. Your work and home responsibilities both require time and resources that quite often pull you in different directions. It is up to you to find a balance between the two. Working toward work/life balance means understanding that both work and home are part of your life, and taking care of one doesn't mean not taking care of the other.

There are many ways and places to work. You may work full-time or part-time, have a flextime job, or work remotely or virtually. Many people work in offices or on job sites. For some, work means driving all day, and for others it means manual labor. Some working people never go to an office. They work at home or in a shared space near home. All jobs have their own challenges, and all workplaces have different policies.

Just as people's work is diverse, home can also mean many different things to different people. You may live alone, or your home can include family. Your home life may also include friends, household responsibilities, community involvement, hobbies, and many other non-work activities.

Work and home life often interact in complex ways. Work affects home, and home affects work. Having a busy, stressful day at work can make you feel fatigued and more likely to pick up fast food on the way home. After work, you may feel physically tired and emotionally run-down. It may feel like there is little left to give at home after a long day at work. Conflict or problems at home can distract people from work and cause things to pile up and make people less productive.

Work/life balance isn't always the same. The needs of work and home change day to day and can tilt one way or the other. You can learn to anticipate the times when your work and life are out of balance and identify ways to get back on track. This will help you be a better self-manager.

Managing Your Time

When your work and life are out of balance, the first step is to identify the problems that are causing the lack of balance. (By now this problem-solving step should sound familiar. If it isn't, review Chapter 2, *Becoming an Active*

Self-Manager.) Effective time management is the most important tool for finding work/life balance. The goal is to make time for home, time for work, and a bit of time for yourself.

Start to pay attention to how you spend your time. Tracking your time (much like you track what you eat or how much you exercise) can help you identify how and where you currently spend your time. Make a list of what you do each day. Break the day down into hours. For each hour, use general categories to describe how you spent that time (for example, work, chores, reading the paper, watching TV, exercising, etc.). Make sure to make a list for at least one workday and at least one non-workday. Figure 12.1 on pages 281 and 282 is a worksheet that you can use. You may find it helpful as you start to track your time. If you want to see how all these activities affect your pain, you can add a pain column.

After a few days, look for patterns. Once you discover your patterns, you may find changes you can make. Think about how you are spending your time. Is this helping you meet your personal or professional goals? Is this a "good" use of your time?

Building Good Habits

People tend to do the same things over and over. Those things become habits. It becomes easy to come home, turn on the TV, or surf the web, and before you know it, a great deal of time has passed. Although it is fine to do the activities that help you unwind and relax, such as watching TV, reading, or shopping, moderation is key. Make sure that those activities are not keeping you from accomplishing your goals. If you find yourself spending more time than you like doing things that don't help you meet your personal or professional goals, consider breaking those time-spending habits.

Changing habits can be hard; it takes effort and time. A good first step is to identify one hour of time that you could spend in a more enjoyable or productive way and make an action plan. Review the discussion of action planning in Chapter 2, *Becoming an Active Self Manager*, pages 33–39. Keep a calendar, and schedule the things that are priorities in your life. Those may include exercise, time for self-care, playing with children or grandchildren, studying a new language, attending a ball game or live theater performance, or anything else.

Managing Pain at Work

Some of the strategies that you have for pain self-management may not be possible to do at work. However, there are ways to manage pain even when you are working.

- Know your limits and what can cause you pain or make your symptoms worse.

- Take breaks and leave your work area. Use the time to meditate or do other relaxation techniques, or just sit quietly and practice deep breathing.

- Be mindful of how you sit or stand at work. Make sure you have good posture, and adjust your workspace as needed. A new office chair, keyboard, hand rest, telephone headset, or mat to stand on may be extremely helpful. Your employer may

Figure 12.1 **Time Management Worksheet**

Write down everything you do in blocks that are each 1 hour long. You may do many tasks in the same hour. For example, from 7:00 to 8:00 in the morning, you may do your stretching exercises, dress, eat breakfast, and commute to work. Decide if the hour's activities are important to you or not and mark that in the priority column. Indicate if you are pleased or disappointed with how you are spending your time for each block in the "Use of time" column.

Time	Task	Priority	Use of Time
7:00 A.M.		☐ High ☐ Medium ☐ Low	☐ Good ☐ Poor
8:00 A.M.		☐ High ☐ Medium ☐ Low	☐ Good ☐ Poor
9:00 A.M.		☐ High ☐ Medium ☐ Low	☐ Good ☐ Poor
10:00 A.M.		☐ High ☐ Medium ☐ Low	☐ Good ☐ Poor
11:00 A.M.		☐ High ☐ Medium ☐ Low	☐ Good ☐ Poor
12:00 P.M.		☐ High ☐ Medium ☐ Low	☐ Good ☐ Poor
1:00 P.M.		☐ High ☐ Medium ☐ Low	☐ Good ☐ Poor
2:00 P.M.		☐ High ☐ Medium ☐ Low	☐ Good ☐ Poor
3:00 P.M.		☐ High ☐ Medium ☐ Low	☐ Good ☐ Poor
4:00 P.M.		☐ High ☐ Medium ☐ Low	☐ Good ☐ Poor
5:00 P.M.		☐ High ☐ Medium ☐ Low	☐ Good ☐ Poor

Figure 12.1 **Time Management Worksheet (*continued*)**

Time	Task	Priority	Use of Time
6:00 P.M.		☐ High ☐ Medium ☐ Low	☐ Good ☐ Poor
7:00 P.M.		☐ High ☐ Medium ☐ Low	☐ Good ☐ Poor
8:00 P.M.		☐ High ☐ Medium ☐ Low	☐ Good ☐ Poor
9:00 P.M.		☐ High ☐ Medium ☐ Low	☐ Good ☐ Poor
10:00 P.M.		☐ High ☐ Medium ☐ Low	☐ Good ☐ Poor
11:00 P.M.		☐ High ☐ Medium ☐ Low	☐ Good ☐ Poor
12:00 A.M.		☐ High ☐ Medium ☐ Low	☐ Good ☐ Poor
1:00 A.M.		☐ High ☐ Medium ☐ Low	☐ Good ☐ Poor
2:00 A.M.		☐ High ☐ Medium ☐ Low	☐ Good ☐ Poor
3:00 A.M.		☐ High ☐ Medium ☐ Low	☐ Good ☐ Poor
4:00 A.M.		☐ High ☐ Medium ☐ Low	☐ Good ☐ Poor
5:00 A.M.		☐ High ☐ Medium ☐ Low	☐ Good ☐ Poor
6:00 A.M.		☐ High ☐ Medium ☐ Low	☐ Good ☐ Poor

provide these to you if they understand your situation.

■ Be prepared. Keep a bag with things that help you manage pain (an ice pack and/or heating pad, water, medications, etc.) at work.

■ Talk with your primary care provider about medications and how they may affect you at work.

Managing Stress and Working

Juggling workloads, family responsibilities, and your health often results in high stress. You can learn more about stress in Chapter 4, *Understanding and Managing Common Symptoms and Problems*, on pages 66–91 and more about stress management in Chapter 5, *Using Your Mind to Manage Pain and Other Symptoms*.

There are things that you cannot change about your job. However, by prioritizing and organizing, you can help control and decrease your stress response at work. The following are useful tips for dealing with workplace stress:

■ Plan regular short breaks to take a walk, chat with a friend, or relax.

■ Establish boundaries. Though it is easy to feel the need to be connected to phones and email 24 hours a day, set up a block of time each day to not deal with work tasks and not think about work. It may take some practice to break the habit of being available 24/7, but lower stress levels will be your reward.

■ Learn to say no. Don't overcommit to things, avoid scheduling things back to ack, and don't be afraid to say no to things that you can't do or things you do not want to do.

■ Prioritize your work tasks, and break projects into small steps. Use action plans and pace yourself to make and reach your small goals. See Chapter 2, *Becoming an Active Self Manager*, and Chapter 6, *Organizing and Pacing Your Life for Pain Self-Management and Safety*.

■ Delegate work tasks when you can, and be willing to compromise.

■ Resist the urge to set unrealistic work goals for yourself. Make sure that your goals are achievable.

■ Reduce negative talk and focus on the positive. Find something in your job that you enjoy and focus on that.

■ Take time off!

Finally, if these small tips are not working, you may need to think about speaking with your manager, supervisor, or the human resources department about your responsibilities and expectations. If you feel like your stress levels are having an impact on your health or your condition, share this with your health care provider.

Communicating and Working

One of the hardest self-management tasks is talking to others about your chronic pain and how it affects your life. This is even harder when it impacts your work. This section includes some suggestions to make this easier or at least not so frightening.

You do not have to tell anyone about your pain unless you want to. It can be scary to talk about your health at work. Many people fear that they will be treated differently or even lose their job. However, if your pain is impacting the way that you do your job, your attendance at work, or your job performance, it may be time to talk with your supervisor or someone else in the organization. If you choose not to talk, people may make assumptions or jump to conclusions about your job performance.

When communicating with people at work about your chronic pain, it is important to think about:

- **Whom you want to disclose it to.** Should you tell supervisors, coworkers, managers, human resources (HR)?

- **When you want to disclose.** When is the right time for you to bring it up?

- **What you want to disclose.** Will it help you to share this information?

- **How much you want to disclose.** Do they need to know all the details, or will something more general be enough?

Remember, it is always your choice to share!

Deciding When to Share

Talking about your chronic pain can be a very sensitive topic. However, *not* communicating can have consequences as well. You may want to ask yourself the following questions to help make your decision:

- **Do your symptoms interfere with your work duties, assignments, or projects?** Does pain or fatigue cause you to miss deadlines? Does it take longer for you to accomplish tasks because of your symptoms?

- **Do you sometimes need time off because of your condition?** Do you have frequent health care appointments or symptom flare-ups? Does this happen more than once in a while?

- **Do you have pain that is so severe it can affect your mood and the ability to deal with customers or coworkers?** Are you more stressed and have a shorter temper because you are in pain or are fatigued?

- **Does your job impact your symptoms?** Does standing all day make your pain worse? Are you being exposed to something in the work environment that is worsening your condition?

If you answered yes to any of these questions, it may be time to consider saying something to someone at work. People are often afraid of being discriminated against, but without all the information, your supervisor or employer may make incorrect assumptions about you or what is impacting your work. A manager or coworker who knows what you are dealing with is less likely to make false assumptions about you.

Deciding What to Share and Whom to Tell

Remember, communicating about your health needs is different from disclosing your condition. It is possible to discuss the problems you are facing and how your pain is being affected without naming your condition or going into too much detail. How much to share is a very personal decision that you should make based on your circumstances, your job, your supervisors, and your desired outcomes. If you decide to discuss your condition with a supervisor or manager, give some thought ahead of time as to when, how much, and what you will share. Think about your own boundaries—does the idea of sharing make you feel empowered, or would it make you feel exposed? If it makes you feel empowered, then more disclosure may help.

Consider how much you want to share. You may want to only disclose the *symptoms* you experience that are related to your job performance. You can protect your privacy by not sharing details about your condition. Keep the focus on the symptoms and what you want or need. If possible, avoid complaining. Instead offer solutions.

Two key questions to ask yourself are, "What do I want and need from this conversation?" and "How can I make sure this conversation helps me?" You need to be prepared to let your supervisors know what you want and need. They cannot read your mind. Be specific, such as, "I need to walk around every 15 to

20 minutes for a minute or two," or "I need to change my work hours so I do not need to wait long times for public transportation."

Discussing Your Condition at Work

When it is time to discuss your pain with someone at work, it can be helpful if you can control the conversation. Let the person know that you want to discuss something about your health. Explain why you are disclosing this information now (for example, because it explains an absence or justifies why you can't do something related to your job), and keep the focus on the impact of your pain on your work.

Consider this example:

"I know that I am often late. I have rheumatoid arthritis, and in the mornings, I am stiff and have lots of pain. For me to get going in the morning takes several hours. I am wondering if I might come to work a bit later and leave a bit later."

Note that in this example, the person gives information about the problem as well as suggesting a solution.

Clearly set boundaries about the spread of information by saying something like, "I would like this information to stay between you and me." Make sure that what you are sharing provides support for what you want to happen.

Here is another example:

"Hi, I'd like a minute of your time to talk about something important to me. I have been dealing with pain for some time now. Because of this, I will need to take some time for health care appointments, and there may be days when I am unable to come in. I want to be up front with you so that we can discuss how best to handle those days."

Remember, you do not have to share anything with anyone that you do not want to share. Think about what is in your best interest and what will result in a better and healthier work environment for you. In most cases, it is better to be up front and communicate at least the basics than to not communicate at all.

By sharing that you have a condition that may affect you at work, you can become an advocate for yourself. Ask for what you need: adjustments to your workspace, changes to work hours, changing the way you work, and so on. Laws vary between states and countries about workplace responsibilities and accommodations. Know your rights. Check out the laws that apply in your area. Your company's HR department should also have resources.

In the United States, the following two laws protect people with illness and injury in certain ways:

- **The Americans with Disabilities Act (ADA)** requires that employers make reasonable adjustments for disabled workers. For the purposes of ADA, a disability is a physical or mental impairment that substantially limits one or more major life activities. However, employers do not have to provide accommodations if those accommodations would require significant difficulty or expense. Some common accommodations provided by employers are providing parking or transportation, ensuring accessibility, making certain equipment available, restructuring jobs, and modifying the work environment. If you are not sure if you are entitled to accommodations or how to ask for them, you can contact the Job Accommodation Network (https://askjan.org), which is a division of the US Department of Labor. The Equal Employment Opportunity Commission (EEOC) has additional resources about disabilities and your rights under ADA (www.eeoc.gov).

- **The Family and Medical Leave Act (FMLA)** protects employees with a serious health condition and allows employees to take up to 12 weeks off each year for medical or family emergencies, but it does not require that this time be paid. This time can be taken all at once or over the course of the year.

In addition to the federal regulations, many states have specific laws regarding sick leave and accommodations for disabilities. You can learn more about your employer's specific policies and rules by reaching out to a human resources (HR) representative.

Finally, in many work environments, coworkers can be supportive. People spend a lot of time at work and sometimes spend more time with coworkers than with family. Getting some support from those around you can help you get through the tough times. If you do ask for support, do it carefully. If you do not want everyone to know your concerns, share only with the people you trust. One benefit of this sharing is that as someone learns more about you, they are also more likely to share something about themselves. This is the basis of trust and friendship.

In Canada, the Human Rights Act and the Employment Equity Act are federal laws that cover discrimination and equity for people with disabilities working for federally regulated organizations and businesses. The Canadian Human Rights Act requires employers to accommodate an employee with a disability up to the point of "undue hardship," which means it would cost too much or create risk to health or safety. Provincial and territorial human rights laws share many similarities with the Canadian Human Rights Act and apply many of the same principles.

The Canada Labour Code provides up to 17 weeks of sick leave protection to federally regulated employees who have completed three consecutive months of employment with the same employer. The code does not require that this time be paid. Each province and territory has its own Employment Standards Act, and the amount of time employees are entitled to take for sick leave varies.

Some employees may be entitled to cash benefits under the Employment Insurance Act (EI), a federal government program. EI sickness benefits are offered through Employment Insurance Canada to people who have worked and paid into the program and meet the eligibility requirements. Short- and long-term disability coverage may be provided by an employer. Provinces have their own long-term disability income programs based on medical conditions and financial situations.

Communicating about Work at Home

Often, stresses and problems at work show up at home. You may be quiet, not have the energy to help around the house, or snap at your partner or children. As a result, your home life may not be everything you want it to be. You may think, "They just don't understand," or "They should know I am working as hard as I can and appreciate me more," or "There is nothing that can be done." The reason people at home do not "understand" and don't "know" what you are going through is often poor communication.

When work is stressful, communicate with those at home. Find a time to talk with your family about what is going on at work, how they can help, and changes that can be made. When people understand, they are often inventive. Maybe your children can walk the dog, or your partner can prepare lunches for everyone. Family members might even have ideas that you could try at work. At the same time, you might learn that your children have stresses at school and your partner has his or her own concerns. Anytime you find yourself thinking "they don't understand" or "they should," take this as a clue that more communication is needed.

Being Physically Active and Working

Being active has many physical and mental benefits. Chapter 7, *Exercising and Physical Activity for Every Body*, discusses these in more detail. Being active can make you better at your job by improving thinking and memory, increasing your mental stamina, and boosting creativity. Exercise can improve your mood and decrease stress. Despite knowing all of this, many of us think of exercise and physical activity as a luxury—something we would like to do if only we had more time.

Staying physically active when you are working can be a challenge. Getting enough physical activity is often difficult. You may find yourself sitting or standing in one place for most of the workday. Because of job responsibilities, inactivity can be hard to avoid. When you add in commuting time, you can end up spending a large part of your life sitting. Standing or sitting for a long time without a break can have many negative effects. Research has found that being active during leisure time is not enough to make up for sitting down all day.

Being sedentary can be mentally draining and can actually make you feel more fatigued. You may find yourself exhausted at the end of the day so that you also spend your nonwork time in sedentary activities. When you are sitting, your muscles are not working, and when your big muscles (like those in your legs) aren't working, your metabolism slows down, your muscles and joints get stiff, and symptoms such as pain, fatigue, and depression can get worse.

Sitting is not the only problem. Standing is not much better if you are just standing still in one place. The key to being active is moving your big muscles (arms and legs) more and limiting the time that you spend being still. Make a commitment to stand up every 20 minutes and move your big muscles, even if it is just for a minute or two. Set an alarm to keep you on track.

The following are some suggestions for increasing activity and movement at work:

- When you take a break, walk from one side of the room to the other.

- Walk down the hall to talk to a coworker instead of sending an email.

- Use the restroom that is the farthest away from your office or workstation. If possible, take the stairs to the floor above or below.

- Take one or two 10-minute activity breaks at a scheduled time every day.

- Take the stairs instead of the elevator.

- If you are able, have standing or walking meetings. If you do this, be sure that everyone who needs to attend is able to take part.

- Wear comfortable shoes that encourage movement.

- Consider creating a walking group, have challenges with coworkers to see who can walk the most or sit the least, or think up other fitness challenges. One inclusive way to conduct a fitness challenge is for each person to set a weekly goal—say 2,000, 5,000, 7,000, or 9,000 steps a day—and the winners are the people who hit their goals on the most days. This allows the very fit and the not so fit to both "win."

Sedentary (Nonactive) Jobs

Even if you work at a desk, short bouts of physical activity can improve your fitness and cardiovascular health. With some planning, you can get some exercise in between meetings, calls, or other tasks. Though this type of physical activity may not produce dramatic results, it can improve your strength, burn a few extra calories, give you much-needed mental breaks, and keep your muscles and joints from getting stiff. Many of the exercises in Chapter 8, *Exercising to Feel Better*, can be done at your desk or workstation. Again, the key is that more movement is better than less movement.

For more information on general physical activity, developing an exercise routine, and strength and flexibility exercises, see Chapter 7, *Exercising and Physical Activity for Every Body*, and Chapter 8, *Exercising to Feel Better*.

Active Jobs

Many people have active jobs. Food servers, nurses, construction workers, gardeners, and mail carriers are moving and lifting most of their workday. When people exercise during their free time, they can take breaks when they get tired. This is not always true for people with active jobs. They may do the same labor-intensive tasks for hours, with few, if any, breaks.

Moderate physical activity can strengthen the heart and the cardiovascular system. However, when people are very active at work and have limited rest breaks, their heart rate and blood pressure may be high over the whole day. This can put strain on their cardiovascular systems. If the work is very repetitive, it can cause muscle strain and injury that result in pain.

In addition, people with jobs that are physically demanding may not exercise outside of work. They don't do the types of exercise activities that could be beneficial because they are too tired, or they feel that their activity at work is enough. If you are a person with an active job, remember to take breaks during your workday. Be sure to make being active outside of work a priority!

Eating Well and Working

As discussed in Chapter 9, *Healthy Eating and Pain Self-Management,* and Chapter 10, *Healthy Weight and Pain Self-Management*, there is a relationship between what you eat, your health, and your pain. What you eat can affect your pain and also your job performance and mental health.

The following are some tips for healthy eating when you are working. You can learn more about this topic in Chapter 10, *Healthy Weight and Pain Self-Management*.

- **Decide what you are going to eat before you get hungry.** If you wait to decide when you are very hungry, tired, and stressed, you are more likely to make an unhealthy choice.

- **Plan for your meal (usually lunch) at work.** Many of us plan for the meals (usually breakfast and dinner) we eat away from work. Doing the same for our work meal can keep us on track.

- **Plan snacks.** At work, keep healthy snacks such as fruit, cut-up vegetables, nuts, and seeds easily available. This will keep your energy levels up and keep you away from unhealthy snack choices.

- **Choose anti-inflammatory snacks.** These include nuts, seeds, fruits and vegetables, and noncaffeinated teas. (For more details on anti-inflammatory foods, see pages 214–215.) These foods contain nutrients that can improve your health and may reduce pain. Typically, when people eat better, they feel better. High-fat, high-sugar meals can make you tired and cause you to "crash" a few hours after eating.

Healthier Desk Dining

It is estimated that around 70 percent of workers in the United States and 40 percent of Canadians regularly eat at their desks. This can lead to poor food choices, including eating fewer fruits and vegetables and eating more foods that are processed and higher in sugars, fat, and sodium. One of the biggest reasons *not* to eat at your desk is that often people at their desks are distracted by emails, phone calls, or other tasks. If you eat at your desk, you are not fully focused on what and how much you are eating. This encourages overeating. People who eat at their desks tend to snack more and eat more calories. Making it a practice not to eat at your desk has the added advantage of giving you a little exercise and social interaction and a mental break from your work.

Here are some tips for how to avoid eating unhealthily at your desk:

- **Schedule your lunch.** No matter where you eat, give yourself a break and eat before you get too hungry. Set an alarm or calendar reminder.

- **Focus on your food.** Even if it is only for 10 minutes, stop what you are doing and focus on what and how much you are eating. There are very few tasks that cannot wait for a few minutes.

- **Pay close attention to your portions (how much you eat).** More information on

portion and serving sizes can be found on pages 211–212 in Chapter 9, *Healthy Eating and Pain Self-Management.*

- **Bring your lunch to work.** Avoid fast-food, take-out, or drive-through lunches. Plan ahead and bring healthy meals from home. See below for more information on recommendations for packing lunches.

- **Disinfect your desk before you eat.** Your desk or workstation can be covered with bacteria and germs. Wipe down your desk every day.

- **Socialize at lunch when you can.** People who socialize at work are more productive than those who don't. Remember, lunch is about more than consuming calories; it is also a break.

Packing Your Lunch

Lunches you pack at home are usually healthier than fast food or restaurants and can be much less expensive. If you buy your lunches and spend between $5 and $10 each day, that can add up to $200 a month! Try these tips when you are packing your lunches:

- Prepare and pack meals on the weekends or the night before work.

- Repackage leftovers. Use leftover chicken to make a burrito or a sandwich.

- Have fun with basic recipes. By dressing up a sandwich or salad, you can keep your meal interesting and simple at the same time. Buy good quality bread. Spread low-calorie mustard instead of high-calorie mayonnaise. Substitute hummus or avocado for lunch meats. Include things beyond lettuce, tomatoes, and cucumbers in your salads. Add beans, brown rice, nuts, fruit, and small amounts of cheeses. Try out different dressings. Pick up a rotisserie chicken to eat for dinner and toss the leftovers on top of your salad or put them in your soup.

■ Soups can be great lunches. You can cook them in bulk and freeze smaller portions to bring for lunch. If you have never made soup, it is very easy. Find a simple recipe and try it.

  ▶ Search for easy lunch ideas online.

  ▶ Choose healthy frozen dinners.

  ▶ Keep a plate, bowl, and utensils at the office.

  ▶ If your workplace does not have a refrigerator or microwave, ask your employer to install them.

Avoiding Temptations at Work

At work, food is often a distraction or temptation. Many people bring food they want to get out of their house to share at work. There are also endless celebrations in large offices, from birthdays to promotions to baby showers. Almost everyone agrees that it is hard to turn down a donut. Invitations to lunch can be hard to resist, even on days when you bring a healthy lunch from home. Planning ahead, anticipating these distractions, and communicating with your coworkers can help. Follow these tips to manage temptations:

■ Make a pact with office mates to bring healthy items instead of just sweets to share.

■ Ask for and choose healthier options in vending machines and cafeterias.

■ Communicate with your coworkers: "I really appreciate it when you bring snacks in to share, but I am finding it hard to resist them. Please do not offer me food. I promise to tell you if I want something." (Please note the use of "I" messages in this example. See page 253 for more on this important communication tool.)

■ When there is an event such as a potluck, do not expect others to cook with your needs in mind. Rather, be sure to bring something you can eat that will also be enjoyed by others.

■ Have a standing "out for lunch" day. Communicate with your coworkers and ask them not to ask you out for lunch on other days.

Being Unemployed and Managing Chronic Pain

So far, this chapter has been about how to manage pain while working. But not everyone wants to or is able to work. Some cannot work, and others have a hard time finding the right job. When you have pain, you may not be able to work or at least not work at your chosen occupation. Not being able to work may require a major readjustment. This section discusses pain management and unemployment.

Questions like "What do you do for a living?" or "Are you back to work yet?" are common in everyday social conversation. When you are not working due to a problem like chronic pain, questions about employment can be awkward, discouraging, and even maddening. It's natural for others to be interested in your work life, but it's also natural for you to be frustrated by these frequent inquiries.

Many of us define ourselves by our work. Telling others where you work and what you do has become a standard way to introduce yourself and communicate who you are. For example, a new neighbor may introduce himself by saying, "My name is Jose and I'm the manager of Ace Business Products." In this introduction, Jose's roles and interests as husband, father, Boy Scout leader, computer enthusiast, and gardening expert are not even mentioned. They are secondary information. When you are not working, you must define your life more broadly, not just by your place or type of employment.

Unemployment is usually beyond your control. It affects millions of people each year. Restructuring, downsizing, work shortages, changing needs of employers, regional or global issues, pandemics, as well as disability or injury are all causes of unemployment. These factors impact everyone, even those without chronic pain.

Those with chronic pain have special concerns. Chronic pain can affect energy, concentration, and the physical ability to do things. It can become difficult to maintain what is expected of you and sometimes to work at all. If you have lost your job, the challenge is not to blame yourself or be consumed by blaming others. As you restructure your life, you may find the content on problem solving and decision making in Chapter 2, *Becoming an Active Self-Manager*, helpful. Also take a look at the content about challenging negative self-talk on pages 102–104 in Chapter 5, *Using Your Mind to Manage Pain and Other Symptoms*.

Managing the Impacts of Job Loss

Your reaction to losing employment depends on a number of factors, including the ones listed here:

- **How did you feel about the job?** Did you like or dislike the work and environment?

- **How attached were you to your workplace?** How long did you work there? Did you plan to remain long term? How positive were your relationships with coworkers and superiors?

- **Do you have prior experience dealing with crisis?** Have you successfully managed previous periods of unemployment or other obstacles in life?

- **What is the nature or degree of your physical limitation?** Are you able to assume different responsibilities or change positions within your workplace, company, or industry?

- **Do you have advanced or special education or transferable skills?** Can you possibly apply related skills in another position or organization?

- **What is your financial status?** Were you in a short-term or permanent position? Did it have disability benefits or a pension? What are your current financial responsibilities?

Regardless of your reaction to or even the cause of your job loss, unemployment challenges

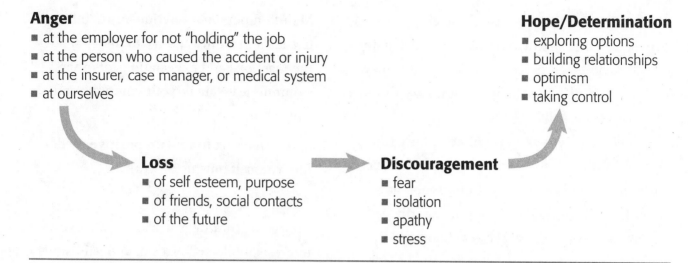

Anger
- at the employer for not "holding" the job
- at the person who caused the accident or injury
- at the insurer, case manager, or medical system
- at ourselves

Loss
- of self esteem, purpose
- of friends, social contacts
- of the future

Discouragement
- fear
- isolation
- apathy
- stress

Hope/Determination
- exploring options
- building relationships
- optimism
- taking control

Figure 12.2 **The Emotional Impact of Unemployment**

your well-being in three areas: emotional, financial, and social.

Emotional Impact of Job Loss

Unemployment has been described as an "emotional roller coaster." It's a time when people may struggle with many issues such as anger, loss, hopelessness, and discouragement, as illustrated in Figure 12.2.

The stages and emotions in Figure 12.2 are felt by anyone who loses their job. It's a time of challenge and, for some, defeat. It is no wonder that emotional reactions are even more complex when you have chronic pain. Job loss for someone with chronic pain often contributes to anger and stress (see Chapter 4, *Understanding and Managing Common Symptoms and Problems*). Identifying your emotions and what is causing them is the first step in managing them. You can use some of the self-management tools in this book to take control and live more positively. If you find that depression, anger, or stress continue or get worse, seek professional help. Some mental health professionals have practices that

focus on helping people with job loss and these sorts of changes.

Financial Impact of Job Loss

The financial impacts of unemployment differ for each person. Reduced finances may prevent you from providing for basic needs such as grocery bills, car payments, rent or mortgage payments, heating bills, and medical bills. Not being able to keep up with the bills can be a great stressor. It can also cause guilt. You may need to depend on your family, friends, or unemployment insurance. In turn, this may affect your family, friendships, and self-esteem. It is important that you do what you can to take care of yourself both physically and mentally as you work your way through these issues. Chapter 5, *Using Your Mind to Manage Pain and Other Symptoms*, has many suggestions and strategies to do this.

Social Impact of Job Loss

Being unemployed often changes your interactions with others. When you are working, you are in contact with coworkers, customers, and clients. It is natural to miss these contacts. It may be a challenge to avoid isolation and remain socially connected. Your former coworkers may see you in a different light, or you may think they see you in a different light.

Unemployment can also affect family roles and responsibilities. When a parent or spouse is "at home," the expectations of everyone in the household changes. This is not necessarily bad; it may be an opportunity to redefine roles in a positive way (for example, you can spend more time with family or be more involved in household tasks, if you pace yourself appropriately). Communication skills can help in these situations. Review the communication strategies and tools in Chapter 11, *Communicating with Family, Friends, and Health Care Providers*.

Self-Management during Unemployment

Managing unemployment requires a range of strategies. Many of the tools to manage pain and other symptoms can also help you take control of life while out of work. You can:

- **Increase your physical abilities** using pain-management strategies such as exercising, using relaxation techniques, sleeping, and activity pacing.

- **Maintain personal relationships.** Talk with friends and family and try to understand the reactions and expectations of others. Communicate about your emotions and expectations.

- **Make an effort to remain positive.** Redefine yourself outside of work.

- **Keep a daily routine.**

- **Engage in volunteer work.** Broaden your interests, build self-esteem, and gain skills and experience.

- **Seek financial counseling.**

- **Explore new friends, hobbies, and interests.**

- **Obtain employment counseling** from an agency that assists persons with special considerations.

- **Consider other options.** Look into a new career, further education, part-time or contractual positions, or self-employment.

Living without work, with all its uncertainty and turmoil, is a challenge faced by many. If you are out of work, you are not alone. However, being unemployed while living with chronic pain can be very difficult. The techniques and skills outlined in this book, along with support from family, friends, and your health care team, can help you meet this challenge.

For a complete list of suggested further readings, useful websites, and other helpful resources, please see

www.bullpub.com/resources.

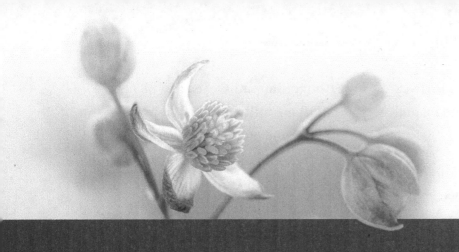

CHAPTER 13

Enjoying Sex and Intimacy

Loving relationships that include intimacy and physical pleasure are an important part of healthy living. Sex and other physical intimacies—including touching, holding hands, hugging, cuddling, and kissing—promote emotional connections that strengthen relationships. Intimacy helps you to build trust, feel valued, and manage life better. Sometimes intimacy involves the physical pleasure of sex with your partner, but mostly it is about creating relationships and making connections with the people you love. These connections in turn positively affect your physical, mental, and emotional health. Intimacy also improves your outlook on life.

295

Over the years, studies have shown that sex and physical intimacy have physical and mental health benefits, including the following:

- **Chronic pain management.** When approached carefully, physical intimacies like touching, cuddling, and sex can help reduce pain by releasing certain hormones and other chemicals in the brain. One hormone called oxytocin increases emotional connection or bonding with other people and promotes a sense of calm and well-being. In addition, oxytocin reduces the effects of stress and the perception of pain. Physical touch also releases other chemicals that contribute to pain relief and improved sense of well-being. These chemicals include serotonin, which serves as nature's antidepressant and plays a role in sleep and mood; phenylethylamine, which stimulates the brain's pleasure center; and endorphins, which act as the body's natural painkillers.

- **Improved heart health.** Sex is a less intense form of endurance exercise. Depending on the individual, sex can provide benefits similar to the benefits of taking a short, moderately intense walk. Sexual activity helps strengthen muscles, burn calories, lower blood pressure, and reduce your risk of heart disease, stroke, and hypertension. Studies also show that people with active sex lives tend to exercise more and eat healthier, which adds to their overall physical fitness, health, and well-being.

- **Stronger immunity.** Sex can increase important antibodies that help you fight off infection and protect you from getting sick. Sex also improves circulation and helps maintain fluid balance, which leads to less bloating and better resistance to minor health problems.

- **Stress reduction and relaxation.** Like any form of physical activity, sex can help reduce levels of the stress hormone cortisol. Cortisol can cause anxiety. Sex and other physical intimacies can also relieve muscular tension. Reduced muscle tension promotes both physical and mental relaxation as well as pain relief by helping to close the pain gate. (Learn more about the pain gate in Chapter 1, *Chronic Pain Self-Management: What It Is and How to Do It*, pages 4–11.)

- **Better quality of sleep.** During sexual activity—especially during orgasm—the body produces beneficial hormones. These hormones, including serotonin, can act like sedatives, calming your nerves and helping to center the mind, helping you to fall asleep and stay asleep during the night. Getting a good night's sleep also helps with overall pain management. (Learn more about pain and sleep in Chapter 4, *Understanding and Managing Common Symptoms and Problems*, on pages 66–91.)

- **Increased sense of well-being and improved mood.** Sex, like exercise, causes the body to release endorphins that not only help relieve pain but make you feel happier and more energetic.

Despite these benefits, many individuals and couples with chronic pain problems find it challenging to maintain this important part of their lives. Emotions, including fear of worsening pain and being unable to perform, can create frustration and decrease desire in one or both partners.

Managing Common Concerns about Sex

For many people with chronic pain, intercourse is difficult because of the physical demands it makes on your body. Intercourse increases your heart rate and breathing. Intercourse can be a challenge if you are in pain or have limited energy due to fatigue, poor sleep, and stress. Having intercourse can also be physically uncomfortable. It can place strain on muscles, tissues, and joints that may already be hurting or sensitive to touch.

For these reasons, it may be more satisfying to spend more time on sensuality or foreplay rather than on actual intercourse. Finding ways to pleasure yourself and/or your partner in a relaxed, comfortable atmosphere will increase your intimacy and satisfaction. Sharing pleasure through physical intimacies such as caresses and kisses can also be gratifying. Using the mind—either by refocusing thoughts, engaging in visualization or fantasy, or concentrating on pleasurable feelings instead of physical discomfort—can also enhance your experience.

Fear or other difficult emotions can also affect intimate relationships for people with chronic pain. For example, someone with angina may fear that sexual activity will bring on a heart attack, so they may avoid sex. People with migraine headaches may worry that orgasms may trigger an episode. People with neck, back, or joint pain may be anxious that sex will spike their pain if they move the wrong way. Their partners may fear that sexual activity might cause these problems. Partners worry about feeling responsible if something bad happens. Some chronic health problems, such as diabetes or just normal aging, can make erections difficult or cause vaginal dryness that makes intercourse uncomfortable or embarrassing. All these worries can hurt the relationship.

Loss of self-esteem and a changed self-image can be sexual barriers as well. Many people with chronic conditions believe that they are physically unattractive. If pain has left you physically changed, unemployed, or not able to contribute to your home life in the way you did in the past, you may think of yourself as "unattractive" or "undesirable" to your partner. Thinking this way can damage your sense of self and may cause you to avoid sex or intimate situations. You just "try not to think about it."

Ignoring the sexual part of a relationship or physically and emotionally distancing yourself from your partner can lead to isolation and depression, which in turn leads to lack of interest in sex and more depression—a vicious cycle. Depression can be treated, and you can feel better. Please refer to Chapter 4, *Understanding and Managing Common Symptoms and Problems*, to learn more about depression and how to deal with it. Sometimes self-management techniques are not enough. Talk to your health care provider or therapist if depression is a concern for you.

When you avoid sex and intimacy, not only are you denying yourself an important, pleasurable part of life, but you probably also feel guilty about disappointing your partner. Also, your partner may feel more fearful and guilty than you do—afraid that he or she might hurt you during sex and guilty for feeling resentful about it. This dynamic can cause serious relationship problems. But as an active self-manager, you do not have to allow this to happen. After all, sex and other types of intimacy are supposed to be joyful and pleasurable, not a cause of worry, discomfort, and more pain!

Fortunately, for humans, intimacy is less about having sex or reaching orgasm and more about sharing ourselves emotionally with our partner or others who are close to us. Remember, making changes enables you to continue doing the things you enjoy. Making changes is one of the tasks discussed in Chapter 2, *Becoming an Active Self-Manager*. If sex and intimacy are a priority in your relationship, make the changes you need to in order to openly communicate with your partner. Discuss with your partner the possibility of exploring and experimenting with different types of physical and mental stimulation to experience more sensuality and intimacy, as well as to manage any fears you may have about sex. This process of exploring and communicating openly with your partner can strengthen your relationship.

For successful intimate and sexual relationships, the most important thing is communication. The best way to address the fears of one or both partners is to confront them. Once the fears are out in the open, then you can find ways to talk about them and use problem solving to address them. Without good communication, learning new positions and ways to increase sensuality are not going to be enough. This is particularly important for people who worry about how their pain and other health problems may make them look physically to others. Often, they find that their partner is far less concerned about their looks than they are.

When you and your partner are comfortable with talking about sex, you can then find solutions to the issues you may have. Often, people start by sharing what kinds of physical stimulation they prefer and which positions they find most comfortable. Then, they might share the fantasies they find most arousing. It's difficult to dwell on fears when your mind is occupied with a fantasy.

To get this process started, you and your partner may find some help with the communication skills discussed in Chapter 11, *Communicating with Family, Friends, and Health Care Providers*, and the problem-solving techniques outlined in Chapter 2, *Becoming an Active Self-Manager*. Remember, if your self-management tools are new, give them a chance before deciding they don't work or giving up. As with any new skill, it takes time, practice, and patience to learn to do them well.

If you decide that you wish to abstain from sexual activity because of your chronic pain or if it is not an important part of your life, that's OK. However, it is important that your partner understands and agrees with your decision. Good communication skills are essential. You may benefit from discussing the situation with a professional therapist. Someone trained to deal with important interpersonal situations can help facilitate the discussion. Don't be embarrassed to be open with therapists; they have heard it all.

Sensual Sex

In our society, sexual attraction has become very dependent on the visual experience. This leads to an emphasis on physical images. Sight, however, is only one of our five senses. When being sensual, you can also appreciate the seductive qualities of your partner's voice, scent, taste, and touch. Sensual sex is about connecting with your partner through all the senses, making love not only with the eyes but with your ears, nose, mouth, and hands as well.

Sensual touch is particularly important because the largest sensual organ of the body is the skin, which is rich with sensory nerves. The right touch on almost any area of our skin can be very erotic. Fortunately, sexual stimulation through touch can be done in just about any position and can be enhanced with the use of oils, flavored lotions, scents, feathers, fur gloves—whatever the imagination desires.

Sensitive areas include the mouth, earlobes, neck, breasts and nipples (for both genders), navel area, hands (fingertips if you are giving pleasure, palms if you are receiving pleasure), wrists, small of the back, buttocks, toes, and insides of the thighs and arms. Experiment with different types of touch. Some people find a light touch arousing; others prefer a firm touch. Many people also become very aroused when touched with the nose, lips, and tongue or sex toys.

Some chronic pain conditions can cause hypersensitivity to even light touch. It is especially important to find out what type of touch pleases you and what does not and to talk to your partner about this. By working together, you can find ways to increase sensual pleasure and decrease your fear and anxiety about being touched in the wrong places or in the wrong ways.

Fantasy

What goes on in our minds can be extremely arousing. Most people engage in sexual fantasy at some time or another. There are probably as many different sexual fantasies as there are people. It is OK to have fantasies. A fantasy may be as simple as an expression you or your partner like to hear during sex. If you discover a fantasy that you and your partner share, play it out in bed.

Engaging the mind during sexual activity can be every bit as arousing as physical stimulation. It is also useful when pain or other symptoms during sex interfere with your enjoyment. But be careful—sometimes fantasy leads to

Misconceptions about Sex

Many sexual attitudes and beliefs are learned—they are not automatic or instinctual. You begin learning these from family, friends, older children, and other adults when you are young. The jokes you hear and the things you read and watch such as magazines, TV, movies, and the internet also influence you. Unfortunately, much of what many people learn about sex are the "shoulds" and "should nots," which reflect society's inhibitions and misconceptions.

To explore sexuality and maximize enjoyment, people often need to break down these inhibitions and misconceptions. Some of the following are common beliefs about sexuality that simply aren't true:

- Older people can't enjoy sex.
- Sex is for people with beautiful bodies.
- A "real man" is always ready for sex.
- A "real woman" should be sexually available whenever her partner is interested.
- Lovemaking must involve sexual intercourse.
- Sex must lead to orgasm.
- Orgasm should occur simultaneously in both partners.
- Kissing and touching should only be done when they lead to sexual intercourse.

unrealistic expectations. Your real partner might not compare favorably to your dream lover. If you regularly fire up your imagination with explicit photos or videos of young, hard bodies that do not match your reality, you may experience decreased sexual satisfaction.

Overcoming Symptoms during Sex

Sometimes people are unable to find a sexual position that is completely comfortable. Other times, pain, fatigue, stress, or even negative thoughts (self-talk) during sex are so distracting that they interfere with the enjoyment of sex or the ability to have an orgasm. This poses some special problems. If you are unable to orgasm, you may feel resentful of your partner. If he or she is unable to orgasm, you may feel guilty about it. If you avoid sex because you are frustrated, your partner may become resentful and you may feel guilty. Your self-esteem may suffer. Your relationship with your partner may suffer. Everything suffers.

One thing you can do to help deal with this situation is to review your medications. It is important to take a pain medication so that it is at peak effectiveness when you are ready to have sex. Of course, this involves planning. The type of medication you take may be an issue too.

For example, medications such as narcotic-type pain relievers, some antidepressants, muscle relaxants, and tranquilizers can dull your sensory nerves along with the pain. Obviously, it is counterproductive to dull the nerves that also give you pleasure. Your thinking may be muddled due to medication, making it more difficult to focus.

Alcohol and marijuana (cannabis), which are used by some people to reduce pain, can also impact sexual functioning. Some medications can make it difficult to have an erection; others can help with an erection. Likewise, there are water-based lubricants that can help women with vaginal dryness.

Ask your doctor, nurse practitioner, or pharmacist about the timing of your medications and any alternative medications that may be available. Your doctor may be able to reduce the dosages of these drugs or prescribe other medications that are effective for treating pain and other symptoms but have less effect on your ability to enjoy sex.

Another way to deal with uncomfortable symptoms is to become an expert at fantasy. This involves practice and training. Create one or more sexual fantasies that you can indulge in when needed, making them vivid in your mind. Then, during sex, you can call up your fantasy and concentrate on it. You can keep your mind distracted with erotic thoughts rather than on your symptoms or negative thoughts.

If you have not had experience with using visualization and imagery techniques such as those in Chapter 5, *Using Your Mind to Manage Pain and Other Symptoms*, you need to practice several times a week to learn them well. Your practice, though, does not need to be devoted only to your chosen sexual fantasy. You can start with any guided imagery tape or script such as the ones in Chapter 5. Work on making the imagery more vivid each time you practice. Start with just picturing the images. When you get good at that, add and dwell on colors. After that, look down to your feet in your mind as you walk. As you become more skilled at this, try listening to the sounds around you. Next, concentrate on the smells and tastes in the image and feel your skin being touched by a breeze or mist. Finally, feel yourself touch things in the image.

Work on each one of your senses at a time. Become good at one sense before going on to another. Once you are good at using imagery, you can invent your own sexual fantasy and picture it, hear it, smell it, and feel it. You might even begin your fantasy by picturing yourself setting your symptoms aside. The possibilities are limited only by your imagination.

Learning these concentration skills can also help you focus on the moment. Focusing on your physical and emotional sensations during sex can be powerfully erotic. If your mind wanders (which is normal), gently bring it back to the here and now.

IMPORTANT: Do not try to overcome chest pain or sudden weakness on one side of the body in this way. These symptoms should not be ignored. If you experience them, consult a physician right away.

Sexual Positions

Finding a comfortable sexual position can minimize pain and fear of injury during sex. This can also reduce other symptoms. Experimentation may be the best way to find the right positions for you and your partner. Everybody is different. No single position is good for everyone. Experiment with different positions that reduce strain, preferably before you and your partner are too aroused.

For example, try using a firm support for your back if the person with back pain prefers to be on the bottom. Other tricks for back pain include placing a small pillow at the curve in the lower spine and another pillow under the knees to help reduce any strain or discomfort. Also, try lying side by side or a sitting position on a chair. If muscle spasms are a problem, try a hot shower before sex to help relax the muscles and then icing the affected area after sex to relieve any discomfort. Remember, the experimentation itself can be sensual and arousing.

No matter which position you try, it is often helpful to do some warm-up exercises before sex. Consider some of the exercises in the Moving Easy Program in Chapter 8, *Exercising to Feel Better*. Exercise can help your sex life in many ways. Becoming more fit is an excellent way to increase your comfort and endurance during sex. Walking, swimming, bicycling, and other activities can benefit you in bed as well as elsewhere by reducing shortness of breath, fatigue, and pain. Exercises also help you learn your limits and how to pace yourself during sexual activity as well as during other physical activities.

During sexual activity, changing positions once in a while may help you to manage pain as well. This is especially true if you start experiencing symptoms or they increase when you stay in one position too long. Changing positions can be done in a playful way so it becomes fun for both of you. During sex, as during any physical activity, pacing yourself and stopping to rest is OK.

Sex and Intimacy: Special Considerations

People who have other health problems in addition to chronic pain may have more specific concerns about sex and intimacy. In this section of the chapter, we address some of these special considerations.

People who are recovering from a heart attack or stroke are often afraid to resume sexual relations. They fear they will not be able to perform, or sex will bring on pain or another

attack or even death. This fear may be even more common in their partners. Fortunately, there is little basis for this fear. Sexual relations can be resumed as soon as you feel the desire to do so. Studies show that the risk of sexual activity contributing to a heart attack is less than 1 percent. This risk is even lower for individuals who regularly exercise. After a stroke, any remaining paralysis or weakness may require that you pay more attention to finding the best positions for support and comfort and identifying the most sensitive areas of the body to caress. There may also be concerns about bowel and bladder control. The American Heart Association (www .heart.org) has some excellent guides about sex after a heart attack or stroke, as does Heart & Stroke (www.heartandstroke.ca).

People with diabetes sometimes report problems with sexual function. Men may have difficulty achieving or maintaining an erection. These difficulties may be caused by medication side effects or other medical conditions associated with diabetes. Women and men with diabetes may also have reduced feeling in the genital area. The most common complaint from women is not enough vaginal lubrication. If you have diabetes, the best ways to prevent or reduce these problems is to maintain good control of your blood sugar, exercise, keep a positive outlook, and generally take care of yourself. Lubricants can help with sensitivity for both men and women. If you are using condoms, be sure to use a water-based lubricant. Petroleum-based lubricants destroy latex. The use of a vibrator can be very helpful for individuals with reduced feeling (neuropathy) in the genital area. Concentrating on the most sensual parts of the body for stimulation may lead to more pleasurable sex. There are also new therapies for men with erectile problems. The American Diabetes Association (www.diabetes.org) and Diabetes Canada (https://diabetes.ca) have more detailed information about sex and diabetes.

People who are missing a breast, testicle, or another body part because of their treatment for cancer or some other medical condition may also have fears about sex and intimacy. This is also true for people with surgical scars or swollen or disfigured joints from arthritis. In these cases, you may worry about what your partner thinks. Will your partner or potential partner find you undesirable? Although this may happen, it happens less often than you think. Usually when you fall in love with someone, you fall in love with who the person is, not that person's breast, testicle, or other body part. Here again, good communication and sharing your concerns and fears with your partner can help. If this is difficult to do, perhaps a couple's counselor or therapist can help. Often the things we imagine or worry about do not become serious problems and can be managed.

Fatigue is another symptom that can undermine sexual desire. Chapter 4, *Understanding and Managing Common Symptoms and Problems*, includes tools to combat fatigue. Here is one additional hint: Plan your sexual activities around your fatigue. That is, try to engage in sex during the times of day and night when you are less tired. This might mean that mornings are better than evenings.

Many mental health conditions and the medications used to treat their symptoms can also interfere with sexual function and desire. Talk with your doctor or nurse practitioner about these side effects so that together you can find alternatives. Sometimes your provider can find another medication, change the dosage and timing of the medication, or refer you to a therapist to help you and your partner learn other self-management strategies to decrease or eliminate symptoms. Individual or couple's therapy can help in dealing with other personal relationship, intimacy, and sexual problems that are not related to your medications.

No matter what your chronic pain or health issue, your health care provider is your first consultant for sexual problems that might be related to it. Don't be shy or afraid to mention intimate topics. It's unlikely that your problem is unique. Your provider has probably heard about it many times before and may have some solutions. Remember, sexual considerations are just another issue associated with your chronic condition, just like the pain, fatigue, and physical limitations. These are the kinds of problems that self-managers can learn to solve.

Chronic health problems don't have to mean the end of sex or intimacy. Through good communication, planning, and problem solving, you can enjoy satisfying sex and deeper intimacy. By being creative and willing to experiment, both your sex life and your relationship may improve.

For a complete list of suggested further readings, useful websites, and other helpful resources, please see

www.bullpub.com/resources.

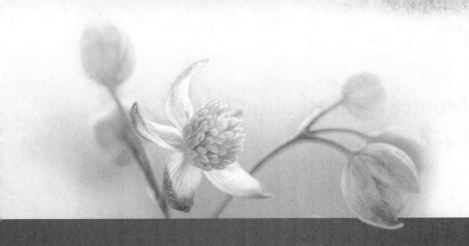

Managing Your Treatment Decisions and Medications

Y OU MAY BE CONSIDERING DIFFERENT TREATMENTS and medications for chronic pain. You may also be taking medications and receiving other types of treatment for other health conditions. Making decisions about your medications and treatments and monitoring them are very important self-management tasks. This chapter gives general guidelines to help you do just that. We recommend that you read this chapter first before reading Chapter 15, *Understanding Medications and Other Treatments for Chronic Pain*, which provides more detailed information.

Evaluating Medical and Health Claims

You hear about new treatments, new drugs, nutritional supplements, and alternative treatments all the time. Not a week goes by without some new treatment making news. There are ads for drugs and nutritional supplements everywhere you look—in newspapers, magazines, on television, and on social media. Emails promise new treatments and cures. Have you noticed that television ads tell us the benefits of these treatments in a slow, upbeat voice, while the side effects are delivered so rapidly, we can barely understand them? Your health care providers may also recommend new procedures, medications, or other treatments. Drug companies spend billions of dollars advertising and marketing to physicians and patients. Imagine if such marketing powers were used to promote self-management skills. There might be far less chronic illness and less need for medications, surgery, herbs, supplements, and alternative medicine offerings.

What can you believe? How can you decide what might be worth a try? Managing your own health involves being able to evaluate these claims. You must make an informed decision before trying something new. It is easy to hope that a special diet, new medication, or trendy treatment may be the answer to chronic pain. Everyone wants that "magic bullet" to take the pain away. Unfortunately, there are few magic bullets when it comes to treating chronic pain. This chapter gives you information to make informed decisions to manage your treatment and medications more effectively. If you can gather the right information, you are one step closer to making better decisions and being a successful self-manager.

Asking Questions about Treatments for Chronic Pain

There are treatments out there that may help you manage your pain better. But before exploring these options, it is important to learn about any treatment, whether it is a mainstream medical treatment or a complementary or alternative approach. When evaluating what you hear and read, ask yourself these important questions before making a decision so you know you are making an informed decision.

Where did you learn about this treatment?

Was the treatment reported in a scientific journal; a supermarket tabloid; an online, print, or television ad; a website; social media; or a flyer you picked up somewhere? Did a friend, neighbor, or family member suggest it? Did your doctor recommend it?

The source of the information is important. Results that are reported in a respected scientific journal are more believable than those you might see in a supermarket tabloid or in advertising. Results reported in scientific journals are usually from research studies. Scientists carefully review these studies before publication. Although bias, errors, and fraud can still occur in mainstream scientific publications, they are far less likely and there are ways to correct errors. Many alternative treatments and nutritional supplements have not been studied scientifically.

If you are told there are studies supporting a treatment but you cannot find them by searching online or in a library, be suspicious. If the science is good, the studies are almost always published. Testimonials, anecdotes, unsupported claims, and opinions aren't the same as objective, evidence-based information. If it sounds too good to be true, it's probably not true. One quick way to look up studies is to search the name of the treatment on Google Scholar.

Are the people who used this treatment and got better similar to you?

It is important to find out if the people whose pain improved are like you. Are they members of the same age group, sex, and race? Did they have the same chronic pain conditions as you do? Do they have similar lifestyles? If the subjects of the study aren't like you, you may not have the same results that they did.

Could anything else have caused the positive changes attributed to the treatment?

Consider this example. A woman returns from a stay at a spa. She reports that her chronic pain improved dramatically thanks to the special diet, herbs, and supplements she received. But could it be that the warm weather, relaxation, and pampering caused her improvement? This example shows that it is important to look at everything that has changed since someone started a treatment. Did the person who improved start another medication or treatment at the same time? Are they under less stress than they were before they started the treatment? Can you think of anything else that could have affected their health? It is common to take up a generally healthier lifestyle when starting a new treatment—could that be playing a part in the improvement?

Does the treatment require extreme diet changes or that you stop other medications or treatments?

Is a magic food or supplement being promoted? If the treatment requires that you change your eating habits, be sure you don't sacrifice important nutrients (see Chapter 9, *Healthy Eating and Pain Self-Management*). The phrase "alternative care" means a treatment is used *in place of* conventional medicine. The phrase "complementary care" is used *along with* conventional medicine. When you choose a complementary care treatment, you may be getting treatment from your doctor or other health care provider while you also use additional therapies to manage the same condition. For example, you may be taking medication for arthritis pain and avoiding foods that may cause inflammation. In contrast, an alternative treatment requires you to stop taking other medical treatments. Be cautious before choosing any alternative treatment that requires you to change any other treatment you already use. Talk with your health care provider before stopping any treatment or making a change.

Is the treatment safe and effective?

All treatments have side effects and possible risks. Only you can decide if the potential problems are worth the possible benefit. Many people think that if something is "natural" or "organic," it must be good for them. This may not be true. When something is strong enough to have an effect, it's also strong enough to have side effects. "Natural" isn't necessarily better or safer than a manufactured product. Just because it comes from a plant or animal instead of a laboratory does not mean it is harmless. The heart medication digitalis comes from a plant, but it can be deadly if the dose is not right. And know that some treatments, herbs, or even vitamin supplements that may be safe in small doses can be dangerous in larger doses.

Just because many people use a product or practice or it has been used for many years also doesn't mean that it's safe or effective. Some traditional practices, such as meditation, have proven health benefits and little or no risk. Other traditional methods may not be safe for certain people to use. And others simply don't work or haven't yet been proven.

The US Food and Drug Administration (FDA) regulates over-the-counter and prescription drugs. It does *not* regulate herbs or other supplements. In Canada, Health Canada's Health Products and Food Branch (HPFB) regulates, evaluates, and monitors the safety, quality, and effectiveness of therapeutic and diagnostic products available to Canadians. In the United States, herbs and supplements do not have to meet the same standards for safety, effectiveness, and manufacturing that over-the-counter and prescription drugs must meet. Scientific tests of some supplements have found striking differences between what's listed on the label and what's in the bottle. Some products were found to not even contain the active ingredient they advertised. And some were found to be contaminated with metals, unlabeled prescription drugs, pesticides, microorganisms, or other substances. Research the company selling the product before you try it. Ask your health care provider or pharmacist before adding any supplement to your medication regime, even if it is "natural" or herbal.

What is the "cost" of the new treatment?

There are many costs to consider when thinking about treatments, including financial, physical, and emotional costs. Do you have the money to spend on this treatment for the time it will take to produce an improvement? Is your health strong enough to maintain this new regimen? Will you be able to handle it emotionally? Will this put a strain on your ability to function at home or work? Some of the newer medications available today are both very effective and very costly. If you think you cannot afford a medication, ask your health care provider or health insurance company for suggestions. Many pharmaceutical companies offer discounts or even take care of copayments, but to take advantage of these offers, you must contact their patient or consumer services people.

Learning More about Treatments

Just because something is commonly done doesn't mean it is always the best thing to do. Sometimes it is wise to say no to standard medical treatments. After reviewing the medical evidence, various medical specialty organizations have recommended that many common treatments should *not* be used. They also recommend tests and treatments you *should* have but may not be getting. To learn more about this, see www.choosingwisely.org. (Canada's equivalent website is www.choosingwiselycanada.org.) For example, you may not need X-rays or MRIs for back pain, antibiotics for sinus infections, whole-body scans for early detection of illness, CT scans for uncomplicated headaches, and so on. At the same time, there may be tests that are not being offered to you that are good options for you. The US Preventive Services Task Force and the Canadian Task Force on Preventive Health Care provide evidence-based, critical reviews of various screening tests and medical treatments for both providers and consumers.

Where can you get more information about treatments to make good decisions about them? The internet can provide information about new treatments and can be a resource for up-to-date information. But be cautious—especially when you are on sites that are selling products or services. Not every piece of information on the internet is correct or even safe. Seek out the most reliable sources by noting the author or sponsor of the site and the site's internet address (also called its URL). Addresses ending in .edu, .org, and .gov are generally more objective and reliable. These URLs originate from universities, non-profit organizations, and governmental agencies, respectively. Some .com sites can also be good, but because they are maintained by commercial or for-profit organizations, their information may be biased in favor of their own products. Review Chapter 3, *Finding Resources*, to learn how to find reliable sources of information. The following list provides some sites to explore. You can find updated URLs for these sites at www.bullpub.com/resources under the topic headings "Making Treatment Decisions" and "Medications, Herbs, Supplements & Other Treatments."

- **National Center for Complementary and Integrative Health** is a government agency providing research-based info from A to Z (acupuncture to zinc), including up-to-date, reliable information about chronic pain and complementary treatments.

- **Natural Medicines Comprehensive Database** (consumer version) reviews clinical

data on approximately 90,000 herbal products, dietary supplements, vitamins, minerals, homeopathic products, Ayurvedic (Indian) medicines, complementary alternative medicines, integrative therapies, alternative treatments (such as acupuncture), traditional Chinese medicine products, and other natural remedies. It also provides an Interaction Checker that shows how natural products interact with prescription and over-the-counter medications.

- **ConsumerLab** provides independent testing on nutritional products.

- **Consumer Reports** reviews and evaluates both alternative and conventional treatments and products.

- **Canada regulates natural health products** and maintains a natural health products webpage.

- The government of Canada also maintains the **Licensed Natural Health Products Database (LNHPD)**. It contains information about natural health products that have been issued a product license by Health Canada. It includes information on vitamin and mineral supplements, herb- and plant-based remedies, traditional Chinese medicines, traditional Ayurvedic medicines, homeopathic medicines, and many everyday consumer products.

Making decisions about new treatments can be difficult. A good self-manager uses the questions raised in this chapter and the decision-making steps in Chapter 2, *Becoming an Active Self-Manager*, to make informed personal decisions. If you ask yourself all the questions in this chapter and decide to try a new treatment on your own, it is very important to inform your health care providers about it. You and your provider are partners, and you need to keep your partner informed on your progress during the time you are taking the treatment.

General Information about Medications

Medications are heavily advertised. These ads are aimed at making you believe that if you just use a certain pill, your symptoms will be cured and life will be better. It seems like there is a pill for every ill. As you review these claims, keep in mind that your body is often its own healer, and given time, many common symptoms and conditions improve. The prescriptions filled by the body's own "internal pharmacy" are frequently the safest and most effective treatments. Patience, careful self-observation, and monitoring are often excellent choices.

It is also true that medications can be a very important part of managing chronic pain. In Chapter 15, *Understanding Medications and Other Treatments for Chronic Pain*, you can learn about specific medications to treat chronic pain. Here we share some information about medications in general. Although most medications do not cure chronic pain, they can do the following:

- **Relieve symptoms.** For example, a nitroglycerin tablet expands the blood vessels to relieve chest pain. Acetaminophen (Tylenol®) may relieve pain. An antidepressant can reduce depression and improve mood, which may help lessen pain.

- **Prevent further problems.** For example, blood thinners can help prevent blood clots, which cause strokes and heart and lung problems. Anti-inflammatory drugs used to treat diseases, including rheumatoid arthritis, help prevent destruction of joints and surrounding tissues.

- **Improve or slow the progress of the disease.** For example, nonsteroidal anti-inflammatory drugs quiet the inflammatory process of arthritis. Antihypertensive medications can lower blood pressure. Sometimes even if medications do not stop symptoms, they help prevent future symptoms by slowing the underlying condition or illness.

- **Replace substances that the body is no longer producing adequately.** This is why people with diabetes take insulin and why thyroid medication is prescribed for underactive thyroid.

As these examples show, many medications for chronic health problems lessen the consequences of the condition or slow the disease process. Some medications act in different ways to address different conditions.

When you take medications like these, you may not feel anything. You may think that the drug isn't working. However, even though you may not feel its effects immediately, the drug may be preventing complications or keeping you from getting worse. For this reason, it is important to continue taking your medications and discuss medication use with your health care provider when you have questions.

Medications can be very helpful, but we pay a price for having such powerful tools. Besides being helpful, medications have side effects. Some of these effects are predictable and minor, and some are unexpected and life-threatening. As many as 5 to 10 percent of all hospital admissions are due to drug reactions. At the same time, not taking medications as prescribed is also a major cause of hospitalization. Many thousands of people a year die from overdoses of prescription opioids and other prescription drugs.

Using Mind Power: Expecting the Best

Medication affects your body in two ways. The first is determined by the chemical nature of the medication. The second is triggered by your beliefs and expectations. Your beliefs can change your body chemistry and your symptoms. Your beliefs can change how *any* medication or treatment works. Perhaps you have heard of a placebo. A placebo is given as medicine, but it does not contain an active substance meant to affect health. The placebo effect refers to what happens when people take a so-called sugar pill and their symptoms improve even though the pill does not contain any medicine. The placebo effect is an example of how closely the mind and body are connected.

Many studies have shown the power of the placebo—the power of mind over body. The point is, every time you take a medication, you are swallowing your expectations and beliefs as well as the pill. You can learn to take advantage of your powerful internal pharmacy along with taking medications. *Expect the best!*

Consider the following ways to use your mind to get the most out of your medicine:

- **Examine your beliefs about the treatment.** If you tell yourself "I'm not a pill taker" or "medications always give me bad side effects," how do you think your body is likely to respond? If you don't think the prescribed treatment is likely to help your symptoms or condition, your negative beliefs undermine the ability of the pill to help you. You can change these negative images into more positive ones. To practice this strategy, review the discussion of positive thinking in Chapter 5, *Using Your Mind to Manage Pain and Other Symptoms.*

- **Think of your medications the way you think of vitamins.** Many people associate healthful images with vitamins—more so than with medications. Many people, when they are taking a vitamin, think that they are doing something positive to prevent disease and promote health. If you regard your medications as health restoring and health promoting, like vitamins, you may see more benefits.

- **Imagine how the medicine is helping you.** Develop a mental image of how the medication is doing its job inside of you. For example, when taking a pain medication, tell yourself it is finding its way through your central nervous system and closing the pain gate. Or think of an antibiotic as a broom sweeping germs out of your body. For many people, forming a vivid mental image is helpful. Don't worry if your image of what's happening inside of you is not chemically or medically accurate. Your belief in a clear, positive image is what counts.

- **Keep in mind why you are taking the medication.** You are not taking your medication just because your health care provider told you to. You are taking your medication to manage your condition and help you live your life. It is important to understand and remind yourself how the medicine is helping you manage your chronic pain. You can use this information to help the medicine do its job. For example, suppose a man with lower back pain is given an antidepressant medication to improve his pain and mood. He has been told it will make him feel drowsy and dizzy, and it will cause him to have a very dry mouth. This knowledge may worsen his side effects. But suppose he is also told that the side effects will likely only last a few days and that it means that the medicine is building up in his body. In a few weeks he should start to experience an improvement in his pain and mood. The presence of side effects can sometimes be proof that the medicine is working. He can then take actions to manage these side effects and have an easier time tolerating them. (See Chapter 15, *Understanding Medications and Other Treatments for Chronic Pain*, page 324, for more tips on how to get the most out of pain medications.)

Taking Multiple Medications

People with chronic pain often have other health problems, which means they often take many medications. For example, a person might take a medication to lower blood pressure and cholesterol, a drug to help arthritis pain, a medication to manage depression, and an antacid for heartburn. They might also take vitamins, herbs, and other over-the-counter (OTC) remedies. The more medications you are taking, the greater the risk of side effects. Not all drugs play well together. When you take multiple medications together, they sometimes cause problems.

Fortunately, it is often possible to take fewer medications and lower the risks. However, you should not do this without the help of your health care providers. Most people would not just change the ingredients in a recipe or throw out a few parts when fixing a car. It is not that these things can't be done. It is just that if you want the best and safest results, you may need expert help.

The goal of treatment is to get the most benefits with the fewest risks. This means taking the fewest medications, in the lowest effective doses, for the shortest period. (Note that some medications need to be taken for life.) Making sure your medications are helpful often depends on being informed about your medications, communicating about your medications with your health care providers, and taking your medications as directed.

Communicating with Your Health Care Provider about Medications and Other Treatments

How you respond to any medication depends on your age, daily activity, symptoms, chronic conditions, genetics, and frame of mind. To make sure you get the most from your medications, your health care team depends on you. You need to report what effect, if any, the drugs you take have on your symptoms. You also need to report any side effects. Based on this information, your provider continues, increases, discontinues, or changes your medication. In a good provider-patient partnership, information flows in *both* directions.

Unfortunately, this communication often does not happen. Studies show that fewer than 5 percent of patients getting new prescriptions ask any questions. Doctors tend to think that if their patients are silent, it means they understand and will take the medications properly. Problems often result when patients do not get enough information about medications or do not understand how to take them. In addition, consumers often do not follow instructions. Safe, effective drug use depends equally on your provider's expertise and on your understanding of when and how to take the drug. You must ask questions to get the information you need.

Some people are afraid to ask their provider questions. They are afraid that they will seem foolish or stupid or that the doctor will think they are difficult. Asking questions is a necessary part of a healthy provider-patient relationship. See Chapter 11, *Communicating with Family, Friends, and Health Care Providers*, for more on this important communication skill.

Things to Tell Your Provider before Tests, Procedures, and New Medications or Treatments (Even If Your Provider Doesn't Ask!)

As we have noted in this chapter, communication is key. Your health care provider needs to know about the following issues even if he or she doesn't ask about these things:

If you are taking other medications

Report to your physician (and your dentist) all the prescription and nonprescription medications you are taking. Include birth control pills, vitamins, aspirin, antacids, laxatives, alcohol, and herbal remedies. An easy way to do this is to carry a list of all medications and the amounts you take (dosage). Many electronic medical records (EMRs) have a complete list of your medications that you can download or copy. You can also ask your primary care provider for a list of all the medications they have in your electronic record. Your record may include medications there that you are no longer taking. If it does, let your provider know. The important thing is that you and your health care team have current, accurate information about what you are taking. If you don't have a list and cannot put one together, gather together all your medications and take them to your medical appointments. Saying that you are taking "the little green pills" isn't very helpful.

If you are seeing more than one provider, each one may not know what the others have prescribed. Unless you know that all your providers use the same medical record, always bring a list of your medications and supplements each time you visit.

It is necessary for your provider to know about every medication you take. They need this information to correctly diagnosis and treat you. For example, if you have symptoms such as nausea or diarrhea, sleeplessness or drowsiness, dizziness or memory loss, or sexual dysfunction or fatigue, a drug side effect rather than your chronic pain or other illness may be the cause. If health care providers do not know all your medications, they cannot protect you from drug interactions.

If you have had allergic or unusual reactions to any medications

Describe any symptoms or unusual reactions caused by medications, anesthetics, or X-ray contrast materials. Be specific: describe which medication you took and exactly what type of reaction you had. A rash, fever, or wheezing that develops after taking a medication is often a true allergic reaction. If any of these happened in the past, let your provider know. If any of these develop after a treatment or taking a new medication, call your provider at once. Nausea, diarrhea, ringing in the ears, light-headedness, sleeplessness, and frequent urination are likely to be side effects rather than true drug allergies. You also want to mention these when you discuss medications or treatments with your provider.

If you have other medical conditions in addition to chronic pain

Some medical conditions can make a drug less effective or increase the risks of side effects. Your kidneys or liver control how the body uses and breaks down a drug, so it is important

your provider knows about how your organs are functioning. Your health care provider may also avoid certain medications if you have ever had high blood pressure, peptic ulcer disease, asthma, heart disease, diabetes, or prostate problems. Be sure to let your provider know if you have a history of bleeding or are possibly pregnant or are breastfeeding. Many drugs are not safe in those situations.

If you tried other medications or treatments in the past to treat your condition

It is a good idea to keep your own records of medications or treatments that were used in the past and what the effects were. You can also usually find some of this information online in your electronic medical record (EMR). But also, be sure to record self-care, self-prescribed, over-the-counter, and alternative treatments, herbs, and supplements. Knowing what has been tried and how you reacted informs the recommendation of any new medications or treatments. However, the fact that a medication did not work in the past does not necessarily mean that it can't be tried again. Chronic pain and other conditions change, and a medication that did not work the first time may work the second time.

Things to Ask Your Provider Before Tests, Procedures, and New Medications or Treatments

Ideally, you should ask the following questions before any test, treatment, or surgical procedure or before you take a new medication. Realistically, you probably want to save the time and effort and ask these only before more significant or risky interventions. Remember, except for in extreme emergencies, when a doctor "orders" something, this "order" is really just a recommendation for you. *You* make the final decisions.

Do I really need this test, treatment, procedure, or medication?

Some doctors and other health care providers prescribe medications or order tests not because the tests are necessary but because they think patients want and expect them. Doctors often feel pressure to do *something* for the patient, so they prescribe a new drug. Don't pressure your doctor. Many new medications are heavily advertised. Some are later found to be so hazardous that they are withdrawn from the market. So be cautious about requesting the newest medications. If your doctor doesn't prescribe a medication, consider that good news.

Instead of asking for new medications, ask about nondrug alternatives. In some cases, lifestyle changes such as exercise, diet, and stress management may have better results than medications for chronic pain. When any treatment is recommended, ask what may happen if you postpone treatment. Would your pain likely get worse or perhaps better with time? Sometimes the best medicine is none. Sometimes the best option is taking a powerful medication early to avoid permanent damage or complications.

When it comes to medical tests, ask, "What happens if the result is not normal?" and "What happens if the result is normal?" If the answers are the same, then you probably do not need the test. If you have already had a similar test or medication, let your provider know. Providing information about past treatment and medication can sometimes prevent unnecessary care and risk.

What are the risks and benefits of this test, treatment, procedure, or medication?

No test, procedure, or medication is without risk. Weighing the possible risks and benefits can be difficult, but it is very important. You are the one who will live with the results. Side effects and complications range from minor, common, and reversible to major, rare, and permanent. Reading about all the possible side effects on patient information inserts can be scary. Talk with your health care provider or pharmacist to help sort out your risks. *Remember, there may also be risks associated with not taking necessary and helpful medications.*

Your doctor may have to try several medications before finding the one that is best for you. You need to know what symptoms to look for and what action to take if they develop. Should you seek immediate medical care, discontinue the medication, or call your doctor? Though the doctor cannot be expected to tell you every possible side effect, the most common and important ones should be discussed. Unfortunately, a recent survey showed that 70 percent of people starting a new medication did not recall being told by their physicians or pharmacists about precautions and possible side effects.

Like medications, there can also be a risk with medical tests, surgeries, and procedures. A "false positive" result incorrectly says you are ill. A "false negative" test is a test result that fails to identify you are sick. Such inaccuracies can lead to anxiety, delayed diagnosis, and further risky testing. When it comes to surgery, the skill and experience of the surgeon and surgical team can make a significant difference in successful outcomes and risk of complications.

Being aware of and avoiding unnecessary risks is important, but there is another side to this story. Some tests such as mammograms, pap smears, prostate exams, and colonoscopies (examination of the rectum and colon) are somewhat unpleasant and can be embarrassing. Some treatments, such as chemotherapy, have side effects. However, these are not reasons to avoid these tests, treatments, and medications. They can be lifesaving. As a self-manager, you must weigh the risks and benefits. Your health care team can help.

What can I expect from this test, treatment, procedure, or medication?

If your provider prescribes a new medication, you need to know its name, how much to take, how you should take it, for how long, and when you can expect to feel better. Is the medication intended to prolong your life, completely or partially relieve your pain and other symptoms, or help you function better? Some medications help prevent problems in the future and other medications treat acute problems today.

For example, if you are given a medicine for high blood pressure, the medication is usually given to prevent later complications (such as stroke or heart disease) rather than to stop a headache. On the other hand, if you are given a pain reliever such as ibuprofen (Motrin®, Advil®), the purpose is to help ease a headache.

You also need to know how soon you should expect results. Drugs that treat infections or inflammation may take several days to a week to show improvement. Antidepressant medications and some arthritis drugs typically take several weeks or even months to start providing relief.

Taking medication properly is vital. Yet nearly 40 percent of people report that their doctors fail to tell them how to take the medication or how much to take. If you are not sure about your prescription, contact your doctor or pharmacist. Even if you get your drugs by mail order or online, you can still contact your local pharmacist with questions.

Does "every 6 hours" mean every 6 hours while awake or every 6 hours around the clock? Should the medication be taken before meals, with meals, or between meals? What should you do if you accidentally miss a dose? Should you skip it, take a double dose next time, or take it as soon as you remember? Should you refill and continue taking the medication until you have fewer symptoms or until you finish the current medication? Some medications are prescribed on an as-needed ("PRN") basis. Others need to be taken regularly. Some medications need lab tests to check for side effects. If you are taking one of these medications, work with your health care provider to make sure you are getting the necessary lab tests.

If a surgical procedure is recommended, it is important that you discuss the options for anesthesia and how to prepare for the operation. For example, before the procedure should you continue taking medications? Stop eating and drinking? When? Can you drive yourself to the procedure and then drive home? Ask how long recovery is likely to take and when you can resume normal activities. You will probably be given medications to relieve pain, but also ask about some of the nondrug pain-relief tools in Chapter 5, *Using Your Mind to Manage Pain and Other Symptoms*.

How much does this test, treatment, procedure, or medication cost?

Ask for an estimate in advance of the cost for tests, procedures, and medications. Ask if there are less expensive tests, treatments, or procedures that your insurance may cover instead.

Discuss less expensive alternative or generic medications as well. Every drug has at least two names: a generic name and a brand name. The generic name is the medication's scientific name. The brand name is the name given to the drug by its developer. When a drug company develops a new drug in the United States, it is granted exclusive rights to produce that drug for 17 years. In Canada, patent terms are currently 20 years. In the United States, after this 17-year period, other companies may market chemically identical versions of that brand-name drug. These generic medications are generally considered as safe and effective as the original brand-name drug but often cost much less. In rare cases, your physician may have a special reason for preferring a brand name instead of a generic version. Even so, if cost is a concern, ask your health care provider if a less expensive but equally effective medication is available.

You may also be able to save money by knowing how to best use your insurance. For example, your copayment may be less if you get your medications from a company designated by your insurer or if you order refills online and receive them by mail. Also, many national pharmacies have discount programs for seniors and individuals with low income. It pays to ask and then ask again. And it is wise to shop around. Even in the same town, different stores sell the same medication at different prices. Big box stores with pharmacies are often a good option.

Under the Canada Health Act, prescription drugs administered in Canadian hospitals are provided at no cost to you. Outside of the hospital setting, provincial and territorial governments are responsible for the administration of their own publicly funded drug plans. The public drug plans determine which prescription drugs are listed and under what conditions for eligible recipients. Most Canadians have some access to insurance coverage for prescription drugs through a patchwork of public and private insurance plans. The federal, provincial, and territorial governments offer varying levels of coverage and decide who is covered and what you and your plan pays. The publicly funded drug programs generally provide drug plan coverage for those most in need based on age, income, and medical condition. Many Canadians and their family members have drug coverage linked to employment, and some Canadians may have no effective drug coverage and pay the full cost of prescription drugs.

Is there any written or online information about the test, treatment, procedure, or medication?

Your health care provider may not have time to answer all your questions. You may not remember everything you hear in a possibly rushed appointment. Fortunately, there are many other good sources of information. For example, pharmacists are experts on medications and can answer questions in person, over the phone, via email, or through a secure web portal. In addition, many hospitals, medical schools, and schools of pharmacy have medication information services that you can call to ask questions.

As a self-manager, be sure to also consult nurses, package inserts, pamphlets, books, and websites. Review Chapter 3, *Finding Resources*, and for a complete list of suggested further readings, useful websites, and other helpful resources, please see www.bullpub.com/resources.

Managing Your Medications

Medicine doesn't work if you don't take it! Sounds obvious. Yet nearly half of all medicines are not taken as prescribed. Sometimes this is referred to as "the other drug problem." There are many reasons why people don't take their prescribed medication: forgetfulness, lack of clear instructions, complicated dosing schedules, side effects, and cost. Whatever the reason, if you are having trouble taking your medications as prescribed, discuss this issue with your health care team. Often, simple changes can make it easier. For example, if you are taking many different medications, sometimes one or more can be stopped. If you are taking one medication three times a day and another four times a day, your doctor may be able to prescribe medications you only need to take once or twice a day.

If you are having trouble taking your medications, read the following questions and discuss the questions you answer yes to with your doctor, pharmacist, or other health care provider.

- Do you tend to be forgetful?

- Are you confused about the instructions for how and when to use the medications?

- Is the schedule for taking your medications too complicated?

- Do your medications have bothersome side effects?

- Is your medicine too expensive?

- Do you feel that your condition is not serious enough to need regular medications? (With some diseases such as high blood pressure, high cholesterol, or early diabetes, you may not have any symptoms.)

- Do you feel that the treatment is unlikely to help?

- Are you denying that you have a condition that needs treatment?

- Have you had a bad experience with the medicine you are supposed to be taking or another medication?

- Do you know someone who had a bad experience with the medication, and are you afraid that something similar will happen to you?

- Are you afraid of the medication's effects or becoming addicted to it?

- Are you embarrassed about taking the medication? Do you view taking it as a sign of weakness or failure, or do you fear you'll be judged negatively if people know about it?

- Do you need to review the benefits of the medication when taken as prescribed?

Reading a Prescription Label

Prescription labels can be a great source of information on your medication's name, dose, appearance, how to take it, precautions, and more. Figure 14.1 is a guide for reading the labels on your prescriptions.

Remembering to Take Your Medicines

If forgetting to take your medications is a problem for you, here are some suggestions to help you remember:

■ **Make it obvious.** Place the medication or a reminder next to your toothbrush, on the breakfast table, in your lunch box, or some other place where you're likely to "stumble across" it. (Be careful where you put the medication if there are children in your household.) Put a reminder note on the bathroom mirror, toothbrush, refrigerator door, coffee maker, television, or some other obvious place. If you connect taking the medication with some well-established habit such as mealtimes, brushing your teeth, or watching your favorite television show, you'll be more likely to remember.

■ **Use a checklist or an organizer.** Make a weekly or monthly medication calendar or chart listing each medication you are taking and the time when you take it. Check off each medication on the calendar as you take it. There are websites that have charts you can print to help you track your medications. You can also buy a medication organizer online or at a drugstore. A medication organizer is a container that separates pills according to the time of day they should be taken. You can fill the organizer once a week so that all your pills are ready to take at the proper time. A quick glance at the organizer lets you know if you have missed any doses and prevents double dosing. Some pharmacy services will sort and prepackage your medications for each day in "blister" packs.

■ **Use an electronic reminder.** Get a watch or mobile phone that you can set to beep at

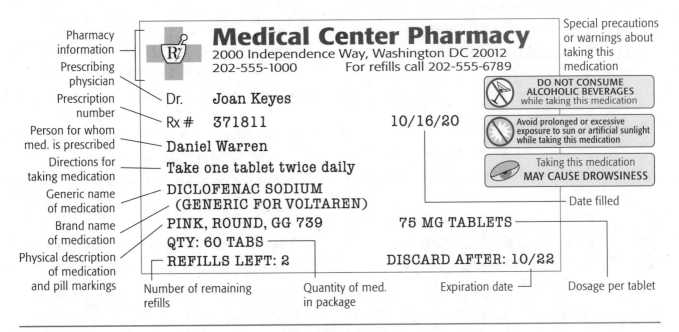

Figure 14.1 **How to Read a Prescription Label**

pill-taking time. There are also electronic medication containers that beep at preset times to remind you. You can also download smartphone apps that remind you to take your medication at the right times.

- **Have others remind you.** If you are having trouble managing your medications, consider asking members of your household to remind you at the right times.

- **Plan ahead so you don't run out.** Don't let yourself run out of your medicines. When you get your prescription filled, add a reminder to your calendar on the date one week before your medications will run out (or two weeks if you get your medications by mail). This will remind you about your next refill. Don't wait until the last pill is taken to order refills. You can sign up with most mail-order pharmacies for automatic refills so your medications arrive when you need them.

- **Plan before you travel.** Before you travel, put a note on your luggage reminding you to pack your pills. Always pack medications in your carry-on luggage. Don't put them in your checked bags. Also, bring a copy of your prescription(s) in your carry-on bag in case you lose your pills. To be extra sure, also put a few days of medication in your luggage. That way if you forget and leave your medications somewhere, you will not get caught short.

Taking Nonprescription or Over-the-Counter (OTC) Medications

More than 200,000 nonprescription drug products are for sale to the public in the United States. These drugs include about 500 active ingredients. In Canada, more than 15,000 nonprescription drugs and over 43,000 natural health products are available.

You may take nonprescription or over-the-counter (OTC) medications or herbs. In the United States, 81 percent of adults use OTC products as their first choice for treatment of minor illnesses and symptoms. Many OTC drugs are highly effective and may even be recommended by your health care provider. If you take nonprescription medicines and supplements, you should know what you are taking, why you are taking it, and how to use these substances wisely.

Many people learn about OTC drugs online or from TV, radio, newspaper, and magazine advertising. The message of drug advertising is that for every symptom, every ache and pain, and every problem, there is a medication solution. Although many OTC products are effective, many are a waste of your money. OTC medications may also prevent you from managing your condition in other less medication-centered ways. They may interfere or interact badly with your prescription medications.

Whether you are taking prescribed medications or using over-the-counter medications or herbs, here are some helpful suggestions:

- **If you are pregnant or nursing, have a chronic condition, or are already taking multiple medications, consult your health care provider before self-medicating.**

- **Always read labels and follow directions carefully.** Reading the label and reviewing the individual ingredients may prevent you from taking medications that have caused problems for you in the past. It may also prevent double dosing on medications that you may already be taking. For example, aspirin and acetaminophen are popular medications for pain. And aspirin and acetaminophen are also ingredients in over-the-counter products such as cold remedies. If you don't understand the information on a product's label, ask a pharmacist or doctor before buying or using the product.

■ **Do not take more than the recommended dose or take it for longer than recommended** unless you have discussed this plan with your health care provider.

■ **Be careful if you are taking other medications.** Over-the-counter and prescription drugs can interact, either canceling or exaggerating the effects of one or all medications. Ask your doctor or pharmacist before mixing medicines.

■ **Try to select medications with a single active ingredient rather than combination ("all-in-one") products.** If you use a product with multiple ingredients, you are likely to get drugs for symptoms you don't even have. Why risk the side effects for medications you don't need? Single-ingredient products also allow you to adjust the dosage of each medication separately for the best symptom relief with fewest side effects.

■ **Learn the generic names for active ingredients and look for generic products.** Generics contain the same active ingredient as the brand-name product, usually at a lower cost.

■ **Never take a drug from an unlabeled container or a container that has a label you cannot read.** Keep medications in their original labeled containers or transfer them to a labeled medication organizer or pill dispenser. Do not mix different medications in the same bottle.

■ **Do not take medications that were prescribed for someone else**, even if you have similar symptoms.

■ **Do not share your medications.** The largest source of prescription opioid misuse is drugs that are borrowed or stolen from family or friends.

■ **Drink at least a half glass of liquid with your pills** and remain standing or sitting upright for a short while after swallowing. This can prevent the pills from getting stuck.

■ **Store your medications where children, young adults, and others cannot find them.** Poisoning from medications is a common and preventable problem. The main sources of recreational drugs used by teens and young adults are the prescription medications of relatives or the relatives of friends. Despite its name, the bathroom medicine cabinet is not usually an appropriate place to store medications. A locked kitchen cabinet or toolbox with a lock is far safer.

Using Alcohol and Recreational Drugs

The use of alcohol and recreational drugs (illegal or prescription medications used for nonmedicinal purposes) has been increasing in recent years, particularly among people over the age of 60. These drugs, whether legal or illegal, can cause problems. They can interact with prescription medications, making them less effective or even causing harm. They can fog judgment and cause problems with balance. This can in turn cause accidents and result in injury to you and others.

In some cases, alcohol or recreational drugs can make existing long-term conditions worse. Alcohol use is associated with higher risk of hypertension, diabetes, gastrointestinal bleeding, sleep disorders, depression, erectile dysfunction, breast and other cancers, and injury.

"At risk" alcohol use for women is drinking more than seven drinks per week or more than three drinks per day. For men, "at risk" alcohol use is drinking more than 14 drinks per week or more than four drinks in a day. Women of any age and anyone over age 65 should average no more than one drink per day, and men under 65 should have no more than two drinks per day on average. In Canada, the recommendation is no more than 10 drinks a week for women, with no more than two drinks a day most days, and no more than 15 drinks a week for men, with no more than three drinks a day most days.

One alcoholic drink equivalent contains 0.6 fluid ounces (17 g) of pure alcohol, which is equivalent to 12 fluid ounces (355 mL) of regular beer (5% alcohol), 5 fluid ounces (148 mL) of wine (12% alcohol), or 1.5 fluid ounces (44 mL) of 80 proof distilled spirits (40% alcohol). Note that these guidelines may change with new evidence.

Avoiding alcohol altogether may be best depending upon your medical conditions, history, and how you react to alcohol. If you are at the "at risk" level for alcohol or are regularly using recreational drugs, consider reducing or stopping their use. Talk to your doctor or other health care provider about your use of these drugs. Doctors are often hesitant to raise the issue because they don't want to embarrass you. So, it is up to you to bring up the subject. Doctors will be very willing to talk about it. They have heard it all, and they will not think less of you. An honest conversation may save your life.

■ ■ ■

Medications and other treatments can help or harm. What makes the difference is your knowledge about medications and treatment, the care you exercise when taking medications, and clear two-way communication with your health care team about medications and treatment.

For a complete list of suggested further readings, useful websites, and other helpful resources, please see www.bullpub.com/resources.

CHAPTER 15

Understanding Medications and Other Treatments for Chronic Pain

MEDICATION FOR CHRONIC PAIN WORKS BEST when combined with exercise, mind-body approaches, and other techniques and treatments. Pain medications and other pain treatments may help you use and benefit from the self-management tools in this book. For example, if a medication lessens your pain, it may allow you to become physically active again, and being physically active is critical to long-term pain management. In this chapter we discuss specific pain medications as well as other types of pain treatments, from acupuncture to injections, from physical therapy to psychological therapies.

Please review Chapter 14, *Managing Your Treatment Decisions and Medications*, before you read this chapter. Chapter 14 has important general information on making

Special thanks to Sean Mackey, MD, PhD, Redlich Professor and Chief of the Division of Stanford Pain Medicine, and Beth Darnall, PhD, Associate Professor and Director of the Stanford Pain Relief Innovations Lab, for their contributions to this chapter.

decisions about medications, taking multiple medications, communicating with your health care team regarding medications and treatments, and self-medicating. Chapter 14 also provides tools to help you be actively involved in treatment decisions and use of pain medications.

After reading Chapter 14, you will be better able to apply the information in this chapter about specific medications and pain treatments. In Chapter 16, *Managing Specific Chronic Pain Conditions*, you will learn more about other medications that treat specific disease conditions.

Taking Medicines for Chronic Pain

Pain medicines (often called analgesics) and other medications are helpful for some but not all people with chronic pain. Medications alone rarely stop pain completely. And each person responds differently to medications. In fact, for some people, pain medicines may worsen pain or other symptoms. For others, medications may cause unpleasant or serious side effects. That's why it is important to balance the risks and benefits of pain medication. It is also the reason why medication is just one tool for managing chronic pain.

Getting the Most Out of Pain Medications

Recall that expecting the best from your medicines is important, as we discuss in Chapter 14, *Managing Your Treatment Decisions and Medications*. If you believe that pain medicines are not for you, speak to your doctor or other health care provider. Your pain medicines are unlikely to work well if you have negative beliefs about them. Instead, focus on the many other ways to manage your pain and symptoms.

Most pain medications are taken on a regularly scheduled basis. Others are prescribed on an as-needed basis. If you have medicine to take as needed when your pain is starting to worsen,

don't put off taking it. It takes less medication to *prevent* severe pain from coming back then it does to *treat* pain that has gotten out of control.

All medications have side effects. Your provider can decrease these effects by starting with a low dose and slowly increasing it. When starting a new pain medication, try to put up with these early side effects, unless very severe, for at least one to two weeks before giving up. Do not drive or do other things needing close attention such as operating equipment if you are feeling drowsy after a recent medication or dosage change.

Understanding Your Type of Pain

Some chronic pain is the result of a known disease process. Rheumatoid arthritis is an example. The underlying cause of the pain is well understood, and there are established treatments for that condition. Medication taken to treat the disease process may also reduce the pain from the disease.

But chronic pain is not always the result of disease or injury (as we discuss in Chapter 1, *Chronic Pain Self-Management: What It Is and How to Do It*, on pages 8–9). Chronic pain itself can be the "disease" or the condition. For these types of pain problems, medicines do not treat a specific disease but can help reduce pain, increase comfort, manage other symptoms, and improve everyday life.

When health care providers prescribe medication for pain, they first need to decide what most likely caused the pain. Pain may be due to tissue damage or injury (called nociceptive pain). For example, inflammation may result when tissues such as the skin, muscle, tendons, joints, or bones are damaged. Inflammation is a normal response of the body to injury. It occurs because your body sends more blood to an injured area and releases chemicals that stimulate nerve endings. This makes the area more sensitive and painful. In addition, fluid accumulates, causing swelling and pressure. This inflammation response is the body's natural way of healing. However, if the inflammation does not get turned off, pain can continue. Inflammation can cause certain types of back pain, neck pain, and arthritis.

Pain may also be nerve related (called neuropathic pain) and result from damage of the nerves that transmit pain signals. Nerve-related pain can occur when there is damage or injury to the nerves, spinal cord, or brain itself. Nerve-related pain may involve the abnormal firing of nerves anywhere between the tips of your fingers or toes to the top of your head. Some examples of this type of pain result from nerve damage after surgery or traumatic accident, strokes, shingles, and diabetic neuropathic pain. Phantom limb pain is also a form of nerve-related pain.

Some people experience a combination of tissue damage and nerve-related pain after surgeries or other injuries. This combination can also develop when pain from damaged tissues persists for a long time. It may lead to changes in the central nervous system and brain so the body interprets even normal sensation as painful. This kind of response can happen even after the original injury has healed and is called central nervous system amplification. The term *amplification* refers to adding to or increasing.

Understanding the type of pain you have— whether it's due to tissue damage, nerve damage, or central nervous system amplification—can help you better understand why your health care provider suggests certain medications and not others. Patients often have mixed or chronic overlapping pain conditions. In addition, other medical conditions, mood, and mental well-being can increase pain and affect how you respond to medications. As discussed in Chapter 4, *Understanding and Managing Common Symptoms and Problems*, and Chapter 5, *Using Your Mind to Manage Pain and Other Symptoms*, depression and anxiety can also affect how a person responds to pain. Even if depression or anxiety did not appear until the pain condition started, these mental health conditions need treatment and should not just be left to "get better" when the pain gets better. It is essential to talk with your health care providers about how you are feeling emotionally, how the pain is affecting you physically, and any other chronic medical conditions you might have.

Depending on the source and mechanism of pain, there are several kinds of drugs that your provider could prescribe to treat any given problem. It is very difficult to predict exactly who will respond to what drug or what combination of drugs. For this reason, it may be necessary to try a variety of drugs and combinations to see what works best for you. For severe chronic pain, it may take two or three medications used in combination to get the best pain relief with the fewest side effects. Sometimes combining two drugs at a low dose brings more effective relief than increasing the dose of one of them.

Work with your health care providers to achieve the best result. And remember that there is evidence that the nondrug approaches described throughout this book can also lessen pain with or without use of medications.

Pain Medications

Research on medications and treatments is rapidly progressing, and drug names and treatment options you encounter may differ from the information in this chapter. Consult your physician, a pharmacist, or recent online drug references for the latest information. These sources are also the best place to start when you have specific questions about specific medications. Remember, the latest treatments are not always more effective. There may be less research on new treatments and their safety and interactions with other drugs. Medications that have been in use for many years may be more established as safe and effective.

Nonprescription Over-the-Counter Medicines and Natural Products

Over-the-counter (OTC) medicines are those you can purchase without a prescription. A natural product is a chemical compound or substance produced by a plant or animal rather than a medication made in a lab. Recall from Chapter 14, *Managing Your Treatment Decisions and Medications*, that products that are "natural" are not necessarily better or safer than a manufactured product. It is important to *always* read the labels on all medicines and know the ingredients. Many over-the-counter medications

contain ingredients that are the same as or similar to those contained in prescription medications. For example, many cold remedies also contain acetaminophen (Tylenol®), aspirin, ibuprofen (Motrin®, Advil®), or naproxen (Aleve®). Ibuprofen, aspirin, and naproxen are nonsteroidal anti-inflammatory drugs (NSAIDs). These popular pain drugs block the production of certain body chemicals that cause inflammation and pain. (We will discuss them in more detail later.) Some natural products for pain contain things like willow bark extract, which is the original source of aspirin (acetylsalicylic acid). To prevent or minimize drug interactions or the potential for overdose of some substances, your health care provider and pharmacist need to know *all* the medications, natural products, and supplements you are taking.

Topical Pain Relievers

Topical pain-relieving medications are applied directly to the skin as creams, lotions, ointments, gels, sprays, and patches. Some work by stimulating nerve endings to cause feelings of warmth or cold to block pain signals. Some even promote irritation or itching! Mild irritants such as methyl salicylate, menthol, or camphor are the active ingredients in brands like Bengay®, Icy

Hot®, Salonpas®, and Thera-Gesic® The topical product Zostrix® contains capsaicin from hot chili peppers. This chemical causes a burning sensation that can decrease levels of substances that transmit pain signals. Other topical medications, such as the local anesthetic lidocaine, numb the nerves of the skin to reduce pain. These numbing medications may be available in skin patch form or as a cream or gel.

When some topical medications are absorbed on your skin, they can cause effects throughout your body. For example, some contain nonsteroidal anti-inflammatory drugs (NSAIDs), such as diclofenac (in Voltaren®) or aspirin-like substances called salicylates. (Recall that NSAIDs are popular pain drugs that block the production of certain body chemicals.) Always read the label, as you should with all medications. If you are already taking aspirin or NSAID tablets or pills—either prescription or over the counter—talk to your health care provider. Using both oral and topical NSAID or aspirin pain relievers may lead to taking too much.

Do *not* apply *any* topical medication to a wound, broken skin, or your face or eyes unless you are specifically told to do so by your health care provider. After applying a topical medication, be sure to carefully wash your hands to avoid getting these products in your eyes.

Nonprescription (OTC) Acetaminophen and Anti-inflammatory Medications

Many pain-relieving medications are available over the counter (OTC) in pill form. These include analgesics such as acetaminophen (Tylenol®, Panadol®) as well as nonsteroidal anti-inflammatory drugs (NSAIDs) such as aspirin, ibuprofen (Motrin®, Advil®), and naproxen (Aleve®). NSAIDs are helpful drugs if your pain is due to inflammation. NSAIDs can also sometimes help with other types of pain.

Even though analgesics and NSAIDs are easy to purchase, they have potentially serious side effects, including stomach upset and bleeding. They can also interfere with blood clotting. Always take NSAIDs with food, and always report stomach upset to your health care provider right away. Sometimes a provider may give you an additional medication to protect your stomach when prescribing these drugs. If you have a history of stomach ulcers, kidney problems, or risk factors for heart disease or are taking blood thinners, you need to be careful with these medicines. In addition, if you smoke, drink alcohol, or are over 65 years of age, you also need to be careful taking aspirin or any NSAID. Talk to your health care provider or pharmacist about safe dosages.

If you take acetaminophen, limiting the amount you take is extremely important. Too much can cause liver problems. Carefully read labels. More than 500 available combination medications also contain acetaminophen! Current guidelines recommend that adults take no more than 3,000 mg of acetaminophen daily or up to 4,000 mg if advised by a doctor. Discuss the amount you should take with your health care provider.

Prescription Anti-inflammatory Drugs

To use some non-steroidal anti-inflammatory drugs (NSAIDs), you need a doctor's prescription. These medications are usually given for mild to moderate pain due to injuries or inflammation. Examples include diclofenac (Voltaren®), meloxicam (Mobic®), and indomethacin (Indocid®, Indocin®). You need to take the same precautions with these medications that you take with over-the-counter NSAIDs. If you are older or have had stomach ulcers, kidney problems, high blood pressure, or risk for heart disease, use these medications with caution. As noted earlier, you should always take NSAIDs with food, and report stomach upset to your doctor. A doctor may suggest an additional medication to protect your stomach when taking these drugs.

COX-2 inhibitor drugs are a newer group of prescription NSAIDs. Celecoxib (Celebrex®) is a COX-2 inhibitor drug that appears to have less risk of causing stomach ulcers than other NSAIDs. However, celecoxib has also been shown to increase the risk of cardiovascular problems such as heart attack. Your doctor should assess your risk of cardiovascular problems before prescribing this drug.

Muscle Relaxants

Painful muscle spasms can be a problem with some conditions, including chronic neck or lower back pain and fibromyalgia. Spasms can also add to the discomfort for people with multiple sclerosis or spinal cord injuries. Muscle relaxant medications such as baclofen (Lioresal®), cyclobenzaprine (Flexeril®), tizanidine (Zanaflex®), methocarbamol (Robaxin®, OTC Robaxacet®), and others may provide some relief from muscle spasm, and some have pain-reducing effects as well. For people with musculoskeletal pain, such as neck and back pain, these medications may be most helpful for acute

flare-ups. They are not generally recommended for chronic pain.

Muscle relaxants do not work directly on the muscles. Instead, they act as "brain relaxants" that cause drowsiness and dizziness. So avoid driving, operating machinery, or other activities that require alertness until you know how you will respond to these drugs. Muscle relaxants should be taken with caution, especially if you take opioids. Some muscle relaxants such as carisoprodol (Soma®), like opioids and benzodiazepines, can also lead to problems with abuse and dependence.

Tramadol and Tapentadol

Tramadol (Tramacet®, Ralivia®, Zytram®, Tridural®) is similar to opioid pain relievers (see the discussion of opioids in this chapter on pages 329–333). Tramadol is a prescription pain reliever that is available with or without acetaminophen. It has been available internationally for almost 30 years and is prescribed for many types of moderate to severe pain, including lower back pain, osteoarthritis, fibromyalgia, and some other types of pain. The side effects of tramadol are mainly drowsiness, nausea, and headaches. If you are taking tramadol, contact your health care provider or call 911 right away if you experience serious side effects such as seizures or muscle rigidity. The risk of addiction is low for tramadol, and it does not pose a risk to your stomach, liver, heart, or kidney as NSAIDs or acetaminophen.

Tapentadol (Nucynta®, Nucynta® ER) is a prescription drug that works similarly to opioids and some antidepressant medications. It may be used to treat moderate to severe chronic pain.

Short-Acting and Long-Acting Medications

Tramadol, tapentadol, and some opioid pain medications come in two forms: short acting and long acting. Short-acting drugs relieve pain within 15 to 30 minutes and have their best effect within 1 to 2 hours. To continue relieving pain, you must take these drugs every 3 to 4 hours. Doctors usually prescribe short-acting pain medicines for acute pain and for moderate to severe chronic pain to test whether the drug works before prescribing a long-acting medicine.

Long-acting (also called slow-release) pain medicines release the active drug slowly into the body. Most of these drugs provide steady pain relief for 8 to 12 hours, and some provide relief up to 24 hours or even days. Doctors usually prescribe long-acting drugs to be taken at regularly scheduled times, such as once every 12 hours or once daily. Long-acting pain medications are sometimes prescribed to people who have continuous moderate to severe chronic pain. Long-acting drugs that come in pill form should be swallowed whole and not broken, chewed, dissolved, or crushed. Tampering with a slow-release pill can lead to rapid release of the drug in your body and a potentially fatal dose.

Opioids[*]

We have all heard of opioid pain medications. Many of us have been prescribed opioids or know somebody who has been prescribed opioid medication. Like all prescription medications, opioid medications are useful and essential for some people, but for other people they can cause serious problems.

Until recently, many health care providers overprescribed opioids for pain. Opioids were prescribed too often, too quickly, and without providing other options for managing pain. Opioid prescribing has changed. These drugs are now prescribed far less often. Due to concerns about overuse, some people who need opioid medications for pain may have difficulty getting them. Risk for opioid addiction is low in the overall population but higher for some people who have a history of addiction in the family or other risk factors.

What are opioid pain medications?

Opioids are still widely used prescription pain medications. In the United States, medical use of opioids requires a prescription, and you cannot purchase opioids over the counter. Examples of prescription opioids include:

- acetaminophen/hydrocodone (Vicodin®, Norco®)
- acetaminophen/oxycodone (Percocet®)
- oxycodone (Oxycontin®, Roxicodone®)
- oxymorphone (Opana®)
- fentanyl (Duragesic®, Abstral®)

---

[*]The section on opioid medication is adapted with permission from Beth Darnall, PhD, *Less Pain, Fewer Pills: Avoid the Dangers of Prescription Opioids and Gain Control over Chronic Pain* (Boulder, CO: Bull Publishing, 2014).

- hydromorphone (Dilaudid®, Exalgo®)
- morphine (MS Contin®)

How can opioids be useful?

Opioids are particularly useful for treating acute pain that is the result of illness, injury, or surgery. Opioids may also be helpful in treating certain types of pain associated with cancer. Once healing starts, usually after a few days, the pain starts getting better and opioids are no longer needed. In most cases, when one stops taking opioids after an acute incident, there is still pain, but it is less intense. This pain can typically be handled with an over-the-counter pain reliever, such as acetaminophen, ibuprofen, naproxen, or aspirin.

Just as our bodies need time to heal, pain needs time to lessen. This does not happen all at once. For this reason, some discomfort may be present during the healing process. Although nobody should suffer in pain, it is also not realistic to expect to be pain-free right away. Expecting zero pain can lead to overuse of medications, so it is important to use many different ways to manage pain.

When opioids are taken for more than a few weeks, on average they reduce pain by about 25 to 30 percent. Rather than taking more, speak with your health care provider about other low-risk pain treatments such as sleep, physical therapy, cognitive behavioral therapy, exercise, social activity and engagement, and relaxation. A combination of treatments can help you need less medication and have better pain control. We describe many of these effective options in this book.

What is wrong with long-term opioid use?

There are many side effects and problems with long-term opioid use. Opioid overdose deaths occur every day. That is why there is so much concern about this issue. The problems associated with opioid use include:

- poor sleep (review Figure 1.2, The Vicious Cycle: Chronic Pain Symptoms, on page 10; a lack of sleep can actually increase your pain)
- poor mood/depression (which also can increase pain)
- fatigue (another pain increaser!)
- drowsiness and foggy thinking
- constipation
- low estrogen for women and low testosterone for men, which lead to lessening of sexual desire and ability and can also cause irritability, mood swings, and body changes

For some people, opioids may even worsen pain over time. So, despite the concern that reducing opioid doses will increase pain, some people find that their pain is substantially improved by reducing or stopping opioid use. For these people, the solution is not taking more opioids but stopping opioids and treating the pain differently.

Opiod use is a complex issue. Opioids do work for some people and can enhance functioning and well-being. For other people, they cause problems and even more pain in the long run. For this reason, it's important to use lower-risk medications first. When opioids are used, monitor your response closely, and communicate often with your health care provider. However, there is no shame in needing opioids for pain management if they work for you and are not causing problems.

How do I know if I am tolerant or addicted, and why does this matter?

If you use opioids long term, your body adjusts to the medication and becomes tolerant to it. Tolerance means the medication works less well, so you may need more medication to gain pain relief (tolerance is different than addiction). This can lead to higher and higher doses over time, which may or may not give better pain relief. Tolerance to prescription medication does not mean a person is misusing medication. Every person is different. While some people may require opioids long term, and even at doses that seem high, this is not generally the case. If this is the case for you, you should discuss it with your health care provider.

Almost everyone who is taking opioids several times a day for more than a few weeks experiences withdrawal symptoms if the opioids are suddenly stopped or if a dose is missed. *Withdrawal symptoms do not mean a person is addicted.* Instead, withdrawal symptoms are a natural indication that the body has become dependent on opioids (or other medications), and the medications are needed to prevent withdrawal symptoms.

Again, tolerance is not addiction. Withdrawal is not addiction. Needing opioids is not addiction. Even taking opioids daily for many years is not addiction. Addiction is a condition that results when a person takes a substance (such as an opioid) and cannot stop despite wanting to, or despite the substance use having many negative effects on their life and relationships. It is possible to become addicted to opioids even if they have been prescribed by a doctor for medically related pain. A person's life may begin to revolve around opioids. The focus is exclusively on getting opioids, taking them, and thinking about them. For many people, the continued use of opioids can begin to interfere with day-to-day life, such as work, school, relationships, and health. Often, people who are addicted are not aware that they are causing harm to themselves as well as friends and family. Addiction is a serious medical condition, not simply a moral weakness, that needs professional treatment and aid.

Many people think that they cannot become addicted if they take opioids exactly as prescribed. This is not true. Using prescribed opioids can be a slippery slope for some people who are in pain. Physical pain and emotional pain are very closely related. It is easy to begin taking opioids for a physical problem but end up taking more to treat the emotional aspects of a health condition or other stressful parts of life. People who have a history of addiction to cigarettes, alcohol, or drugs are at increased risk for opioid addiction. In addition, people with depression, a family history of addiction, and early childhood traumas are at increased risk.

How can I cut down on opioid use without having terrible symptoms?

Many people who are not addicted to opioids want to reduce their use of opioids because they do not like being dependent on them. It is common for people to think that they cannot cut down or stop opioids because they will experience more (and worse) pain or withdrawal. But that does not have to happen. For most people, opioids can be reduced or "tapered" without increasing pain if it is done the right way.

Research shows that when opioids are reduced sensibly, many people do not have increased pain and many experience *less* pain.

To achieve these positive results, opioids must be tapered very slowly. This is done by making small reductions in the dose over long periods of time. This tricks the body into not noticing that any change in medication is occurring. The body has time to adjust, and this prevents withdrawal symptoms. Using a slow, gentle taper method, people can successfully taper off opioids even if they have been on high doses for many years.

If you want to reduce your opioid use, *do not try tapering at home by yourself.* Talk to your health care team and find out what's right for you. This is a relatively new area of medicine. If your provider does not know much about tapering, bring in this information and ask that they access the following resource from the US Department of Health and Human Services: *HHS Guide for Clinicians on the Appropriate Dosage Reduction or Discontinuation of Long-Term Opioid Analgesics.*[*]

Tips for Reducing Opioids

- **Partner with your doctor or prescriber.** Share with your doctor your desire to reduce your opioids very slowly over time.

- **Think big picture.** It may take at least three to six months or more to reduce your opioids by 50 percent.

- **Go slow.** Give your body the time it needs to adjust to a dose decrease. It is OK to "pause" an opioid taper if you have symptoms or are going through a stressful time.

- **One thing at a time.** Try not to make other medication changes during an opioid taper.

- **Use mind-body skills each day.** Use your relaxation skills daily to help manage any fear or stress you have about reducing your opioids. (See Chapter 5: *Using Your Mind to Manage Pain and Other Symptoms*). Good stress management helps keep your pain low.

- **Start (or continue) a gentle exercise program.** Exercise can help with stress management and your overall health. If you are not already doing this, it is a good time to start. (Try the Moving Easy Program on pages 173–189 in Chapter 8, *Exercising to Feel Better.*)

- **Be kind to yourself and very proud.** You are doing something really important that will benefit your health and well-being for years to come.

Practicing Opioid Safety

Opioids are dangerous if they fall into the wrong hands, are combined with certain other medications or alcohol, or if too large a dose is taken. Follow these steps to keep yourself and others safe:

- **Lock opioids up.** Keep your opioid medication in a locked box, cabinet, or safe. Doing so prevents your medication from being stolen or accessed by children, family members, or visitors to your home. Even one pill can kill a child.

---

[*] Available online at https://www.hhs.gov/opioids/sites/default/files/2019-10/Dosage_Reduction_Discontinuation.pdf.

- **Keep to your prescribed dose.** Never take more opioid medication than is prescribed to you.

- **Your medication is yours.** Never give your opioid medication to others, and never take another person's opioid prescription.

- **Tell any doctor who prescribes opioids to you about all other medications you are taking,** especially sedative hypnotics or antianxiety medications like benzodiazepines. Only one doctor should be prescribing you opioids.

- **If you drink alcohol at all, share this with your doctor.** Your life may depend on it.

- **Make sure your doctor knows about all your medical conditions,** especially respiratory conditions such as asthma or chronic obstructive pulmonary disease (COPD). Opioids can affect breathing.

- **Ask your doctor or pharmacist about preventing constipation.** Opioid-induced constipation is a common side effect since these medications slow down the contractions of the bowel.

- **When you travel,** keep your opioids in their original container with you in carry-on luggage, and bring a letter from your doctor documenting your need for opioids, especially if you are traveling outside your state, province, or country.

Other Medications Used to Treat Pain

Some medications used to treat various conditions have been found to be helpful in treating certain types of pain. This can sometimes be confusing. For example, your health care provider may prescribe an antidepressant medication to treat your pain, not depression. Or a provider may prescribe a medication used to treat epilepsy to treat your pain even if you don't have seizures. Government agencies have approved the use of a number of medications for several different disorders, including chronic pain. In this section, we discuss some of these so-called adjuvant pain medications. Those used for specific conditions are discussed in Chapter 16, *Managing Specific Chronic Pain Conditions: Arthritis, Neck and Back Pain, Fibromyalgia, Headache, Pelvic Pain, and Neuropathic Pain Syndromes.*

Antidepressants

Certain antidepressant medications called tricyclics (TCAs) and serotonin norepinephrine reuptake inhibitors (SNRIs) can lessen pain in addition to treating depression. Neurotransmitters involved in depression are also involved in some forms of chronic pain. If you are prescribed one of these drugs for your pain, it does not mean you are clinically depressed or that your physician believes your pain is "only in your head." When prescribed for pain, TCAs and SNRIs are usually prescribed at a lower dosage than when they are used to treat depression. Common TCAs include amitriptyline (Elavil®), nortriptyline (Aventyl®), and desipramine (Norpramin®). These drugs can be helpful for people suffering from neuropathic pain, shingles, fibromyalgia, and some types of headache, facial pain, and lower back pain. TCAs are also useful for sleeping problems. Chronic pain itself can make sleeping more difficult, and poor-quality sleep can make chronic pain worse. To read more about pain and sleep, see pages 69–74 in Chapter 4, *Understanding and Managing Common Symptoms and Problems.*

Common SNRIs include venlafaxine (Effexor®), duloxetine (Cymbalta®), and bupropion (Wellbutrin®). These medications restore balance of chemical neurotransmitters in the brain to block transmission of pain signals.

A third common class of antidepressants is selective serotonin reuptake inhibitors (SSRIs). SSRIs have not been found to be very effective as pain relievers as TCAs and SNRIs. Still, if you have both pain and depression, your provider may prescribe them to treat the depression.

Antidepressant medications may take weeks to work. Be patient. The dosage for most antidepressants used to treat pain starts low and is increased slowly until either the dosage is effective or an intolerable side effect occurs. Side effects of antidepressants include drowsiness, dizziness, nightmares, confusion, dry mouth, and constipation.

Antiepileptic Drugs (AEDs)

The antiepileptic family of medications (also called anticonvulsant drugs) was initially developed to treat epileptic seizures ("convulsions"). Doctors discovered that AEDs also help some people with a variety of nerve-related pain such as diabetic neuropathic pain, persistent pain after a shingles outbreak, and fibromyalgia pain. The two AEDs that doctors most often prescribe today are gabapentin (Neurontin®) and pregabalin (Lyrica®). AEDs may help to alleviate

symptoms of anxiety in addition to pain symptoms. Side effects may include drowsiness, dizziness, weight gain, and leg swelling. Other AEDs that are sometimes used are carbamazepine (Tegretol®) and valproic acid (Depakene®). Newer AEDs include topiramate (Topamax®, sometimes prescribed for migraine prevention), lamotrigine (Lamictal®), oxcarbazepine (Trileptal®), and levetiracetam (Keppra®).

Medical Marijuana (Cannabis)

Some state governments have approved the use of marijuana (cannabis) for medical use. Many people with pain believe that cannabis will lessen their pain. Some people believe that cannabis will reduce their reliance on opioids. Some people may believe both. Unfortunately, the current evidence on how cannabis affects pain and opioid use is uncertain. A recent large review of studies found there are few if any studies on cannabis use that meet the standards for good research. However, researchers are beginning to conduct high-quality studies and should have better answers in a few years.

Research is also progressing on isolating the individual compounds in cannabis. For example, cannabidiol (CBD) is one of the individual compounds found in cannabis. Another individual compound found in marijuana is the psychoactive compound tetrahydrocannabinol (THC). When isolated, some of the compounds in cannabis, such as CBD, may be found to be valid medical treatment options that do not produce the "high" that the THC produces. Products containing cannabidiol, such as CBD oils, topical pain-relief treatments, edibles, and other nonsmoking applications, are now available.

Since 2001, medical cannabis has been a legal treatment option in Canada for certain health conditions. Medical cannabis is not a Health Canada–approved treatment. If you are living in Canada, talk to your health care provider about the benefits and risks of using medical cannabis to decide if it is right for you. Your provider will give you instructions on what type of medical cannabis to try, how much to use, how to take it, and how often to take it. In Canada, it is a good idea to become a registered user for medical cannabis to make sure you get the right dosage and that you are purchasing products that are government regulated for safety and consistency standards. If you register with Health Canada, you can grow your own cannabis for medical purposes or designate someone to do this for you. If you have side effects or think you have a problem with cannabis use, contact your health provider.

Some experts are concerned about negative effects of marijuana on memory and mental ability, increased incidence of accidents, as well as damage to the lungs from smoking. If marijuana is bought on the street, there is no way to know for sure how strong it is and what chemicals may have been sprayed onto the plants as they grew. Processes are underway to better regulate the growing, dispensing, and quality and content of the drug. Before using cannabis products in any form, have an honest discussion with your health care provider.

Other Treatments for Chronic Pain

In addition to medicines, your primary doctor, pain specialist, or other health care provider may suggest other types of interventions to treat your chronic pain, including physical, psychological, and medical therapies, as well as self-management tools.

Acupuncture

Acupuncture is the practice of inserting thin, solid needles into one or more of 361 specific points in the skin that lie along "meridians"—lines of energy flow in the body. The areas where the needles are inserted are stimulated when a practitioner twirls the needles for brief periods. The needles are so thin that virtually no pain is felt when administered by a qualified practitioner.

Acupuncture originated in China and has been used for thousands of years. Scientists are not exactly sure how it works, but they think that the needle stimulation may release endorphins and other pain-relieving substances to close the pain gate in the spinal cord. Endorphins are neurochemicals that serve as the body's natural painkillers. (See the discussion of theories of pain and neurochemicals in Chapter 1, *Chronic Pain Self-Management: What It Is and How to Do It*, on pages 5–11.) Acupuncture may also activate the immune system and improve blood flow. Another contributing factor to the effectiveness of acupuncture may be the person's belief that it will help them. (See the discussion of mind power in Chapter 14, *Managing Your Treatment Decisions and Medications*, pages 311–312.)

Much research on acupuncture has been conducted in the United States, Canada, China, and Europe over the past 40 years. There is now solid evidence that the procedure can help some people with chronic back and neck pain, shoulder pain, osteoarthritis pain, and chronic headache pain. It is not known if acupuncture is helpful for fibromyalgia pain. Acupuncture is now routinely used in the United States military for pain management. As with any treatment, if you decide to have acupuncture, be sure to seek a qualified practitioner.

Exercise

Exercise is an essential component of chronic pain treatment for everyone. Various types of movement, physical activity, and exercise are discussed in Chapter 7, *Exercising and Physical Activity for Every Body*, and Chapter 8, *Exercising to Feel Better*. Effective exercises include the gentle Moving Easy Program, balance exercises, aerobic activity such as walking, biking, and water aerobics, as well as resistance or weight training, yoga, and tai chi. There are many people who can help you develop a physical activity program that is right for you. Review these chapters to incorporate exercise into your overall pain treatment plan.

Heat and Cold

Cold therapy (cryotherapy) and heat therapy (thermotherapy) are inexpensive self-treatment approaches with minimal risks. Although there are some individuals who find cold helpful for chronic pain conditions, it is mostly utilized for acute injuries when there are damaged superficial tissues that are inflamed and swollen. Heat is more helpful for chronic muscle pain.

Electrical Stimulation

Your health care provider might suggest techniques for pain management that you can do at home. One of the most common is transcutaneous electrical nerve stimulation (TENS). In TENS therapy, a small battery-powered machine about the size of a pocket radio transmits electrical impulses that counteract pain. You connect two electrodes from the machine to your skin in the area where you are feeling pain. When the machine is turned on, you feel a tingling sensation or vibration that may block pain signals. Though this treatment does not help everyone, it is easy to learn, safe, inexpensive, and within your control. The machine can be set for different wavelength frequencies and intensities so that you can experiment with the setting that works best.

Manual and Other Physical Therapies

Manual (hands-on) therapies include massage, mobilization, and manipulation. Manual therapists may also use high-frequency ultrasonic waves or sound waves applied to the overlying skin, though the effectiveness of this approach to managing chronic pain is not clear.

Massage is a form of hands-on therapy that works on the muscles and other soft tissue. Massage has been extensively studied, and it has few risks. There are many kinds of massage therapy, including Swedish massage, sports massage, lymphatic drainage, and massage that focuses on trigger points. Massage can help relax muscles and tissues and improve blood flow to an area. It is helpful for people with chronic lower back pain, chronic neck pain, and osteoarthritis pain in the knee, and it may also help reduce depression. It may temporarily reduce pain, fatigue, and other symptoms for people with fibromyalgia. Self-massage can also be helpful. (See Chapter 4, *Understanding and Managing Common Symptoms and Problems,* page 62).

Mobilization involves gently moving a joint through its existing range of motion. Manipulation is a more forceful movement of a joint. Both mobilization and manipulation can improve the range of motion of a joint, allow increased movement and activity, and reduce pain. Spinal manipulation has been studied and found to be helpful for chronic lower back pain. It may also be helpful for chronic tension-type headaches, neck-related headache, and the prevention of migraines. Research studies have shown that spinal manipulation can be a more effective treatment for chronic back pain than bed rest, traction, topical gels, or no treatment. Although spinal manipulation is safe for most people if performed by a qualified practitioner, there are some risks. If you decide to seek this sort of treatment, make sure to educate yourself and evaluate the risks.

Manual therapy can be conducted by a variety of licensed health care providers, including physical therapists, chiropractors, osteopaths, and registered massage therapists. As with any treatment, be sure to seek a qualified practitioner, and check with your state or provincial certification boards.

Injections, Nerve Blocks, and Surgeries

Other pain treatment options include injecting medications into painful areas of the body, injecting medications around certain nerves, surgically inserting electrical devices or medication pumps into the spinal canal, or surgically cutting nerves.

Trigger point injections are injections of anesthetic (a medication that blocks pain) into trigger points, which are painful hard knots of muscle, ligaments, or tendons. Trigger points can be caused by direct pressure on a muscle, chronic muscle tension, abnormal posture, or prolonged muscle fatigue. Injecting trigger points with anesthetic can result in temporary relief of pain. This pain relief can in turn allow the person to stretch and exercise to improve their function. Trigger points can also be managed with massage, exercise, and relaxation techniques.

A nerve block is an injection of an anesthetic (a medication that produces a loss of sensation, including pain) or steroid (a medication used to relieve swelling and inflammation) into an area of the body such as a sore joint or into the space around the spinal cord. Nerve blocks have been used for more than 50 years for lower back pain, neck pain, and arthritis. Results are varied; some people experience pain relief while others do not. If there is relief, it can last from hours to days to weeks, but the effect is usually temporary. Nerve blocks are sometimes done with the help of an X-ray or CT scan to be sure they are placed correctly.

For more severe pain problems, surgeons may insert an electrical device called a spinal cord stimulator around the spinal canal that runs through the vertebrae and contains the spinal cord. A spinal cord stimulator reduces pain signals going to the brain. Another surgical option is to implant a small pump that delivers pain medications (such as local anesthetic and opioids) directly into the spinal fluid. Both of these techniques are very expensive and do not help many who undergo the procedures. When neck or back pain is associated with certain types of nerve damage, surgery may be recommended, especially if all other treatments have been tried. Surgery to cut nerves or relieve pressure on nerves is usually a treatment of last resort in patients who have severe pain.

Psychological Therapies

Treating the body is only one part of managing chronic pain. You also need to be sure your mind and your emotions are supporting your treatment. In addition to psychological self-management skills, you may need professional help dealing with your thoughts, emotions, and feelings. (See Chapter 4, *Understanding and Managing Common Symptoms and Problems*, and Chapter 5, *Using Your Mind to Manage Pain and Other Symptoms*.) Psychologists are highly trained therapists who specialize in human behavior and emotional health. Talk to your health care providers about how you are feeling.

They can ask questions to determine if you may have an underlying depression or other disorder that can be treated. If you need help dealing with your emotions and stress, your provider can help you locate a qualified health psychologist in your area. Alternatively, you can contact your state or provincial licensing body to find a psychologist with expertise in chronic pain.

One of the most frequently used therapies for chronic pain is cognitive behavioral therapy, or CBT. This approach is based on the idea that what you think and feel influences how you behave, and how you behave influences your thoughts and feelings. CBT helps people think realistically about their pain by encouraging them to change their thoughts, feelings, and behavior, including their stress responses. Researchers have found that CBT reduces depression and anxiety, disability, and negative or catastrophic thinking and improves everyday functioning in people who suffer from many kinds of chronic pain. This includes people who have pain conditions, including lower back pain, headaches, arthritis pain, mouth or face pain, and fibromyalgia pain. Experts now recommend CBT as a "first-line" treatment for some chronic pain conditions. (See Chapter 4, *Understanding and Managing Common Symptoms and Problems*, pages 77–78.)

Pain Clinics and Rehabilitation Programs

Pain clinics offer a variety of treatments and education. Some clinics are staffed only by pain physicians who offer expert advice on medications and other medical procedures, such as

trigger point injections and nerve blocks. The most comprehensive programs have a multidisciplinary team that may include psychologists, physical and occupational therapists, social workers, nutritionists, pharmacists, specialist nurses, exercise specialists, and others. Multidisciplinary pain programs use a combination of the treatments and techniques described in this book. Although these programs are usually for people with severe chronic pain, there are also pain-assessment services and short programs for people who are less affected by their chronic pain.

Ask your health care provider if a pain clinic is an option for you. They should be able to refer you to one that addresses your specific pain problem. Pain clinics are in most US states and Canadian provinces. If your provider is not able to help, try contacting your local hospital, medical school, or pain-related organizations.

■ ■ ■

Chronic pain affects everyone differently. There are a variety of medicines, treatments, and resources to help you. Finding the right combination takes patience and persistence. Work closely with all your health care providers so that you can find ways to manage your pain and do the things you want to do every day.

For a complete list of suggested further readings, useful websites, and other helpful resources, please see

www.bullpub.com/resources.

CHAPTER 16

Managing Specific Chronic Pain Conditions:

Arthritis, Neck and Back Pain, Fibromyalgia, Headache, Pelvic Pain, and Neuropathic Pain Syndromes

THIS CHAPTER WILL HELP YOU UNDERSTAND specific conditions where chronic pain is often a major symptom. These include arthritis, chronic neck and back pain, fibromyalgia, headache, chronic pelvic pain, and neuropathic pain syndromes (including diabetic peripheral neuropathy and chronic regional pain syndrome). Although each of these can occur on their own, they often occur together. In addition to pain, these conditions also cause fatigue, loss of strength and endurance, and negative emotions such as stress and depression. As we discuss in Chapter 1, *Chronic Pain Self-Management: What It Is and How to Do It*, the healthy way to live with chronic pain is to work at managing the physical, mental, and emotional challenges of your particular condition. Becoming a chronic pain self-manager helps

Special thanks to Sean Mackey, MD, PhD, Redlich Professor and Chief of the Division of Stanford Pain Medicine, for contributions to this chapter.

341

helps you function at your best, achieve the things you want to do, and get pleasure from life.

This chapter includes detailed discussions of several conditions that cause chronic pain. Although each condition is different and has different causes, the self-management skills are usually the same. Therefore, you can apply the advice given throughout this book regarding exercise, nutrition, and so on for all the conditions in this chapter.

Arthritis

The term *arthritis* commonly refers to any kind of inflammation or damage to a joint. Arthritis can result in cartilage loss in the joint as well as damage to nearby bone, ligaments, and tendons. Cartilage covers and cushions the ends of bones, tendons attached to muscles move the joints, and ligaments stabilize the joints. Recall that inflammation occurs as a natural response to damage when your body sends more blood to an area and chemicals are released that stimulate nerve endings. In some types of arthritis, such as rheumatoid arthritis, there is much more inflammation than other types, such as osteoarthritis. When a joint lining is inflamed or the joint is swollen or deformed, those tendons, ligaments, and muscles can be affected. The tendons, ligaments, and muscles may become inflamed, swollen, stretched, displaced, thinned out, or even torn. In this way, arthritis of any kind does not simply affect the joint; it can affect all the structures in the area around the joint. Although most forms of arthritis cannot be cured, if you have arthritis, you can learn to reduce your pain, maintain your mobility, and slow down the progress of the disease.

Understanding Arthritis

Osteoarthritis (OA) is the most common type of arthritis. It generally affects people as they age. Symptoms include knobby fingers (especially the joints near the tips), hip pain, swollen knees, and back pain. In osteoarthritis, the cartilage that cushions the ends of bone wears away, as do the ends of the bones. Ligaments that hold bones together and tendons that connect muscles to bones may also be damaged. This damage can lead to pain and loss of function. The medical community does not know the exact cause of osteoarthritis, but research has shown that activity such as walking helps protect joints and even lessens pain.

Although osteoarthritis is not caused by inflammation, inflammation causes many other kinds of chronic arthritis. In some forms of arthritis, inflammation occurs when your own immune system attacks your joints, as in rheumatoid arthritis and psoriatic arthritis. In gout, crystals in the joints cause the inflammation. In rheumatoid arthritis, the thin membrane lining the joint (synovium) becomes inflamed and swollen and makes extra fluid. As a result, the joint becomes swollen, warm, red, tender, and painful, and some movements are painful or difficult. If it continues, arthritis can also result in destruction of cartilage and bone. If this destruction is not stopped, it can ultimately lead to deformity and loss of function. Today, rheumatoid arthritis and other types of arthritis in which inflammation is a major problem can be slowed or stopped by the use of medications.

Managing Arthritis

Although arthritis can have damaging effects, you can do a lot to offset or eliminate these effects. Exercising, using medications properly, and managing your emotional well-being are self-management tools that can help you lead a productive, satisfying, and independent life.

Important goals of arthritis self-management are to maintain the maximum possible use of affected joints and to maintain good posture. Unless you use your affected joints, they will slowly lose mobility, and the surrounding muscles and tendons will weaken. Good posture is important to reduce the strain on other parts of the body. For example, if arthritis affects the joints of one leg, that leg may be favored during walking. This can strain other body areas and result in even more pain.

The key to joint mobility and good posture is exercise, an essential part of any chronic pain self-management plan. Exercise when done properly does not make arthritis worse. In fact, the most dangerous thing to do is avoid activity and exercising. Failing to exercise can increase arthritis symptoms because of loss of joint mobility, loss of muscle strength, and overall reduction in physical conditioning. To maintain joint mobility and healthy cartilage, you need to move your affected joints through their full range of motion several times a day. Consult with a health care provider, such as a physical therapist, to learn the best way to move your joints safely. A physical therapist can also examine your posture and provide

ideas on improving your posture when doing different activities.

Gentle flexibility exercises are good ways to start increasing your activity. You can start with the Moving Easy Program (MEP) and balance exercises in Chapter 8, *Exercising to Feel Better*. The MEP can also help with stiffness that can occur after periods of rest, such as sleeping and prolonged sitting. You can find appropriate guidelines for activity pacing and exercise programs discussed in earlier chapters.

Because the pain of arthritis is often felt in one area of the body, self-management approaches such as the use of heat or cold can be helpful for joint pain and stiffness. Another important area of arthritis self-management is nutrition and maintaining a healthy weight. If you are overweight, losing even a few pounds can reduce the strain on joints in your hips, knees, and feet.

If your joint function is limited, you may find assistive technology helpful. Many types of devices are available, including braces, canes, special shoes, grippers, and reachers. Chapter 6, *Organizing and Pacing Your Life for Pain Self-Management and Safety*, has helpful information on these topics. If you need help making decisions about devices that could be most useful to you, consult an occupational therapist. They have specialized knowledge in this area and can help make daily living easier for you.

Because there are more than 100 different types of arthritis, your medical treatment will be specific to your arthritic condition. Your health care provider may prescribe medications to prevent or control inflammation, swelling, and pain and to improve your physical function. The most commonly prescribed medications for the pain of osteoarthritis and some other rheumatic diseases are acetaminophen and mild or strong anti-inflammatory drugs (NSAIDs). See Chapter 15, *Understanding Medications and Other Treatments for Chronic Pain*, for information on these and other medications you may be prescribed, including antidepressants.

If you have rheumatoid arthritis or other form of arthritis with major inflammation, your health care team may also prescribe such strong medications as "disease-modifying" drugs, corticosteroids, and methotrexate and newer "biological drugs" derived from substances produced by living organisms. These drugs include:

- tocilizumab (Actemra®)
- certolizumab (Cimzia®)
- etanercept (Enbrel®)
- adalimumab (Humira®)
- anakinra (Kineret®)
- abatacept (Orencia®)
- infliximab (Remicade®)
- rituximab (Rituxan®)
- golimumab (Simponi®)

These medications may stop or greatly slow the destruction caused by inflammatory types of arthritis. Today, these medications are used early in the disease to avoid permanent joint damage. However, these medications are powerful and need to be closely monitored. Take the time to develop a good relationship with your pharmacist and health care team so that you have all the information you need to manage your medications safely.

Sometimes, despite self-management and drug treatments, joints are damaged by arthritis to the point where they no longer work effectively. Fortunately, modern surgical techniques allow for replacement of many types of joints. Joint replacement surgery can greatly relieve pain and improve function. This is especially true for hip and knee replacements.

Chronic Back and Neck Pain

If you have chronic back or neck pain, you are not alone. Back and neck pain are very common medical conditions. Over two dozen bones, collectively called the vertebrae, make up your spinal column. The spinal column has several regions: the neck or cervical area, the middle or thoracic area, the lumbar or lower back area, the sacrum, and the coccyx (a group of bones fused together at the base of your spine). See Figure 16.1.

A healthy back is strong, flexible, and able to support everyday activities. Muscles attached to the spinal bones support the bones of the back. The muscles in your abdomen and pelvis also support your spine. Spinal bones or vertebrae are separated from each other by jelly-like cushions called intervertebral discs. These discs act as shock absorbers as your body moves. The vertebrae surround and protect your spinal cord, which contains the many nerves that travel to and from your brain.

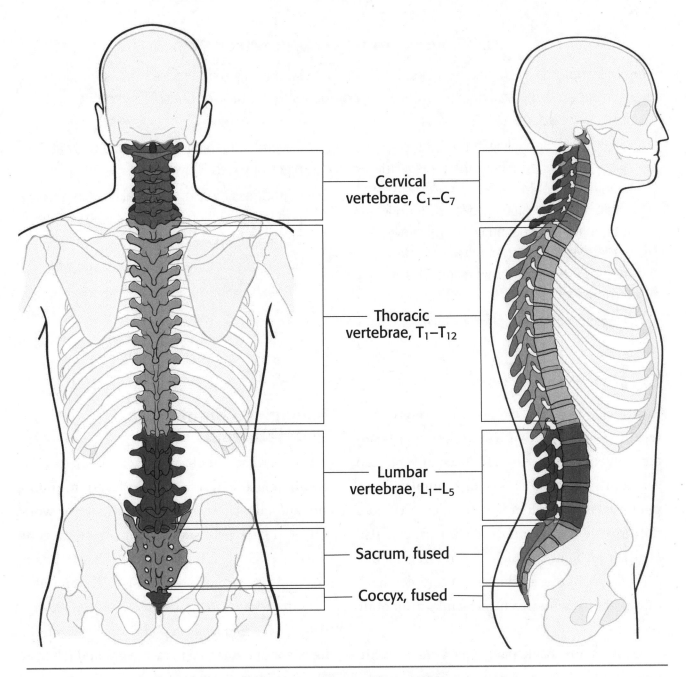

Figure 16.1 **The Spinal Column**

Understanding Chronic Back and Neck Pain

Pain can develop anywhere along the spine. The two most common areas for pain to occur are the neck and the lower back. Pain can be located in a single small area or can spread to a wider area. For example, neck pain can spread to the shoulders and upper back. Similarly, lower back pain can spread to the buttocks and down one or both legs.

Nearly everyone has back or neck pain sometime in their life. It can be caused by many things, including poor posture, weak back or abdominal muscles, lifting heavy objects

Red Flags: Chronic Back and Neck Pain

Rarely, symptoms of chronic neck and back pain are warning signs of a more serious problem. Seek immediate medical help if you have any of the following new or unusual symptoms with your neck or back pain:

- Numbness or tingling in the buttocks, groin, and inner thighs (the parts of the body that would contact a saddle if you were riding a horse) and/or sudden loss of control of urination or bowel movements. This may mean that important nerves are being compressed. This is an emergency.

- Unexplained weight loss or fever

- Severe worsening of pain, especially at night or when lying down

- Numbness, tingling, or weakness in arms and hands (if you have neck pain) or legs and feet (if you have lower back pain)

- Severe pain in the chest or between the shoulder blades

incorrectly, twisting, excess body weight, and repetitive activities that require lifting or bending. Sometimes the reason for neck or back pain is a poorly designed desk—for example a computer that is too high or low, or a chair that does not provide back support. Back pain can also result from motor vehicle or other accidents. An example of this is whiplash, a common neck injury that results from rear-end automobile accidents.

Most acute back pain gets better within one month. But for a small number of people, back pain becomes chronic. Most people with chronic back pain have "nonspecific" back pain that is related to the muscles and ligaments that surround and support the spine and not the spine itself. As with most chronic pain, changes occur in the brain and nervous system that can prevent back pain from stopping even after an injury has healed. But you can take action to calm your nervous system to reduce your pain and improve your life.

Managing Chronic Back and Neck Pain

The experience of chronic back and neck pain is different for everyone. The location, intensity, and impact on everyday activities and work varies. If back pain starts when you are in your thirties or forties, it may affect job and financial security. Job change and job loss are difficult challenges. Review Chapter 12, *Managing Pain During Employment and Unemployment*, for more about managing pain at work and job loss.

Even though your neck or back may cause severe pain, there are many ways you can manage the pain and live a full, satisfying life. The most effective approach is to combine self-management techniques, such as the ones in this book, and care from your health care providers. Research has shown that staying physically active and developing a regular exercise program improves pain and function in people with chronic back and neck pain. Being inactive and lying in bed or on the sofa can weaken muscles and make chronic pain worse. Although exercising can sometimes hurt a bit, remember that as long as you are exercising in a safe manner, "hurt" does not equal "harm." Once the muscles and ligaments of your neck and back have already healed, being involved in regular physical activity will not harm them further unless you overdo it. So go slow. Consult with your health care provider about the type of exercise to avoid before beginning an exercise program. There are specific suggestions about exercise and chronic neck and back pain in Chapter 7, *Exercising and Physical Activity for Every Body*, and Chapter 8, *Exercising to Feel Better*. You may also find the Moving Easy Program exercises, which are explained in detail in Chapter 8, helpful.

Negative emotions and depression can make chronic back and neck pain harder to deal with. It is important to learn and use the self-management skills and relaxation techniques in Chapter 5, *Using Your Mind to Manage Pain and Other Symptoms*.

Healthy eating and weight management are other key self-management goals. Excess weight can impact your back pain by increasing the stress on muscles in your back and abdomen and on your joints. Research findings are consistent about smoking being a risk factor for many types of chronic musculoskeletal pain problems, including back pain. This is true especially if you are under the age of 50. If you smoke, talk to your health care provider about ways to stop.

Heat and cold applications, acupuncture, and massage, especially when combined with physical activity and self-management skills, have been shown to help people with chronic back pain. More studies are being done on chiropractic and other spinal manipulation treatments. Some studies have shown a positive impact from spinal manipulation, while others have not. In addition to these types of treatments, your health care provider may prescribe medications such as acetaminophen, mild anti-inflammatory medicines, low-dose antidepressants, muscle relaxants, and other more powerful medications if your neck or back pain is severe. Please see Chapter 15, *Understanding Medications and Other Treatments for Chronic Pain*, for more specific information about pain medications and treatments.

Fibromyalgia

The term *fibromyalgia* is made up of three root words: "fibro" means fibrous or connective tissue, "myo" means muscle, and "algia" means pain. Fibromyalgia literally means pain in muscle and connective tissue.

Understanding Fibromyalgia

People with fibromyalgia feel pain, tenderness, or both even when there is no injury or obvious inflammation. People are typically diagnosed with fibromyalgia when pain and tenderness last longer than three months and involve muscles and soft tissue throughout the body—both sides as well as above and below the waist. If you have fibromyalgia, you may have times when you hurt more, followed by times when symptoms happen less often, hurt less, or disappear. Sometimes fibromyalgia involves "trigger points," which are sensitive areas over muscle that are painful when touched.

Fibromyalgia symptoms may also include fatigue, poor sleep, problems with thinking and memory (called "fibro fog"), depression, and anxiety. You might also experience headache, irritable bowel or painful bladder syndrome, painful menstrual cycles, or other painful concerns.

Fibromyalgia is twice as common in women as in men. It can develop at any age, including childhood. The cause of fibromyalgia is not known but is likely due to multiple factors, including genes, as well as psychological or physical trauma. Fibromyalgia also involves abnormalities in neurotransmitters and how pain signals are processed, which amplify pain, disrupt sleep, and affect mood.

Managing Fibromyalgia

You can manage fibromyalgia. Your goals are to manage symptoms, be as healthy as possible, and maintain or improve physical and social functioning. The latest evidence indicates that regular physical activity is the cornerstone of fibromyalgia treatment. No one specific type of exercise is recommended; you can engage in a combination of aerobic, strengthening, flexibility, and balance exercises. Your exercise options can be very gentle, such as slow walking, the Moving Easy Program (pages 173–189), gentle yoga, or tai chi. Once you build up your stamina, you can include more vigorous endurance exercise. Your exercise can be done in water or on land, either at home or in a group. The best exercise to choose is the one that you will do.

"Fibro fog" describes the problems with thinking and memory that can happen with fibromyalgia. You can best manage fibro fog by pacing your activities and taking some of the specific actions described in Chapter 6, *Organizing and Pacing Your Life for Pain Self-Management and Safety*.

Headache

Headache is one of the most common pain conditions. The World Health Organization recently reported that 47 percent of adults worldwide have had a headache in the past year. For many people, headaches are infrequent, brief, and not severe. Others deal with headache pain on a regular basis—daily, weekly, or monthly. Persistent or chronic headache can wear you down, make you depressed and anxious, and negatively impact your quality and enjoyment of life.

Understanding Headache

Headache is often quite different for different people. Headache is pain that occurs in any area of your head. It can be on one or both sides, on the top or back of your head, or both. It can also be widespread or in a specific spot. If your pain is located in your face, mouth, or jaw, your provider may refer to it as orofacial pain. Headache pain can be sharp and jabbing, throbbing and pounding, or dull and achy. It can be mild, or it can be so severe that it is disabling. It can come on gradually or suddenly and can be gone in an hour or last for many days at a time. Depending on the type of headache, you may have other symptoms such as nausea, extreme sensitivity to light and noise, or flashing lights in your eyes.

Physicians classify headache into two types: primary or secondary headache. Primary headaches are caused directly by activity in your blood vessels, muscles, and nerves in your head and neck, as well as changes in brain chemical activity. Common examples of primary headache are tension headaches, migraine, and cluster headaches. A secondary headache is a symptom of another health condition that stimulates the pain-sensitive nerves in your head. Many conditions can cause secondary headache, including dehydration, fever, and infection such as a cold or flu.

More serious problems can also bring on secondary headache, including high blood pressure, stroke, blood clots, head injury, arthritis in your neck, tumors, or other pain conditions in your face or jaw. Most of these more serious conditions have other associated symptoms in addition to headaches that can offer clues to the underlying condition (see *Red Flags: Headache*, page xxx). A common but not well understood cause of secondary headache is the overuse of pain medicines. These headaches are sometimes called "rebound headache." Ask your health care provider to take a careful medical history from you and perform tests if indicated to rule out any disease-related causes for your headaches.

If you have diabetes, headaches can be a sign of low blood sugar (hypoglycemia). Drinking juice or a sugary drink, not a diet drink, should help. Follow this by eating a regular meal within about an hour. Talk to your diabetes health care team, as hypoglycemia can be a serious condition but is usually easily treated.

Managing Headache

Though you may not be able to get rid of your headaches entirely, the self-management strategies in this book can help reduce their number and severity.

One of the first things you can do is identify triggers that might bring on your headaches or make them worse. Become a "headache detective" and keep a diary for at least two weeks or, even better, for a month. Your headache pain diary can be like Figure 4.2, Your Behavioral Worksheet, on page 57. When you get a headache, stop and take a few minutes to write down the events or actions that led to the beginning of your pain. Consider what might have triggered it or made it worse. Note how severe the headache is and how long it lasts.

Many things can affect headache. You may have sensitivities to certain foods, alcohol, or other beverages or to strong odors or bright or flickering lights. Chapter 9, *Healthy Eating and Pain Self-Management*, lists some of the most common food triggers (see page xxx). Emotions and events can be triggers too. Are you angry, sad, or under increased stress? Have you skipped meals or changed your activity pattern? Are there any changes to your posture—resulting from a change in the chair or desk you use, for example—that might cause neck or shoulder tension? Are you fatigued or sleeping poorly? Are you going through hormonal changes? Does the weather seem to be a factor? In addition to identifying triggers, it is important to note what

Red Flags: Headache

Occasionally, headache symptoms signal a new serious health problem. Do not wait: Some headache symptoms can be symptoms of a stroke. Immediate medical attention can mean the difference between life and death or between a normal life and a life of disability. Seek immediate emergency care if you experience an unusual sudden severe headache, the worst headache of your life, or a headache with one or more of the symptoms below if they differ from your usual headache pattern:

- confusion or trouble understanding speech
- trouble speaking
- changes in vision
- trouble walking
- dizziness or fainting

- numbness, weakness, or paralysis on one side of the body
- high fever, greater than 102°F to 104°F (39°C to 40°C)
- stiff neck
- unexplained nausea or vomiting

you do when you get a headache. Record the self-management strategies you try, including medications, and whether they help.

After you have recorded information in your headache symptom diary or behavioral worksheet for a few weeks, begin to look for patterns. Remember, sometimes a combination of things can trigger pain. If you identify some possible triggers, divide them into triggers you can avoid (for example, certain foods or drink), triggers you can't avoid but can learn to manage (for example, stress, emotional reactions, fatigue, poor posture), triggers you can minimize (for example, missed meals, late nights), and triggers that are not in your control (for example, hormonal or weather changes). Being aware of the triggers that can be controlled, even partially, can be an important step in managing your headaches.

Once you have a sense of your headache patterns and triggers, you can start planning

how to avoid, manage, or minimize your triggers. To learn more about methods to self-manage stress, strong emotions, fatigue, poor sleep, and other factors that might impact your headache, review the many self-management skills discussed in earlier chapters. Pacing, for example, can help you balance your activity and rest and stay below your headache "threshold." Your headache threshold is the point when you start to feel a headache coming on. You may find that if you take action (for example, going for a short walk, doing a relaxation or breathing exercise, taking medication, etc.) as soon as you feel signs of a headache, you can prevent or reduce its intensity.

Living an overall healthy lifestyle is also important for headache self-management. Regular moderate exercise can give you an overall sense of well-being, reduce stress and anxiety, lift your mood, and reduce the frequency of headache attacks. If you suffer from migraine headaches, you may need to be careful when you exercise. Work out at a moderate pace, not too fast or too hard. Stay hydrated, and don't exercise if you have not eaten.

Eliminating food triggers and eating a healthy diet with regular meals is also important. Also, be sure to communicate with your family, friends, and coworkers about how they can support you when you do get a headache.

Medications can be effective in managing headache, but they need to be taken with care. Review information on pain medications in Chapter 15, *Understanding Medications and Other Treatments for Chronic Pain*. Over-the-counter medicines such as aspirin, acetaminophen (Tylenol®, Panadol®), and anti-inflammatory medicines (Advil®, Motrin®) can be taken. But they should not be used for more than 14 days in a month. This is because, as we mentioned previously, the overuse of pain medications can be the cause of daily or frequent "rebound" headaches in some people. This is not addiction but a side effect of taking too much. If you take multiple medications or high doses for headache and have frequent or daily headaches, talk to your health care provider about the possibility of medication overuse and how you can reduce the amount of medications you take. If you suffer from severe migraine or cluster headaches, your health care provider may prescribe other types of medicine to prevent or treat them. There are some very promising new medications, including some that target calcitonin gene-related peptide (CGRP), a protein that inflames nerve endings and is involved in the development of migraines. These newer medications to prevent migraine include erenumab (Aimovig®), fremanezumab (Ajovy®), and galcanezumab (Emgality®). They are taken by self-injection once a month or once every three months. Some patients with migraine may also benefit from injections of Botox® in the head, face, and neck areas.

Chronic Pelvic Pain

Pelvic pain is pain in the lower part of the abdomen and pelvis. This pain affects the area directly below your belly button down to your hips. The pelvis includes organs involved in reproduction and sexuality such as the womb or uterus, the vagina, the vulva, the penis, testicles, and prostate gland. The pelvis also includes the bladder, bowel, and many muscles, nerves, bones, and soft tissue. Chronic pelvic pain can occur in any of these structures as well as in the lower back, buttocks, or thighs.

Understanding Chronic Pelvic Pain

There are many possible reasons for pelvic pain. Normal menstruation can cause some pelvic pain. Other reasons for pelvic pain include infection, abnormal tissue growth, and diseases of the urinary tract or bowel. Pelvic pain can also be caused by damage to nerves, tissues, or bones, or injury that causes tender, tight, or weakened muscles in the lower abdomen, lower part of the pelvis (called the pelvic floor muscles), or the buttocks. Chronic pelvic pain can also be caused by prostatitis (inflammation of the prostate gland). If your pelvic pain is due to a known cause, treatment is specific to that cause. Treatments can include various medications to cure the infection or disease or to manage troublesome symptoms; surgery to remove a growth, cyst, or tumor; and physical therapy and exercise to stretch tight muscles and ease trigger points.

Sometimes the cause of pelvic pain is complex and specific treatments do not work. The pain persists and becomes chronic. Like other kinds of pain, chronic pelvic pain may be due to abnormal nerve activity patterns in the pelvic region, the central nervous system, and the brain.

Chronic pelvic pain is different for everyone. It can be mild to severe. It can feel dull, sharp, burning, or cramping. It might be there all the time, or you might only notice it at certain times such as when having a bowel movement, passing urine, during sexual activity, or after you sit for long periods of time. It may not be very bothersome most days, or it may frequently interfere with sleep, work, and enjoyment of life.

People with chronic pelvic pain may find it difficult to discuss the pain with other people, even health care professionals. The relationship of pelvic pain to sexual, urinary, or bowel functions can cause embarrassment, curb conversation, and make you want to hide it from others. Pelvic pain is often surrounded by a "culture of secrecy." Just like anyone who experiences any kind of chronic pain, people with chronic pelvic pain need supportive relationships and need to be taken seriously. Secrecy means that you may not talk openly to friends, family, or even

your health care provider about your pain problem. Urinary or bowel incontinence as well as vaginal discharge can lead to fear of embarrassment or undermine your self-confidence. If you decide to avoid social events, these issues can add to social isolation and depression.

Managing Chronic Pelvic Pain

Although chronic pelvic pain is complex and challenging, there are many things you can do to improve your quality of life. Your role in the management of pelvic pain begins with open communication. Open communication will help you build a trusting relationship with members of your health care team so that you feel comfortable talking with them. You will likely be referred to medical and other specialists. You may be asked about any past or current sexual or physical abuse, because for some people abuse is associated with pelvic pain. Prepare for health care visits by reading Chapter 11, *Communicating with Family, Friends, and Health Care Providers*, pages 263–270. If you are a victim of abuse, it may be hard to talk about these things, but it is very important that you do. Not doing so may mean that you will not get the proper help you need. Health professionals are not mind readers. Chronic pelvic pain has been described as an emotional roller coaster of anger, depression, guilt, anxiety, frustration, and fear. Sometimes, the cause of pelvic pain results in infertility (not being able to conceive a baby) and related feelings of loss and grief. You may be able to better manage these difficult emotions using the self-management tools in earlier chapters. Sometimes, self-management is not enough, and you may require additional help to deal with your emotions. A support group or professional counseling may be helpful. Talk to your health care provider about your feelings, and seek emotional support from family and friends. Sexual concerns are common with pelvic pain. To learn more about sexuality and chronic pain, see Chapter 13, *Enjoying Sex and Intimacy*.

Your health care provider may recommend analgesics and other medicines to manage your symptoms. Your provider may also suggest other forms of treatment or products.

When you have chronic pelvic pain (or any chronic condition), you need to pay attention to your overall health, including issues relating to nutrition, weight, and exercise. Eating well, maintaining a healthy weight, and getting enough physical activity will improve your overall sense of well-being, increase your energy, and improve many other symptoms.

In addition to a flexibility and aerobic exercise program, you may be referred to a physical therapist for assessment and treatment of pain in the muscles and tissues of the lower abdomen and pelvic floor. Ask if there are specific exercises you should not do or exercise machines you should not use. For example, to reduce nerve irritation, you may be advised not to do abdominal "crunches," not to use an elliptical machine, and to avoid bicycling or to use a well-padded seat or padded clothing if you do bicycle. You may also be given special pelvic floor and abdominal exercises that will help relax and strengthen muscles in this area.

Neuropathic Pain Syndromes

Pain may be nerve-related. This type of pain is called neuropathic pain. Nerve-related pain can occur when there is damage or injury to the nerves, spinal cord, or brain itself. Nerve-related pain may involve the abnormal firing of nerves anywhere in the body. Some examples of this type of pain result from nerve damage after surgery or traumatic accident, strokes, and shingles. Neuropathic pain syndromes also include diabetic neuropathy and complex regional pain syndrome (CRPS), which we discuss here.

Managing Diabetic Peripheral Neuropathy

Diabetes can cause damage to the nerves. This damage is referred to as neuropathy. Diabetes can cause a burning or tingling sensation, numbness, or severe pain, especially in the feet. Over time, high blood sugar levels from diabetes can damage nerves throughout the body. The higher your blood sugar levels, the more likely you are to have nerve damage. So, controlling your blood sugar throughout your life is very important.

The key to managing the pain caused by diabetic neuropathy is to maintain healthy blood glucose levels as much as possible. You also need to take special care of your feet which may lose sensation (or may become numb) to prevent injuries and infections. In addition, your health care provider may recommend one or more medications to reduce the uncomfortable or painful sensations in your feet.

Managing Complex Regional Pain Syndrome (CRPS)

Complex regional pain syndrome (CRPS) is a difficult chronic pain condition. It is also known as causalgia or reflex sympathetic dystrophy (RSD). This rather rare syndrome can be quite disabling. CRPS usually affects an arm, hand, finger, leg, foot, or toe, but it can also occur in other parts of the body. If you have CRPS, you may feel a continuous burning or "pins and needles" type pain in the affected limb and increased sensitivity to even light touch and cold. The skin in the painful area can change color and look pale, shiny, blotchy, blue, or very red. The painful area can feel cold or very warm compared to normal areas. There can also be changes to fingernails and toenails and even changes in hair growth in the area. You might also have abnormal sweating near the painful area. Muscles and joints in the affected area can become stiff and spasm. In some people, CRPS moves up the limb and spreads to the opposite limb.

The exact cause of CRPS is not known. There is often a triggering event that starts the pain. The most common initial causes are crushing injuries, sprains (even mild ones such as a twisted ankle or wrist), bone fractures, or surgery. It is also associated with other causes such as heart attack, stroke, or infection. A key finding is that the pain is much more severe than expected from the original injury or illness. CRPS results from damage to nerves that travel from the limbs to the central nervous system in the spinal cord and brain. The nerves in your limbs are part of the sympathetic nervous system. Among other things, the sympathetic nervous system controls the flow of blood to limbs, skin temperature, and our response to stress. The skin changes in CRPS can be caused by damage to nerves in the sympathetic nervous system.

Managing CRPS involves a learning process for both you and your health care team. You may need to undergo multiple tests, procedures, and treatments before finding some pain relief. Review your role in managing medications and other treatments for chronic pain in Chapter 14, *Managing Your Treatment Decisions and Medications*. Because CRPS is difficult to manage, it is very important for you to work closely with all members of your health care team and keep them informed about what is working and what is not improving your quality of life.

CRPS can trigger negative thinking, heightened emotions, and fear or avoidance of movement. These reactions can make the pain of CRPS much worse. The sympathetic nervous system that controls our response to stress is directly involved in CRPS. That is why managing emotions and monitoring your stress levels is so important when you have CRPS. Read more about management of depression, anger, and stress in Chapter 4, *Understanding and Managing Common Symptoms and Problems*.

Learning and practicing self-management techniques to reduce stress and quiet the mind and the nervous system can really help with the stress that accompanies CRPS. Excessive negative thinking, sometimes called catastrophic thinking, happens when you can't stop thinking about pain and how bad it is. To help manage negative thinking, use distraction, positive realistic thinking, and relaxation. If these techniques do not work for you, talk to your health care provider and seek professional help.

People with CRPS may fear or avoid movement. Because the affected limb is often very painful, you may want to protect it by moving as little as possible. But not moving the affected limb will cause many problems, including muscle wasting, weakness of muscles and bones, joint stiffness, and contractures (shortening and hardening of muscles that can lead to deformed and rigid joints). It will also decrease your ability to function on a daily basis. Seeking the help of a physical therapist (PT) as soon as you are diagnosed with CRPS is important. A PT can help you start a program of exercise to maintain the function of your affected limb as well as help you develop an exercise program for your overall health.

■　■　■

Your health care team may have additional recommendations for self-management and treatment of the specific pain syndromes discussed in this chapter. In addition, these specific conditions may overlap. Fortunately, many of the self-management skills in this book can help you relieve pain resulting from more than one pain condition.

For a complete list of suggested further readings, useful websites, and other helpful resources, please see

www.bullpub.com/resources.

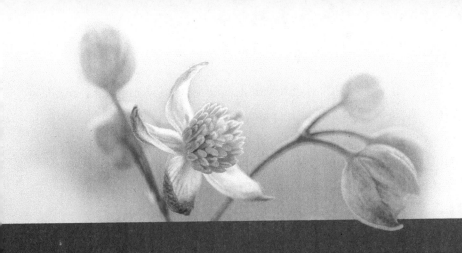

CHAPTER 17

Planning for the Future: Fears and Reality

CHRONIC PAIN OFTEN CHANGES OUR LIVES, and sometimes chronic pain is a symptom of a disease that gets worse over time. Also, people with chronic pain, just like all people, may develop additional conditions as they age. If you have chronic pain, you may worry about what will happen to you if your condition becomes disabling or life-threatening. You may fear that at some time in the future you may have problems managing your condition and your life. Sometimes you may not fear this for yourself but for a partner, family member, or friend.

The challenges you face in the future depend on your pain condition, other health conditions you have, and your age. Your personal challenges also depend on other important factors such as your family and friends and your resources. One way to deal with fears about the future is to take control, problem-solve, and plan. The way to start planning for an uncertain future is to examine your important fears, name each one,

357

and then look at them one by one and decide if each fear is realistic. If you are not sure which fears are realistic and which are not, you may want to consult with a family member, friend, or health professional. You may never need to put your plans into effect, but it is still good self-management to figure out your fears and put a plan in place. You will be reassured knowing that you will be in control if the events you fear happen. In this chapter, we examine the most common concerns and offer some suggestions to help you feel more in control.

Problem Solving about Your Living Situation and Care Needs

No matter how healthy you are or you feel, you may, like most people, fear becoming helpless and dependent. This fear is a common one for everyone and is even greater among people with potentially disabling chronic pain and other health problems. This fear is complex. Often it is not only fear about how to manage physical changes over time but also about financial, social, and emotional concerns.

As your health condition changes, you may need to consider changing your living situation. You may consider either hiring someone to help you in your home or moving to a place that provides more help. The decision you make depends on your physical needs as well as your financial, social, and emotional needs. In this part of the chapter, we walk through the problem-solving steps using a common future planning example: what to do about taking care of yourself as your abilities change.

Start by evaluating what you can do for yourself. What tasks affect your pain and health? Do you need help with any activities of daily living (ADLs) such as getting out of bed, bathing, dressing, preparing and eating meals, cleaning house, shopping, and paying bills? Most people can do these activities, even though they may have to do them slowly, with some modifications, or with some help from assistive devices. In addition to taking care of yourself, you may be responsible for helping someone else with their ADLs. Whether for you or someone else, evaluate which of these tasks you can continue to do and which are becoming too difficult.

You may find that you can do one or more of these tasks without help but you need help for others. For example, you may still be able to fix meals but can no longer do the shopping. Or if you have problems with dizziness or have fallen several times, you might need to have someone

Problem-Solving Steps

1. Identify the problem.
2. List ideas to solve the problem.
3. Select one idea to try.
4. Check the results.
5. Make changes as needed.
6. Use other resources.
7. Accept that the problem may not be solvable now.

around all the time to help. You may find that some activities you enjoyed in the past, such as gardening, are no longer pleasurable.

Use the problem-solving steps discussed in Chapter 2, *Becoming an Active Self-Manager*, to identify and write down a list of the potential problems. (This is step 1: identify the problem. Review the steps of problem solving on page 358.) Once you have listed your concerns, you can then try to solve the problems one at a time. For each problem on your list, write down every possible solution you can think of. (This is step 2: List ideas to solve the problem.) For example:

Problem: Can't Go Shopping

Possible solutions:

- Ask a family member to shop for me.

- Find and sign up for a volunteer shopping service.

- Shop at a store that delivers.

- Ask a neighbor to shop for me.

- Shop for groceries online and have them delivered.

- Get home-delivered meals.

Problem: Can't Be by Myself

Possible solutions:

- Hire in-home care.

- Move in with a relative.

- Get an emergency response system, such as from Lifeline®.

- Move to a retirement community.

- Move to an assisted living facility, board-and-care home, or skilled nursing facility.

When you have listed your problems and the possible solutions, choose one solution for each problem that is workable, acceptable, and within your financial means. (This is step 3 of problem solving.) Your solution choices will depend on your finances, your family, other resources available to help, and how well you think the potential solutions will solve your problem. Sometimes one solution may be the answer to several problems. For instance, if you can't shop and can't be alone and household chores require help, you might consider a retirement community that offers meals, regular housecleaning, and transportation for errands and medical appointments.

As you begin to make changes in your life, go slowly, one step at a time. You don't need to change your whole life to solve one problem. Remember, you can always change your mind. Just be careful not to make a major change in your life that you cannot reverse.

For example, if you are thinking of moving out of your own place to another location (a relative's, a retirement community, or elsewhere), don't give up your current home until you are sure you want to stay in your new home. If you think you need help, hiring help at home is a less drastic solution than moving. If you can't be alone and you live with a family member who is away from home during the day, then going to an adult or senior day care center may be enough to keep you safe and comfortable while your family member is away. In fact, adult day care centers are ideal places to find new friends, and they often provide activities geared to your abilities.

Figuring out what to do when you need help and can't manage on your own anymore is a complex issue. Throughout this chapter, we discuss the issues relating to changing your living situation. For example, you can learn more about hiring in-home help on pages 364–367 and more about moving to a new residence on pages 367–370. As you think about solutions and future planning, remember that a good self-manager makes use of multiple resources. (This is step 6 of problem solving). Your local hospital, senior center, or center for people with disabilities can provide information about resources in your community. You can read more about using other resources in the section *Using Other Resources for Future Planning* on pages 361–362.

Problem Solving about Employment

Let's consider another future planning challenge. How can you plan for the possibility you won't be able to do your job in the same way you have in the past? The first thing to do is return to problem solving. Seldom is life all or nothing. There may be many alternatives to doing things the way you do them now. There may be options such as working part-time or doing another job with the same employer. Another option is to go on disability. One advantage of long-term disability in the United States is that when you do so, you can also go on Medicare and have health insurance. If you have been injured on the job, you may be eligible for workers compensation.

Being open to new plans and adapting as the future unfolds can lead to a better future. Consider the example of Julio, who had a back injury. Julio worked in a job helping others. His job required that he be on his feet all day and do a lot of lifting. After months of rehab and trying to go back to his job, Julio realized that he would have to find some other way to earn a living. He was both very sad and angry. He loved his job. After a lot of thought and help from his family and friends, he realized he had always been a spiritual person. Someone suggested that maybe he would like to be chaplain. He did some research and discovered that he did not have to become a minister to be a chaplain. Rather, he could take a year-long chaplaincy training program. He did this, was hired by a hospital, and has found a new profession and meaning in life.

It may be that like Julio, you will need to change occupations. Look at this as an opportunity. The following are some steps to help you make this change if needed.

- **Think about your interests, values, and skills.** Review what you have done in the past that you enjoyed, such as volunteer work, special projects, or other jobs. Then identify the skills you used for those activities.

- **Look into other career options.** Are there things that you have always wanted to do? Start a small business, teach children, or be a designer? Start by researching all the careers you have considered interesting. Then list ideas for more career options.

Ask family, friends, and others who work in various jobs about their jobs. If you have difficulty coming up with ideas, meet with a vocational or career counselor for advice. You can find one through government employment offices, the US Department of Veterans Affairs, workplace human resources departments, or local community colleges. Part of this counseling often includes career interest and ability testing. What you learn from this testing might send you in directions you have never thought about.

- **Learn more about interesting options.** Find out as much as you can about these different jobs. Do an online search of jobs that interest you. Contact people you know in different fields. Find a human resources department or a college career center or alumni organization that can help you schedule informational interviews. Ask about the possibility to observe or "shadow" people who have a job that interests you to see what it is like.

- **Try out new job possibilities.** Look for volunteer opportunities related to your interest. For example, if you are interested in working with animals, volunteer at the local animal shelter. If you think you might want to teach, ask to volunteer or work as a teacher's aide in a classroom at a local school or teach for your church or temple's children and youth ministries.

- **Take a class or find other ways to improve your skills.** If a new job you are interested in requires skills you do not have, you might need additional school or training. Consider taking courses offered online or through the local community college, a union, or a future employer. Take seminars related to the skills needed for this job. Find ways to develop new skills in your current job to prepare for a change. For example, offer to do or help with a project outside your current job description, or sign up for training classes offered by your company. This may even help you find a new job within your same company or in the same type of industry.

Using Other Resources for Future Planning

It may help to discuss your wishes, abilities, and limitations with a trusted friend, a relative, or a professional such as a social worker or occupational therapist. Sometimes this other person can identify things you overlook or would like to ignore. Seeking ideas from others and using other resources are important parts of becoming a good self-manager. (These are also part of step 6 in the problem-solving process.)

A vocational counselor or social worker at your local senior center, center for people with disabilities, or hospital social services department can help by providing you with information about resources in your community. This person can also give you some ideas about how to deal with your care needs. There are several kinds of professionals who can help.

Social workers are good for helping you decide how to solve financial and living arrangement problems and for locating appropriate community resources. Some social workers are also trained in counseling and can assist you in dealing with emotional and relationship problems that may be associated with your health condition or advancing age.

Another helpful professional is an occupational therapist (OT). An OT can assess your daily living needs and suggest assistive devices or changes you can make at home or work to make life easier. They can be especially helpful for people with chronic pain who have limited movement. OTs can also help you figure out how to keep doing enjoyable activities.

If you have been hospitalized, you can use the hospital's resource center for help. Most hospitals also have a discharge planner on staff. This person, usually a nurse or social worker, will see patients before they go home and check that the patient and/or family members know what to do at home. If necessary, they will help find resources so that when you leave the hospital you are safe and continue to heal. It is very important that you be honest with this person. If you have concerns about your ability to care for yourself, say so. Solutions are almost always available. However, the planner can help only if you share your concerns. Many hospitals also have chaplains; they might know about resources within your own religious or spiritual community.

Financial planners and attorneys are also very useful resources. Financial planners not only provide advice on investing and managing your money, they can also help you plan for your retirement and discuss your options, including the future need for different types of insurance such as disability or long-term care. If you use a financial planner, be sure that they are not being paid by investing your money. Look for Certified Financial Planners—they are formally recognized as experts in their field.

Attorneys are also important resources. They can help you set your financial affairs in order. They can help you to protect assets, prepare a valid will, and execute durable powers of attorney (DPAs) for health care and financial management. (A general durable power of attorney deals with financial matters, while a durable power of attorney for health care, which is discussed in detail on pages 374–379, is for health care decisions only.)

Making Decisions and Staying in Charge of Your Life

In addition to practical and financial concerns, there are the emotional aspects of needing help. Most people leave childhood wanting and reaching for independence—your driver's license, your first job, your first credit card, the first time you go out and don't have to tell anybody where you are going, and so on. In these and many other ways, you demonstrate to yourself and others that you are "grown up." You are in charge of your life and able to take care of yourself.

If you realize that you can no longer manage completely on your own, it may feel like a return to childhood. This may seem like a loss of independence. You again find yourself with somebody else in charge of parts of your life. This can be painful and embarrassing.

Some people faced with this situation become depressed and can no longer find any joy in life. Others deny their need for help. They may even place themselves in danger, making life difficult for those who want to be helpful. Still others give up and expect others to completely take care of them. They may demand attention and services from their children or other family members. If you are having one or more of these reactions, you can help yourself and develop a more positive response.

The idea of "changing the things you can change, accepting the things you cannot change, and knowing the difference" is key to staying in charge of your life. Take a hard and realistic look at your situation. Identify the activities that you need help with (such as going shopping and cleaning house) and those that you can still do yourself (such as getting dressed, paying bills, and cooking light meals). Another way to approach this is to ask for help from others for the things you least like to do. This gives you time and energy to do the things you like.

Figuring out what kind of help you need means making decisions. And if you are making the decisions, you are in charge. It is important to make decisions and take action while you are still able to do so. Don't let events force someone else to make your decisions. You must be realistic and honest with yourself. Use the decision-making tools on pages 31–33 in Chapter 2, *Becoming an Active Self-Manager*.

Even though you are the decision maker and the manager, you don't need to figure it all out alone. Some people find that talking with a sympathetic listener—either a professional counselor or a sensible close friend or family member—is comforting and helpful. A thoughtful listener can often point out options you may have overlooked. Hearing from someone with a new viewpoint may help you see things in a new light.

Choose your advisers carefully, and be cautious when you take advice. Don't take advice from somebody who is selling something. There are many people whose solution to your problem is whatever they are selling—this can include things like health or burial insurance policies, annuities, special and expensive furniture, "sunshine cruises," special magazines, or health foods.

When talking with family members or friends, be as open and reasonable as possible. At the same time, try to make them understand that you are the one who decides to accept or not accept help. To gain their cooperation, use "I" messages. For example, "Yes, I do need some help with _____, but I still want to do _____ myself." You can learn more about communicating with "I" messages and other communication tips in Chapter 11, *Communicating with Family, Friends, and Health Care Providers*.

Asking for help does not mean giving up your right to choose. Insist on being asked about all the important decisions that affect you. Early on, lay the ground rules with your helpers. Ask to be presented with options when it is time to make choices. Seriously consider good suggestions. Do not dismiss everything that isn't your own idea. If you learn to be a good decision maker, people will see that you make reasonable decisions and will continue to give you the opportunity to do so.

Be appreciative. Recognize the goodwill and efforts of people who want to help you. When you need help, you can maintain your dignity by gracefully accepting help. If you are unable to come to terms with your increasing needs for help from others, talk with a professional counselor. Find a counselor who has experience with the emotional and social issues of people with disabling health problems. Your local agency providing services to the disabled, your senior center, the Area Agency on Aging, or online resources such as the Canadian Seniors Directory can refer you to the right person. Organizations serving people with your specific health condition can also direct you to support groups and classes. In the United States, good resources are organizations such as the American Cancer Society, American Lung Association, American Heart Association, American Diabetes Association, and Alzheimer's Association. In Canada, reach out to organizations such as the Canadian Cancer Society, Canadian Lung Association, Heart and Stroke Foundation of Canada, Diabetes Canada, and Alzheimer Society of Canada. You can locate the agency you need on the internet or in telephone book Yellow Pages under the listing "social service organizations."

When you know you cannot do something yourself, reach out to family and friends. If you cannot turn to close family or friends, turn to helpful agencies. Case managers can make it easier to get help. They assess your needs and then work with you to organize community services to meet those needs. There are at least two situations where case managers might be helpful: when you cannot rely on friends or family but need help, or when you are trying to help someone who refuses help. You can find case managers through your local social services department's "adult protective services" program or organizations like Family Service Association. Religious service organizations such as Jewish Family Services or Catholic Charities also have case managers. In Canada, publicly subsidized home and community care is available through provincial/territorial governments. The social services department in your local hospital can also put you in touch with the right agency.

Finding In-Home Help

If you find that you cannot manage alone, the first option is usually to hire help. There are many different types of people and organizations that offer in-home help. Here we discuss the process of exploring and securing in-home help.

Types of In-home Help

The following list describes the various kinds of help you might want and need.

- **Housekeeper/yard worker.** This is someone who can assist with indoor and/or outdoor chores, including housecleaning, doing the laundry, ironing, or seasonal chores such as lawn care or shoveling the snow.

■ **Personal assistant or care companion.** A personal assistant or care companion can help you or someone you are caring for by doing a variety of tasks, including:

▸ running errands

▸ driving you or a family member on errands, for social outings, or to medical appointments

▸ grocery shopping

▸ cooking and/or preparing healthful prepared meals to freeze

▸ performing light housekeeping duties such as laundry, vacuuming, and kitchen and bathroom cleaning

▸ organizing and cleaning closets, drawers, or even the garage

▸ keeping you or another family member company—playing cards or games, helping with hobbies, or just sitting and chatting

■ **Home aide or personal care assistant.** Home aides or personal care assistants provide care that involves physical assistance. They usually have some training and can help with daily living tasks such as:

▸ bathing

▸ toileting

▸ getting dressed

▸ shaving

▸ dental hygiene

▸ nail care

▸ walking

If needed, some personal care assistants also help with driving, shopping, cooking, light housekeeping, and keeping you company.

■ **Live-in caregiver.** Many in-home care agencies can help arrange round-the-clock live-in care. Live-in care caregivers provide care to the person needing it as well as rest for any other family member or friends. You might arrange for one caregiver who lives with you or a set of caregivers who work in shifts throughout the day or different days of the week. To find live-in care, follow the suggestions for finding respite care below and on pages 366–367.

> In Canada, programs are offered through provincial and territorial health ministries and private companies. Check with such resources as the Canadian Seniors Directory or the Canadian government's "Programs and Services for Seniors" page to find out about respite services. The federal government supports the Veterans Independence Program (VIP) through Veterans Affairs Canada. Also, all the provinces and territories offer a limited amount of publicly funded home care services from both public and private agencies. The types of services offered vary across the country.

Hiring In-Home Help

Two types of organizations offer in-home services—these are in-home care agencies and in-home care registries. You can also hire someone directly. Another option is home sharing. These options are explained in this section.

In-home care agencies assume all the employer responsibilities. An agency hires and pays the caregiver, pays Social Security and payroll taxes, and is responsible for caregiver insurance. The agency also provides training and supervision; it may also send a substitute when your usual assistant is unavailable. Be sure to get all the details about each agency's policies, as these can differ from one agency to the next.

In-home care registries are referral services that can help you find different types of in-home care. Most of these agencies supply home aides as well as licensed staff, such as certified nursing assistants (CNAs), licensed vocational nurses (LVNs), or registered nurses (RNs). Unless you are bedridden or require some procedure that must be done by someone with a certain category of license, a home aide is likely an appropriate choice.

The caregivers referred by registries usually have experience and may have the required training. You pay a fee to the registry for their referral service. However, unlike agencies, registries do not employ these care providers. If you hire someone from a registry, that person is *your* employee. They are an independent contractor who works for you. This means you might be responsible for paying taxes and Social Security for this person, and you must buy your own liability insurance. In Canada, you may be responsible for paying taxes, Canada Pension Plan, and Employment Insurance. When you contact a registry, ask about the training and experience of the people they refer and what you are required to do as the employer of an independent contractor.

Another less expensive way to find in-home help is to hire someone recommended by a friend or through a help wanted ad or posting on a website. If you choose this option, know that it involves more time—you will be responsible for checking all references and doing all the screening. A person you find this way can work for you either as an employee or independent contractor. Talk to a lawyer or get some legal advice about both choices when considering such things as employment taxes and insurance.

In Canada, all the provinces and territories offer a limited amount of publicly funded home care services from both public and private agencies. The types of services offered vary across the country.

If you want to hire in-home help directly without an agency or registry, check the Caring.com website (www.caring.com) or CaregiverJobs.ca (www.caregiverjobs.ca) in Canada. These sites provide lists of agencies, reviews from families, and checklists to guide you through the process. Other resources include local senior centers and centers serving the disabled, community bulletin boards, and neighborhood newspapers. They often have listings of people looking for work as home care assistants. The best source of help is usually word of mouth. It is great to get a recommendation from someone who has employed a person or knows of a person who has worked for a friend or relative. Putting the word out through your family and social network may lead you to a jewel.

Home sharing can also be a solution if you are looking for help in your own home. If you have space, you can offer a residence to someone in exchange for help. This works best if the help needed consists mainly of household and garden chores. Some people, however, may be willing, in exchange for a place to live, to provide care, such as running errands and help with dressing, bathing, and meal preparation. Some communities have agencies or government bureaus that help match up home sharers and home seekers.

To find out more about home health care options, contact your local Area Agency on Aging. Every county in the United States has an Area Agency on Aging. In Canada, every province and territory has an agency that offers resources for seniors. You can find yours in the phone book or online through such places as the Canadian Seniors Directory or the Canadian government's "Programs and Services for Seniors" web page. These are also excellent agencies to contact when you are looking for other resources related to your care and well-being.

Moving to a New Residence

The time may come when you or your partner needs to move to a new residence. This might be because your health is declining or due to the increased health needs of your partner. This is a difficult decision to make regardless of the reason, and the problem-solving steps discussed in Chapter 2, *Becoming an Active Self-Manager*, and listed on page 358 as well as the other decision-making tools discussed in Chapter 2 can help. Once you make your decision, you can then begin to look for the type of community that provides the care you need.

If you are not of retirement age, know that many communities accept residents who are 50 or younger. If you are a younger person, the local center for people with disabilities or "independent living center" may be able to direct you to an out-of-home care facility.

When looking for a residence community, consider the levels of care that are offered. These usually include the following:

- **Independent living senior/retirement communities.** These communities typically include both for-sale and rental units that provide a more protected setting with security and emergency response services. These communities usually offer meals in a dining room and weekly housekeeping. They sometimes also offer laundry service and personal transportation. They often host a variety of activities and field trips. This kind of community is an option if you no longer want to cook and clean but do want to be around others every day. These communities do not offer any personal care assistance.

There are almost always waiting lists for this type of community, often even before they are built and ready for occupancy. If you think such a place would be right for you, get on the waiting list right away, or at least a couple of years before you think you want to move. You can always change your mind or decline if you are not ready when a space is offered. To locate these communities in your area, call your senior center or search the internet for senior independent living or retirement communities near you.

If you have friends living in nearby retirement communities, ask to be invited for a visit and a meal. This will help you to get an insider's view. Some communities even have guest accommodations where you can arrange to stay for a night or two before you commit to a lease or contract.

- **Assisted living residences.** An assisted living residence usually offers all the services that independent living residences do, plus some personal care and/or assistance with taking medication. Personal care assistance typically includes help with daily living tasks such as showering and dressing. However, you or your partner must be able to get to the bathroom, in and out of bed, and to the common dining room on your own. You may need to move out of an assisted living residence if either you or your partner needs to move to a skilled nursing facility or the person receiving the care dies.

> In Canada, retirement homes are usually privately run by for-profit and nonprofit organizations. Costs are mainly paid for by the resident. There are few government subsidies.

- **Skilled nursing facilities (SNF).** Sometimes called nursing homes, convalescent hospitals, or long-term care facilities, a skilled nursing facility provides the most complete care for severely ill or disabled people. Skilled nursing facilities provide medically related care for people who can no longer function without such care. For example, these facilities are designed for people who take medications that must be administered by injection or intravenously or monitored by professional nursing staff. A nursing home patient is usually very physically limited, needing help getting in and out of bed, eating, bathing, or dealing with bladder or bowel control. Skilled nursing facilities can also manage the care of feeding tubes, respirators, or other higher-tech equipment. Usually, a person who has had a stroke or a hip or knee replacement will be transferred from an acute care hospital to a skilled nursing facility for rehabilitation before going home. For people who are partially or temporarily disabled, a skilled nursing facility provides physical, occupational, and speech therapy, wound care, and other services.

Not all nursing homes provide all types of care. Some specialize in rehabilitation and therapies, and others specialize in long-term custodial care. Some provide high-tech nursing services, and others do not. Recent studies have shown that almost half of all people over 65 spend some time in a nursing home, many for only a short time during rehabilitation.

Many people have negative feelings about skilled nursing facilities. You might have read or heard negative stories. Unfortunately, these reports and stories help to create anxiety and fear. There are organizations that monitor skilled nursing facilities. Each facility is required by law to post in a noticeable place the name and phone number of the "ombudsman," a person assigned by the state licensing agency to assist patients and their families with problems related to their care. In Canada, provincial ministries of health monitor all care facilities. Although some of these stories may be true, all the excellent care received in skilled nursing facilities never makes the news. These skilled nursing facilities serve a critical need. They provide a type of care and facilities that you may not be able to provide or afford in your current living situation.

When searching for a skilled nursing facility, ask friends, senior center social workers, and hospital discharge planners about good facilities in your area. You may also want to have family or friends visit several facilities and make recommendations.

- **Continuing care retirement communities (CCRC).** These facilities offer all three types of service we have discussed—independent living, assisted living, and skilled nursing—at one site. The advantage to continuing care communities is that if you and your partner need different levels of care, the facility can accommodate both of you. Another advantage is that should the care needs of you or your partner change, you can stay in the same facility.

- **Residential or board-and-care homes.** Board-and-care homes are licensed by the state or county social services agency. Residential care homes are also known as assisted living in Canada. They are usually small homes in residential areas that provide nonmedical care and supervision for individuals who cannot live alone. Small board-and-care homes have around six residents who live in a family-like setting. Each person usually has a private room,

but residents eat together. Larger board-and-care homes may have more residents who live in a boardinghouse or hotel-like setting.

These residential board-and-care homes offer personal care, meals, housekeeping, and sometimes transportation. They differ from assisted living in that they do not offer the wider range of other activities, although larger homes have more staff and might offer some other types of planned activities. Residents in larger board-and-care facilities usually need to be more independent because they will not receive as much personal attention as residents in smaller homes.

In most states, these board-and-care homes are licensed for either "elderly" (over 62) or "adult" (under 62). The adult category is further divided into facilities for those with mental illness, developmental disabilities, and physical disabilities. When considering a residential or board-and-care home, be sure to evaluate the type of residents already living there to make sure they have conditions and needs that are similar to yours.

Although all homes are by law required to provide healthful meals, make sure that the food is to your liking and can meet your needs.

The monthly fees for residential care homes vary, depending on whether they are simple or luxurious. The simpler facilities cost about the same as the government Supplemental Security Income (SSI) benefit and will accept SSI beneficiaries, billing the government directly. The more luxurious the home is with respect to furnishings, neighborhood, and services, the greater the cost. However, even the nicest of these typically costs less than full-time, 24-hour, 7-days-a-week at-home care. In Canada, costs vary from province to province. Government subsidies may be available depending on your income.

Whatever options you consider, moving residences requires a lot of thought and research. It is a big decision. We encourage you again to use the decision-making tools in Chapter 2, *Becoming an Active Self-Manager*, and consider holding a family meeting to discuss this with and get ideas and help from close family members and friends.

Paying for Health Care

Managing chronic pain and related health problems may require expensive medical care and treatment. Many people fear not having enough money to pay for their needs. Also, if you are unable to work, the loss of income or the loss of your health insurance coverage may present an overwhelming financial problem. You can, however, avoid some of these risks by planning and knowing your resources.

Disability Insurance

If you work in the United States, your employer might offer you short-term and long-term disability insurance as a benefit. California, Hawaii, New Jersey, New York, and Rhode Island require that employers offer disability insurance. In addition, many employers in other states offer disability benefits as well. Short-term disability provides compensation or income replacement for non-job-related injuries or illnesses that leave you unable to work for a limited time period. (This is different from workers' compensation, which is a form of insurance payment for employees who are injured at work or become sick due to work.) Long-term disability insurance assists the employee after short-term

disability benefits end, which is usually after three to six months.

If your employer does not offer disability insurance, you may be able to buy it privately. However, it may be expensive. The cost varies and is based on your age and the type of benefits you want. The cost could be between 1 and 3 percent of annual gross income for private disability insurance coverage. That means if you earn $60,000 per year, you could spend between $600 and $1,800 each year on the insurance. It is best to shop around to find the best deal. Also, carefully review the details of the plan before buying. For example, make sure you understand what types of disabilities are covered, what amount you will receive, how often and for how long you will receive it, as well as if your condition is considered preexisting, which could be excluded from coverage. Some disability insurances may cover some preexisting health conditions but not others. These are called exclusions to coverage, and you want to know about these before buying.

In the United States, if you have a disability that makes it impossible to perform some or all of your job duties or perform an alternative

In Canada, the Canada Health Act covers in-hospital and physician services, but other services may not be covered by the public system. It is up to you to find out which health benefits are covered and which are not. In some cases, a person may qualify for more than one disability benefit. In Canada, private insurance such as disability, long-term care, and critical illness is available. Employers may offer short-term and long-term disability benefits. Provincial disability income programs may supplement Canada Pension Plan (CPP) disability benefits. Eligibility depends on the medical condition and financial criteria. CPP provides disability benefits (disability pension and postretirement disability benefit) to people who have made enough contributions to CPP and who are disabled and cannot work at any job on a regular basis. Provinces have their own disability income programs for people who are eligible and do not qualify for other disability income programs. Publicly subsidized home and community care is also available through provincial/territorial governments.

job, you can apply for Social Security Disability Insurance (SSDI). This benefit is for people who have worked and paid into Social Security retirement. It allows you to receive those benefits early if you have become disabled. Also, because you are no longer working, have lost your health insurance, and receive SSDI, you will qualify for Medicare health insurance. If SSDI is not enough or you do not qualify for these benefits, there is another federal program: Social Security Income (SSI) for disabled people with special financial need. Those who qualify for SSI may also meet the eligibility criteria to receive Medicaid health insurance.

Health Insurance, Medicare, and Medicaid

Health care reform continues to bring many changes in Medicare, Medicaid, and private insurance in the United States. These changes can be difficult to understand. Talk to people at your local senior center, Area Agency on Aging, or disability organization to find the most current and trustworthy sources of information.

Your health insurance and Medicare may meet only a part of your care costs. For example, the number of days in skilled nursing that Medicare covers are limited. And even though Medicare seldom covers the cost of all your health care needs, most private "Medigap" insurance policies only pick up the 20 percent that Medicare does not cover. Medigap plans, the insurance policies that help supplement Medicare that are sold by private companies, usually do not cover any procedure or treatment that is not also covered by Medicare. (However, some Medigap policies may pay for certain health services outside the United States that are not otherwise covered by Medicare.)

There are other types of supplemental insurance policies that may provide for care needs not paid for by Medicare and Medigap insurance. These supplemental policies may be available as a benefit from your employer, or you can purchase them directly from an insurance company. Examples of supplemental insurance include long-term care, critical illness, hospital indemnity, and accidental death insurance. If you plan to buy supplemental insurance, carefully read the policy sections about benefits, limitations, and exclusions. A supplemental policy may not cover all the expenses you expect. It may require waiting periods before payments start. Or it may have limits based on how much you paid and for how long. Be sure the policy covers nursing home care at a daily rate that is enough for your community. Make sure you know how the policy will pay for care. Many policies place a cap and may not cover over three months for skilled nursing or rehabilitation facilities. This time period may be briefer if the policy holder is judged to be "not getting better" and in need of "custodial" care.

If you have minimal savings and little or no income, the federal Medicaid program is supposed to pay for medical treatment and long-term skilled or custodial care. The eligibility rules on assets and income differ from state to state. Consult your local social services department to see if you are entitled to benefits. If you have been in the hospital, the social services department in the hospital where you have been treated can advise you about your own situation and the probability of your being eligible for these programs. The local agency serving the disabled also usually has advisers who can refer you to programs and resources for which you may be eligible. Senior centers often have counselors who are knowledgeable about the ins and outs of health care insurance.

If you or your partner is a United States military veteran, check with your nearest Veterans Affairs (VA) facility or the VA website about services. You may be eligible for a range of services at very low or no cost. In Canada, check with Veterans Affairs Canada for services and programs.

If you or your partner own a home, you might be able to get a reverse mortgage. If you take out a reverse mortgage, the bank pays you a monthly amount based on the value of your home. The nice thing is that no matter how long you live, you can never be thrown out of your home. It is usually better to take out a reverse mortgage than to borrow against the assets you have in your house. Be sure to talk to a good financial planner who knows about health and aging-related issues before making any decisions. There are both risks and benefits to reverse mortgages. The National Council on Aging has excellent information on this topic (www.ncoa .org/economic-security/home-equity/).

It is never too soon or too late to start financial planning for both expected and unexpected future events. Even if the idea of discussing the future makes you and your family feel uncomfortable or uneasy, the sooner you begin this process the more secure you will feel knowing there is a plan in place.

Grieving: A Normal Reaction to Bad News

When you experience loss—small losses (such as losing a special keepsake) or big losses (such as losing a life partner or facing life with chronic pain or a disabling or terminal illness)—you go through an emotional process called grieving. Grieving is natural; it helps people to come to terms with loss.

A person with a chronic disabling health problem such as chronic pain experiences a variety of losses. These can include loss of confidence, loss of self-esteem, loss of independence, loss of lifestyle, loss of employment, and perhaps the most painful of all, loss of a positive self-image. This is especially true if your condition has changed your appearance. This can happen with rheumatoid arthritis, Parkinson's disease, paralysis from a stroke, or the loss of a breast due to cancer.

Psychiatrist Elisabeth Kübler-Ross described the stages of grief as follows:

- **Shock,** when you feel both a mental and a physical reaction to the initial recognition of the loss.

- **Denial,** when you think, "No, it can't be true," and proceed to act for a time as if it were not true.

- **Anger,** when you fume "Why me?" and search for someone or something to blame (e.g., "If only the doctor had diagnosed it earlier," "The job caused me too much stress," etc.).

- **Bargaining,** when you promise, "I'll never smoke again," or "I'll follow my treatment regimen to the letter," or "I'll go to church every Sunday, if only I can get over this."

- **Depression,** when awareness sets in, you confront the truth, and you experience deep feelings of sadness and hopelessness.

- **Acceptance,** when you recognize that you must deal with what has happened and make up your mind to do what you must do to move forward.

People do not necessarily pass through these stages one after another. You are more apt to flip-flop between them. Therefore, don't be surprised or discouraged if you find yourself angry or depressed again when you thought you had reached acceptance. This is normal.

Making End-of-Life Decisions

Most people with chronic pain are not at the end of their lives. However, making end-of-life decisions can help relieve a worry and motivate you to think about your values. Decisions about the end of life can be very difficult. People have a hard time facing the future because they are afraid to think about death. Thinking about death means dealing with the idea of your own mortality. As you age, or as you face chronic pain, you may begin to have fears about death. This is especially true when something happens to bring you face-to-face with the possibility of your own death. Losing someone close, surviving an accident, or learning you have a health condition that may shorten your life can make you think about your own passing.

Your attitude about death is shaped by your core attitudes about life. These are the product of your culture, your family, perhaps your religion, and certainly your life experiences. You might wish or pray for yourself or a loved one to be released from suffering, feel guilty about these wishes, or fear dying. Or you may have all these feelings. If you feel some or all of these things, you are not alone. These feelings are common. Many people try to avoid these feelings.

If you are ready to think about your own and your partner's future—about the near or distant prospect that your lives will most certainly end—then the information in the rest of the chapter will be useful. If you are not ready to think about this just yet, put this reading aside for now and come back when you are ready.

Legal Planning

Taking positive steps to prepare for death is useful and healthful. This means getting your house in order by attending to all the necessary details, large and small. If you avoid dealing with these details, you create problems for yourself and for those who love and care for you. You also may lose your ability to make these important decisions.

Whatever you decide about your future, it is important to tell others. What are your wishes about how and where you want to be during your last days? Do you want to be in a hospital or at home? When do you want to stop procedures that prolong your life? At what point do you want nature to take its course? Who should be with you—only the few people who are nearest and dearest, or all the people you care about and want to see one last time? What will happen if you can no longer manage your affairs? Most people have very definite ideas about what they would like.

End-of-life planning is hard and sometimes frightening. People do not like thinking about all the "what ifs." Nevertheless, such planning is necessary for you, your partner, and your family. Good planning protects you and ensures that your wishes are understood and carried out.

If your plans are not written down, and more importantly written into legal documents, your wishes might not be followed. In this section, we discuss the types of legal documents you should have in place. If you are not sure what you have or you do not have any of these, consult a lawyer. Drafting some types of legal documents may not be something you can do yourself. Many people worry that going to a lawyer will be very expensive, but many lawyers offer a free meeting or consultation to discuss your needs. Law offices can give you the price of each service during a consultation. Also, lawyers' fees do vary. Shop around to find one whose fees fit best with what you can afford to pay. Preparing the two documents that we discuss should not be expensive.

If your budget is a concern, ask your local senior center for the names of attorneys and financial advisers who offer free or low-cost services. AARP (formerly known as the American Association of Retired Persons) and CARP (formerly known as the Canadian Association for Retired Persons) are other important resources for finding advice. You might also contact your local bar association. Someone there can refer you to a list of attorneys experienced in this area. These attorneys are generally familiar with the laws applying to seniors and to younger persons with disabilities as well. If you are living with a disability, even if you are not a senior, your legal needs are much the same as those of the older person. The sooner you can plan for these in the present, the better prepared and more in control you will feel about the future.

Prepare legal documents now, not later. This is especially important if your mental abilities are affected by chronic health problems. Attorneys who are consulted about legal end-of-life planning are required by law to determine that a person is "of sound mind" and able to make these decisions for themselves. Therefore, it is best not to wait.

Know that the following discussion is not complete—these are complex issues, and as we state above, it is a good idea to seek professional help with these documents. Also, the laws are different for each state, province, and country. For more complete details, seek legal counsel. The information we share in this chapter is just the basics to prepare you for a deeper discussion with your partner, family, and legal counsel.

Preparing Advance Directives for Health Care

Although none of us has control over our own death, your death, like the rest of your life, is something you can help manage. That is, you can have input, make decisions, and perhaps add quality to your final days. Proper management can make your death easier on family and friends. An advance directive helps you manage some of the medical and legal issues concerning death. It also helps you plan for both expected and unexpected end-of-life situations. You and all other adult family members should prepare an advance health care directive as early

as possible. This is the best plan even for people who do not have any chronic health conditions. Without an advance directive, your wishes about end-of-life situations may not be followed.

Advance directives are written instructions that tell your doctor or other health care provider what kind of care you would like to receive when you are not able to make medical decisions for yourself (for example, if you are unconscious, in a coma, or mentally incompetent). Usually an advance directive describes both the treatments you want and those you do not want. There are different types of advance directives. We describe the most common types of advance directives in the United States here:

- **Living will.** A living will is a document that states the kind of medical or life-sustaining treatments you would want if you were seriously or terminally ill. A living will, however, does not let you legally appoint someone to make those decisions for you. It expresses your desires but is not a legal document.

- **Durable power of attorney (DPA) for health care.** A durable power of attorney for health care (or more simply a power of attorney for health care) allows you to name someone to act for you as your agent. This document can also spell out guidelines about your health care wishes for your agent. If you want, you can let your agent make the decisions without your guidance. Many people, however, prefer to give guidance to their agent. You can address almost anything about your care, including the use or nonuse of aggressive life-sustaining measures. Whereas a living will applies only if you have an illness that will end your life, a DPA for health care applies anytime you are unconscious or unable to make decisions due to illness, accident, or injury.

In Canada, a DPA for health care may be called a substitute decision maker, proxy, mandatary (Quebec), agent, or power of attorney for health or for personal care. We refer to this document as a DPA for health care for the rest of this section, but the discussion applies equally to Canada.

Note that a general DPA deals with financial matters, whereas a DPA for health care is for health care decisions only. It is important to understand that a DPA for health care allows you to appoint someone else to act as your agent for *only* your health care. It does not give this person the right to act on your behalf in other ways, such as handling your financial matters.

In general, a DPA for health care is more useful than a living will because it allows you to appoint someone to make decisions for you as well states your preferences about medical or life-sustaining treatments. A DPA for health care can be used anytime you are unable to make health care decisions. The only time a DPA for health care may not be the best choice is if there is no one you trust to act on your behalf. The next section of this chapter contains more detailed information on preparing a DPA for health care. In most states, you do not need a lawyer to prepare this document.

- **Do not resuscitate (DNR) order.** A DNR is a request that you are not to be given cardiopulmonary resuscitation (CPR) if your heart stops or if you stop breathing. A DNR can be included in a living will or durable power of attorney (DPA) for health care. However, you do not need to have a living will or a DPA for health care to have a DNR order. Your health care provider can put a DNR in your medical chart so that it may guide the actions of the hospital and any health care provider. You can also put a DNR on your refrigerator or somewhere else in your home so that emergency personnel will know your wishes. Without a DNR order, hospital or emergency personnel will make every effort to resuscitate you. DNR orders are accepted in all states in the United States.

- **Advance directive for mental health care.** Although advance directives for health care are generally used for end-of-life situations, they may also be prepared to direct the type of mental health treatment given in the event a person with dementia or mental illness becomes incapacitated due to that illness. Most states may combine advance directives for health care and mental health care in one document and allow you to appoint an agent to act on your behalf for both health and mental health issues. Some states, however, require separate documents, which also allow you to choose different agents, one for health care and another for mental health care. For more information on mental health advance directives and the specific practices in your state, visit the website of the National Resource Center on Psychiatric Advance Directives (www.nrc-pad.org).

- **POLST (Physician Orders for Life-Sustaining Treatment).** Another advance directive form that is increasingly common is a POLST (Physician Orders for Life-Sustaining Treatment). Doctors introduce this form (which is usually pink) to patients during an appointment. Patients fill it out to let the doctor know what kind of care they would like to receive. It is generally only used for people in the final year of life. A POLST is part of your medical record, but it does not appoint someone to act on your behalf, so a DPA for health care is still important.

In Canada, advance directives are called various things across the country, including personal directives, health care directives, advanced care plans, and mandates in case of incapacity. The term *living will* originated in the United States and has no legal status in the US or Canada. In Canada, a health care directive can be created without the assistance of a lawyer. Most provinces and territories in Canada have their own DNR forms for residents to use. The names of these forms and when they can be applied may differ. Practices on mental health care directives also differ by province. For more information in Canada, check with your local health authority or hospital or contact your local branch of the Canadian Mental Health Association (https://cmha.ca). A POLST is not yet available in Canada.

Preparing a Durable Power of Attorney (DPA) for Health Care

Adults (anyone age 18 or older) should prepare and have a durable power of attorney for health care. Unexpected events can happen to anyone at any age. Although each US state has different regulations and forms for advance directives, this information should be useful wherever you live. Although many states recognize durable powers of attorney for health care that are created in another state, this may not always be the case. To be on the safe side, if you move or spend a lot of time in another state, it is best to check with a lawyer in that state to see if documents from another state are legally binding there.

Make sure your primary care provider has a copy of your DPA for health care, and when you go to the hospital, be sure the hospital also has a copy. If you cannot bring it yourself, be sure your agent knows to give a copy to the hospital. This is important because your primary care provider may not oversee your care in the hospital. Do not put your only copy of your durable power of attorney for health care in your safe deposit box. It needs to be available when it is needed.

Choosing Your Agent

The first step in preparing a DPA for health care is to choose your agent. An agent can be a friend or family member, but it cannot be any of the providers who give you care. Your agent should probably live in your area. If the agent is not available on short notice to make decisions for you, the agent will not be much help. Just to be safe, you can also name a backup or secondary

A Good Health Care Agent

Look for the someone who:

- is likely to be available should they need to act for you.
- understands your wishes and is willing to carry them out.
- is emotionally prepared and able to carry out your wishes and will not feel burdened by doing so.

agent who would act for you if your primary agent is not available.

Be sure that your agent thinks like you or at least would be willing to carry out your wishes. You must be able to trust that this person has your interests at heart and truly understands and will respect your wishes. Your agent should be mature, composed, and comfortable with your wishes. Your agent must be someone you know who will carry out those wishes.

Sometimes a spouse or child is not the best agent because this person is too close to you emotionally. For example, if you wish not to be resuscitated in the case of a severe heart attack, your agent must be able to tell the health care provider not to resuscitate. This could be very difficult or impossible for a family member. Be sure the person you choose as your agent is up to this task and would not say "do everything you can" at this critical time. You want your agent to be someone who will not find this job too much of an emotional burden.

Finding the right agent is a key task. This may mean talking to several people. These may be the most important interviews that you will ever conduct. We talk more about discussing your wishes with family, friends, and your health care provider later in this chapter.

Expressing Your Choices

Once you have chosen your agent, spend some time thinking about your choices and decide what you want. Your beliefs and values guide the directions you give your agent. Some health care DPA forms list several general statements concerning medical treatment. These can help you decide on your wishes. The following are some examples of general statements:

If my primary physician finds that I cannot make my own health care decisions, I grant my agent full power and authority to make those decisions for me, subject to any health care instructions set forth below. My agent will have the right to:

A. Consent, refuse consent, or withdraw consent to any of my medical care or services, such as tests, drugs, surgery, or consultations for any physical or mental condition. This includes the provision, withholding, or withdrawal of artificial nutrition and hydration (feeding by tube or vein) and all other forms of health care, including cardiopulmonary resuscitation (CPR).

B. Choose or reject my physician, other health care professionals, or health care facilities.

C. Receive and consent to the release of my medical information.

D. Donate my organs or tissue, authorize an autopsy, and dispose of my body, unless I have said something different in a contract with a funeral home, in my will, or by some other written method.

E. Prolong my life to the greatest extent possible without regard to my condition, the chances I have for recovery, or the cost of the procedures.

If you use a form containing suggested general statements such as these, all you need to do is initial the statements that apply to you.

Other forms make a "general statement of granted authority," in which you give your agent the power to make decisions. However, you do not write out the details of what these decisions should be. In this case, you are trusting that your agent will follow your wishes even though they are not detailed. Since these wishes are not explicitly written, you must discuss them in detail with your agent.

All health care DPA forms include a space for you to write out any specific wishes. You are not required to include specific details, but you may wish to do so. Knowing what details to write is a little complicated. None of us can predict the future or knows the exact circumstances in which the agent will have to act. You can get some idea by asking your health care team what the most likely developments are for someone with your condition. Then you can direct your agent on how to act. Your directions can include outcomes, specific circumstances, or both. If you specify outcomes, the statement should focus on which types of outcomes would be acceptable and which would not (for example, "resuscitate if I can continue to fully function mentally").

There are several decisions you need to make in directing your agent on how to act on your behalf:

■ Generally, how much treatment do you want? This can range from the very

aggressive—that is, doing many things to keep you alive—to the very conservative, which means doing almost nothing to keep you alive except to keep you clean and comfortable.

■ Given the types of life-threatening events that are likely to happen to people with your condition, what sorts of treatment do you want and under what conditions do you want them?

■ If you become mentally incapacitated, what sorts of treatment do you want for other illnesses, such as pneumonia?

At some of the websites listed on the resource page at www.bullpub.com/resources, you will find downloadable forms for durable power of attorney (DPA) for health care.

Sharing Your Wishes about End-of-Life Issues with Friends and Family

Writing down your wishes and having your advance directives for health care in place and a durable power of attorney for health care is not the end of your job. A good self-manager must do more than just write a memo; a good self-manager must see that the memo gets delivered. If you want your wishes carried out, you must share your wishes with your agent, family, and health care team. Often, this is not an easy task.

Before you can have this conversation, everyone involved needs to have copies of your DPA for health care. Once you have completed these documents, have them witnessed and signed. In some locations you can have your DPA for health care notarized instead of having it witnessed. Make several copies of your DPA for health care. You will need copies for your agents, family members, and hospital doctors. Also, give one to your lawyer. Once you complete and share this document, you are ready to talk about your wishes.

People don't like to discuss their own death or that of a loved one. Therefore, it should not surprise you that when you bring up this subject, the response may be, "Oh, don't think about that," or "That's a long time off," or "Don't be so morbid; you're not that sick." Unfortunately, this is usually enough to end the conversation. Your job is to keep the conversation open. There are several ways to do this.

First, plan on how you will have this discussion. Here are some suggestions:

- After you share copies of your DPA for health care with the appropriate family members or friends, ask them to read it and then set a specific time to discuss it. If they give you one of the avoidance responses, explain that you understand that this is a difficult topic but that you must discuss it with them. This is a good time to practice the "I" messages discussed in Chapter 11, *Communicating with Family, Friends, and Health Care Providers*. For example, say, "I understand that death is a difficult thing to talk about. However, it is very important to me that we have this talk."

- Another strategy is to get blank copies of a DPA for health care form for all your family members and suggest that you each fill one out and share them. This could even be part of a family get-together. Present this as an important aspect of being mature

adults and family members. Making this a family project may make it easier to discuss. Besides, it is a valid exercise. It will help clarify everyone's values about death and dying. Even teens can be part of this discussion.

- If the two suggestions we just listed seem too difficult or for some reason are impossible, write a letter or email or prepare a video to send to family members. At the same time, send them a copy of your DPA for health care. In the video or letter, share why you feel your death is an important topic to discuss and tell them that you want them to know your wishes. Then state your wishes. Give reasons for your choices. Ask that they respond in some way or that you set aside some time to talk in person or on the phone.

As mentioned before, when deciding on your agent, it is key that you choose someone with whom you can talk freely and exchange ideas. If your chosen agent is not willing to or is unable to talk to you about your wishes, you have probably chosen the wrong agent. Remember, the fact that someone is very close to you does not mean that this person really understands your wishes or would be able to carry them out. This topic should not be left to an unspoken understanding unless you don't mind if your agent goes against your wishes. For this reason, you may want to choose someone who is not as emotionally close to you. If you do choose someone outside of close family members, make sure your family knows whom you have appointed and why.

Talking about End-of-Life Issues with Your Health Care Provider

From our research, we have learned that people often have a more difficult time talking with their health care providers about their wishes than they do talking with their families about end-of-life issues. In fact, only a very small percentage of people who have written DPAs for health care or other advance directives ever share these with their physician.

Even though it is difficult, you should talk with your provider. You need to be sure that your provider's values are like yours. If you and your provider do not have the same values, it may be difficult for your provider to carry out your wishes. Second, your provider needs to know what you want. This allows your provider to take appropriate actions such as writing orders to resuscitate or not to use mechanical resuscitation. Third, your provider needs to know who your agent is and how to contact this person. If an important decision must be made and your wishes are to be followed, the provider must talk with your agent.

Be sure to give your primary care provider a copy of your DPA for health care so that it can become a permanent part of your medical record. As mentioned earlier, there is another advance directive called a POLST (Physician Orders for Life-Sustaining Treatment). This form is used for people who are in the final year of life or who have an advanced-stage terminal illness or an illness from which they are not expected to recover. Both you and your primary care provider would typically complete the form during an appointment. This allows both you and the physician an opportunity to discuss what could happen and what you want when it does. As noted earlier, a POLST is part of your medical record, but it does not appoint someone to act on your behalf, so it is still important to have a DPA for health care.

As surprising as it may seem, many health care providers also find it hard to talk to their patients about end-of-life wishes. After all, health care providers are in the business of keeping people alive and well. They don't like to think about their patients dying. On the other hand, most health care providers want their patients to have durable powers of attorney for health care (and sometimes a POLST). These documents relieve both you and your health care providers from added stress and worry.

If you wish, plan a time with your primary care provider when you can discuss your wishes. This should not be a side conversation at the end of a regular visit. Rather, start a visit by saying, "I want a few minutes to discuss my wishes in the event of a serious problem or impending death." When put this way, most primary care providers will make time to talk with you. If the primary care provider says that there is not enough time to talk with you, ask when you can make another appointment. This is a situation where you might need to be a little assertive. Sometimes a primary care provider, like your family members or friends, might say, "Oh, you don't have to worry about that; let me do it," or "We'll worry about that when the time comes." Again, you must take the initiative, using an "I" message to communicate that this is important to you and that you do not want to put off the discussion.

Sometimes health care providers do not want to worry you. They think they are doing you a favor by not describing all the unpleasant things that might happen in case of serious problems. You can help your health care providers by telling them that having control and making some decisions about your future will ease your mind. Not knowing or not being clear on what will happen is more worrisome than being faced with the facts, unpleasant as they may be, and dealing with them.

Even if you know all this information, it is still sometimes hard to talk with health care providers. Therefore, it might also be helpful to bring your agent to this discussion. The agent can facilitate the discussion and at the same time meet your primary care provider. This opens the lines of communication so that if your agent and physician must act to carry out your wishes, they can do so with few problems. If you cannot talk with your primary care provider, you should still provide them a copy of your DPA for health care for your medical record.

If you go to the hospital, be sure to take a copy of your DPA for health care with you. If you do not take it, be sure your agent knows to give a copy to the hospital. If you do not have a DPA already prepared, the hospital will ask you to fill out their advance directive form. This is important so the health care providers who oversee your care in the hospital know your wishes.

Again, do not put your durable power of attorney for health care in your safe deposit box—no one will be able to get it when it is needed. And remember, you do not need to see a lawyer to draw up a durable power of attorney for health care. This is one legal document you can do by yourself with no legal assistance.

Now that you have done all the important things, much of the hard work is over. And remember that you can change your mind at any time. Your agent may no longer be available, or your wishes might change. Be sure to keep your DPA for health care updated. Like most legal documents, it can be revoked or changed at any time. The decisions you make today are not forever.

Preparing Yourself and Others

Sharing your wishes about how you want to be treated in case of a serious or life-threatening illness is one of the most important self-management tasks. Here are some other steps to help reduce the emotional burden on your family and friends:

- **Make your will.** A will is a legal document that spells out the distribution of your assets after death. Even if your belongings are few, you may have ideas about who should inherit what. If you have a large estate, the tax implications could be large. A will ensures that your belongings go where you want them to go. Without a will, some distant or "long-lost" relative may end up with your estate. You might also want to consider a trust. (A trust allows a third party, a trustee, to hold and direct assets in a trust fund on behalf of a beneficiary.) Your will should include information about what you want done with your financial accounts and give directions about who can access them and how. Do not put passwords to your accounts in the will. You may want and need to talk with a lawyer about preparing these documents.

- **Plan your funeral.** Write down your wishes, including if you wish to donate your organs or arrange for your funeral and cremation or burial. Your grieving family will be very relieved not to have to decide what you would want and how much to spend. Pre-paid funeral plans are available. You can purchase your urn vault, or burial space in the location you prefer. Be sure that the people you want to handle things after your death are aware of all they need to know about your wishes. This includes your plans and arrangements and the location of necessary documents. Talk to them directly or prepare a detailed letter of instructions. Give the letter to someone you trust to deliver it to the right person at the right time.

- **Organize your papers.** You can purchase (at any well-stocked stationery store) a kit in which you place a copy of your will, your durable powers of attorney (for health care and financial and legal matters; a general durable power of attorney deals with financial matters, while a durable power of attorney for health care is for health care decisions only), other important papers, and information about your financial and personal affairs. Another useful source to help organize this information is "My Life in a Box," which is listed on the "Planning for the Future" tab in the resources section at www.bullpub.com/resources. It includes forms that you fill out about bank and charge accounts, insurance policies, the location of important documents, passwords to your online accounts, where your safe deposit box and its key are, and other related information. This is a handy, concise way to get everything together that anyone might need to know about. If you keep these documents on your computer instead of printing paper files, be sure others can find your passwords and accounts.

- **Finish your dealings with the world around you.** Mend any damaged relationships. Pay your debts, both financial and personal. Say what needs to be said to those who need to hear it. Do what needs to be done. Forgive yourself. Forgive others. (By the way, this is a good idea at any time, not just at the end of life.)

Talking about Death

Most family and close friends are reluctant to start this conversation but will appreciate it if you bring it up. You may find that there is much to say and to hear from your loved ones. If you find that they are unwilling to listen to you talk about your death and the feelings that you have, find someone who will be comfortable and understanding in listening to you. Most hospital and hospice services have chaplains who have these types of conversations daily. You may find it helpful to talk to a person with this experience and training. Your family and friends might be able to listen to you later. Remember, those who love you will also go through the stages of grieving when they think about losing you.

A large part of the fear of dying is fear of the unknown: "What will it be like?" "Will it be painful?" "What will happen to me after I die?" Most people who die of an illness are ready to die when the time comes. Painkillers and the disease process weaken body and mind. The awareness of self diminishes without the realization that this is happening. Most people just "slip away," with the transition between the state of living and that of no longer living hardly noticeable. Think about how a river meets the ocean. Reports from people who have been brought back to life after being in a state of clinical death indicate they experienced a sense of peacefulness and clarity and were not frightened.

People who are dying sometimes feel lonely and abandoned. Many people cannot deal with their own emotions when they are around a person they know is dying. They avoid the dying person's company, or they may engage in superficial chitchat, broken by long, awkward silences. This is often puzzling and hurtful to those who are dying, who are seeking companionship and solace from the people they counted on.

You can help by telling your family and friends what you want and need from them—attention, entertainment, comfort, music, practical help, and so on. A person who has something positive to do is more able to manage difficult emotions. If you can engage your family and loved ones in specific activities, they can feel needed and can relate to you around the activity. This will give you something to talk about, and it will occupy everyone's time in a beneficial way. It helps to define the situation for them and for you.

Considering Palliative Care and Hospice Care

Both palliative care and hospice care are available in most parts of the world. The goal of both palliative and hospice care is to provide comfort. The word *palliative* refers to relieving symptoms, such as pain, associated with a serious illness as well as improving quality of life. The word *hospice* refers to care provided for the terminally ill at home or in the community rather than in a hospital. Palliative care can begin at diagnosis and occur at the same time as treatment. Hospice care begins after treatment of the illness is stopped, when it is clear the illness will

probably end in death. Whereas the primary aim of hospice is to make the patient more comfortable, hospice professionals also help the family prepare for death with dignity; they help the surviving family members with emotional and support services during the dying process. This help can extend after a loved one's death.

There comes a time when regular medical care is no longer helpful, and it is time to prepare for death. Today, people often have several weeks or months, and sometimes years, to make these preparations. This is when hospice care is

Medical Assistance in Dying (MAID) in Canada

In June 2016, the Parliament of Canada passed federal legislation—Medical Assistance in Dying (MAID)—that allows eligible Canadian adults to request medical assistance in dying. Health Canada encourages patients to contact their physician or nurse practitioner (if applicable) for questions about access. Patients may also wish to contact the resources set up within their province or territory to get information on medical assistance in dying and other end-of-life care options.

so very useful. In hospice, medical and other care is aimed at making the patient as comfortable as possible and providing a good quality of life. Studies have shown that—at least for some illnesses—people who receive hospice care live longer than those who receive more aggressive treatment. Most hospices only accept people who are expected to die within six months. Rest assured, however, that this does not mean that you or your loved one will be thrown out of hospice care if you live longer. One of our original self-management leaders lived more than two years in hospice care.

Most hospices are "in-home" programs. This means that patients stay in their own homes and the services come to them. In some places, there are also residential hospices where people can go for their last days. Skilled nursing facilities often bring in hospice care as well, and they oversee the comfort for the last days, for both the person and the family.

One of the problems with hospice care is that people often wait until the last few days before death to ask for it. They somehow see asking for hospice care as "giving up." By refusing hospice care, they often put an unnecessary burden on themselves, family, and friends. The reverse is also often true. The caregiver and family might say they can manage without help. Although this may be true, the patient's life and dying may be much better if hospice cares for all the medical things so that family and friends are free to give love and support to the dying person.

Death with Dignity Acts in the United States

Death with dignity is another end-of-life option that allows certain terminally ill people to voluntarily and legally request and receive a prescription medication to help them die peacefully and humanely. Currently eight states and Washington, DC have laws that allow physician-assisted dying. The process requires that two physicians confirm the patient's diagnosis, prognosis, mental competence and voluntary nature of the request. This prevents the misuse of this option while still allowing the patient to have the right to control their end-of-life care. For more information about death with dignity and laws in your state, visit the website https://www.deathwithdignity.org.

In Canada, palliative care and hospice care refer to the same thing—a specific approach to providing care and comfort. However, some people use hospice care to describe care that is offered in the community rather than in hospitals. Palliative care in the home may be paid for by the provincial health plan as part of a home care program, but the plan may not cover costs of drugs and equipment. People may use private insurance or their own money to pay for those costs, or they might receive support from social agencies and nonprofit organizations. Palliative care in the hospital is usually paid for by provincial health plans and covers most of the drugs and equipment. In long-term care facilities, residents are usually required to pay for some of their palliative care, and costs vary among facilities.

If you, your partner, a family member, or a friend is in the end stage of illness, find and make use of your local hospice. It is a wonderful final gift. Hospice workers are very special people who are kind, thoughtful, and supportive. An added benefit of hospice care is that many hospice services are paid for by regular insurance or Medicare.

■ ■ ■

In closing, we would like to thank you for choosing to become an active self-manager of your health and life and for taking an active role as the most important member of your health care team. Throughout this book, we have shared tips and tools to make these roles easier for you and to encourage you to live a healthy and satisfying life with your chronic pain.

For a complete list of suggested further readings, useful websites, and other helpful resources, please see

www.bullpub.com/resources.

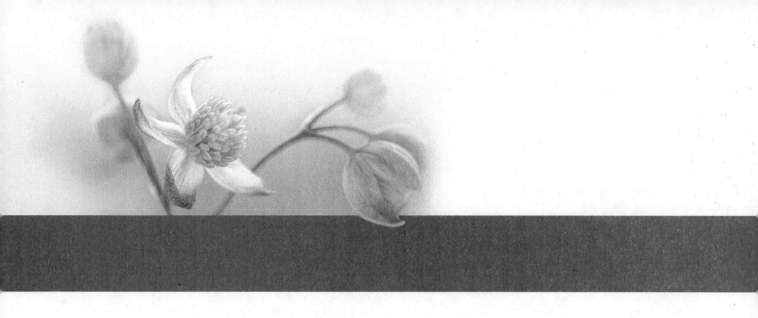

Index

Page numbers followed by f or t indicate a figure or table on the designated page